Blueprints **Notes & Cases**
Neuroscience

Blueprints Notes & Cases

Series Editor: Aaron B. Caughey MD, MPP, MPH

Blueprints *Notes & Cases—Microbiology and Immunology*
Monica Gandhi, Paul Baum, C. Bradley Hare, Aaron B. Caughey

Blueprints *Notes & Cases—Biochemistry, Genetics, and Embryology*
Juan E. Vargas, Aaron B. Caughey, Annie Tan, Jonathan Z. Li

Blueprints *Notes & Cases—Pharmacology*
Katherine Y. Yang, Larissa R. Graff, Aaron B. Caughey

Blueprints *Notes & Cases—Pathophysiology: Cardiovascular, Endocrine, and Reproduction*
Gordon Leung, Susan H. Tran, Tina O. Tan, Aaron B. Caughey

Blueprints *Notes & Cases—Pathophysiology: Pulmonary, Gastrointestinal, and Rheumatology*
Michael Filbin, Lisa M. Lee, Brian L. Shaffer, Aaron B. Caughey

Blueprints *Notes & Cases—Pathophysiology: Renal, Hematology, and Oncology*
Aaron B. Caughey, Christie del Castillo, Nancy Palmer, Karen Spizer, Dana N. Tuttle

Blueprints *Notes & Cases—Neuroscience*
Robert T. Wechsler, Alexander M. Morss, Courtney J. Wusthoff, Aaron B. Caughey

Blueprints *Notes & Cases—Behavioral Science and Epidemiology*
Judith Neugroschl, Jennifer Hoblyn, Christie del Castillo, Aaron B. Caughey

Blueprints **Notes & Cases**
Neuroscience

Robert T. Wechsler MD, PhD
Epilepsy and Clinical Neurophysiology Fellow
Stanford Comprehensive Epilepsy Center
Stanford University School of Medicine
Palo Alto, California

Alexander M. Morss, MD
Resident, Department of Neurology
Resident, Department of Medicine
Massachusetts General Hospital/Brigham & Women's Hospital
Boston, Massachusetts

Courtney J. Wusthoff
Class of 2004
School of Medicine
University of California, San Francisco
San Francisco, California

Aaron B. Caughey, MD, MPP, MPH
Clinical Instructor, Division of Maternal-Fetal Medicine
Department of Obstetrics & Gynecology
University of California, San Francisco
Division of Health Services and Policy Analysis
University of California, Berkeley
Berkeley & San Francisco, California

Series Editor: Aaron B. Caughey, MD, MPP, MPH

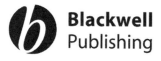

Blackwell
Publishing

Blackwell Publishing, Inc., 350 Main Street, Malden, Massachusetts 02148-5018, USA
Blackwell Publishing Ltd, 9600 Garsington Road, Oxford OX4 2DQ, UK
Blackwell Science Asia Pty Ltd, 550 Swanston Street, Carlton, Victoria 3053, Australia

03 04 05 06 07 5 4 3 2 1

ISBN: 1–4051–0349–3

Library of Congress Cataloging-in-Publication Data

Blueprints notes & cases. Neuroscience / Robert T. Wechsler . . . [et al.].
    p. ; cm. — (Blueprints notes & cases)
  Includes index.
  ISBN 1-4051-0349-3 (alk. paper)
  1. Nervous system—Pathophysiology—Case studies.
  [DNLM: 1. Nervous System Diseases—Case Report. 2. Nervous System Disease—Problems and Exercises. 3. Nervous System—anatomy & histology—Case Report. 4. Nervous System—anatomy & histology—Problems and Exercises. 5. Nervous System Physiology—Case Report. 6. Nervous System Physiology—Problems and Exercises. WL 18.2
  B6585 2003] I. Title: Blueprints notes and cases. II. Title: Neuroscience. III. Wechsler, Robert T. IV. Series.
    RC359.B58 2003
    616.8—dc21
                                 2003014310

A catalogue record for this title is available from the British Library

Acquisitions: Beverly Copland
Development: Selene Steneck
Production: Jennifer Kowalewski
Cover design: Hannus Design Associates
Interior design: Janet Bollow Associates
Typesetter: Peirce Graphic Services in Stuart, FL
Printed and bound by Courier Companies in Westford, MA

For further information on Blackwell Publishing, visit our website: www.blackwellpublishing.com

Notice: The indications and dosages of all drugs in this book have been recommended in the medical literature and conform to the practices of the general community. The medications described do not necessarily have specific approval by the Food and Drug Administration for use in the diseases and dosages for which they are recommended. The package insert for each drug should be consulted for use and dosage as approved by the FDA. Because standards for usage change, it is advisable to keep abreast of revised recommendations, particularly those concerning new drugs.

Contents

I. Brain Anatomy

II. Spinal Cord and Peripheral Nerves

III. Special Senses, Cranial Nerves, and Brainstem

IV. Ventricles, Vasculature, and Meninges

V. Neurophysiology and Neurotransmitters

Reviewers

Umesh A. Dave
Class of 2004
Nova Southeastern University College of Osteopathic
Medicine
Ft. Lauderdale, Florida

Francesann Ford
Class of 2004
Brody School of Medicine—East Carolina
Greenville, North Carolina

Dionne Louis
Class of 2004
Morehouse School of Medicine
Atlanta, Georgia

Christopher Quinn
Class of 2004
Michigan State University College of Osteopathic Medicine
East Lansing, Michigan

Kevin N. Sheth
Preliminary Intern
Brigham and Women's Hospital
Harvard Medical School
Boston, Massachusetts

Jamie L. Steckley, M.Sc
Class of 2004
University of Alberta
Edmonton, Alberta, Canada

Preface

The first two years of medical school are a demanding time for medical students. Whether the school follows a traditional curriculum or one that is case-based, every student is expected to learn and be able to apply basic science information in a clinical situation.

Medical schools are increasingly using clinical presentations as the background to teach the basic sciences. Case-based learning has become more common at many medical schools as it offers a way to catalogue the multitude of symptoms, syndromes, and diseases in medicine.

Blueprints Notes & Cases **is a new series by Blackwell Publishing designed to provide students a textbook to study the basic science topics combined with clinical data.** This method of learning is also the way to prepare for the clinical case format of USMLE questions. The eight books in this series will make the basic science topics not only more interesting, but also more meaningful and memorable. Students will be learning not only the why of a principle, but also how it might commonly be seen in practice.

The books in the *Blueprints Notes & Cases* series feature a comprehensive collection of cases which are designed to introduce one or more basic science topics. Through these cases, students gain an understanding of the coursework as they learn to:

- Think through the cases
- Look for classic presentations of most common diseases and syndromes
- Integrate the basic science content with clinical application
- Prepare for course exams and Step 1 USMLE
- Be prepared for clinical rotations

This series covers all the essential material needed in the basic science courses. Where possible, the books are organized in an organ-based system.

Clinical cases lead off and are the basis for discussion of the basic science content. A list of **"thought questions"** follows the case presentation. These questions are designed to challenge the reader to begin to think about how basic science topics apply to real-life clinical situations. The **answers to these questions** are integrated within the **basic science review and discussion** that follows. This offers a clinical framework from which to understand the basic content.

The discussion section is followed by a high-yield **Thumbnail table and Key Points box** which highlight and summarize the essential information presented in the discussion.

The cases also include two to four **multiple-choice questions** that allow readers to check their knowledge of that topic. Many of the answer explanations provide an opportunity for further discussion by delving into more depth in related areas. An **answer key** for these questions is at the end of the section for easy reference, and **full answer explanations** can be found at the end of the book.

This new series was designed to provide comprehensive content in a concise and templated format for ease in learning. A dedicated attempt was made to include sufficient art, tables, and clinical treatment, all while keeping the books from becoming too lengthy. We know you have much to read and that what you want is high-yield, vital facts.

The authors and series editor for these eight books, as well as everyone in editorial, production, sales and marketing at Blackwell Publishing, have worked long and hard to provide new textbooks to help you learn and be able to apply what you've learned. We engaged in multiple student email surveys and many focus groups to "hear what you needed" in new basic science level textbooks to meet the current curriculums, tests, and coursework. We know that you value this "student to student" approach, and sincerely hope you like what we have put together **just for you.**

Blackwell Publishing and the authors wish you success in your studies and your future medical career. Please feel free to offer us any comments or suggestions on these new books at blue@bos.blackwellpublishing.com.

Acknowledgments

To my parents, Jean and Adriana, for their constant support, and to Casey, Marc, and Audrey. I love you all.
—Robert T. Wechsler

To Laura, for her help and support.
—Alexander M. Morss

Thanks to my sister, Jessie, for everything.
—Courtney J. Wusthoff

To my grandparents, Theodore, who recently passed and Elizabeth, whose vitality at 93 continually inspires.
—Aaron B. Caughey

Abbreviations

5-HIAA	5-hydroxyindole acetic acid	GH	growth hormone
5-HT	5-hydroxytryptamine (serotonin)	GI	gastrointestinal
ACA	anterior cerebral artery	HD	Huntington's disease
ACh	acetylcholine	HIV	human immunodeficiency virus
ACom	anterior communicating artery	HPI	history of present illness
ACTH	adrenocorticotropic hormone	HR	heart rate
ADH	antidiuretic hormone	HSV-1	herpes simplex virus type 1
AICA	anteriorinferior cerebellar artery	HSV-2	herpes simplex virus type 2
AMPA	α-amino-3-hydroxyl-5-methyl-4-isoxazole-propionate	ICA	internal carotid artery
		ICP	intracranial pressure
ATM	acute transverse myelitis	IM	intramuscular
ATP	adenosine triphosphate	INO	internuclear ophthalmoplegia
AVP	arginine vasopressin	IPSP	inhibitory postsynaptic potential
BP	blood pressure	IV	intravenous
BPV	benign positional vertigo	K^+	potassium
C1–C8	cervical spinal cord levels 1–8	kg	kilogram
Ca^{2+}	calcium	L	liter
CA1–CA4	cornu ammonis regions of the hippocampus	L1–L5	lumbar spinal cord levels 1–5
		LGN	lateral geniculate nucleus
Cl	chloride	LH	luteinizing hormone
CN I–XII	cranial nerves I–XII	LMN	lower motor neuron
CN	cranial nerve	MAOI	monoamine oxidase inhibitor
CNS	central nervous system	MCA	middle cerebral artery
COWS	cold opposite, warm same	MEPP	miniature endplate potential
CSF	cerebrospinal fluid	mEq	milliequivalents
CT	computed tomography	mg	milligrams
DDAVP	desmopressin	MGN	medial geniculate nucleus
ECA	external carotid artery	MLF	medial longitudinal fasciculus
ECG	electrocardiogram	mm	millimeters
ED	emergency department	mOsm	milliosmoles
EEG	electroencephalogram; electroencephalography	MPTP	1-methyl-4-phenyl-1,2,5,6-tetrahydropyridine
EHL	extensor hallucis longus	MRI	magnetic resonance imaging
EMG	electromyography	MS	multiple sclerosis
EPP	endplate potential	MSH	melanocyte-stimulating hormone
EPSP	excitatory postsynaptic potential	MTS	mesial temporal sclerosis
FSH	follicle-stimulating hormone	Na^+	sodium
GABA	γ-aminobutyric acid		

NE	norepinephrine		S1–S5	sacral spinal cord levels 1–5
NMDA	*N*-methyl D-aspartate		SaO$_2$	arterial oxygen saturation
NMJ	neuromuscular junction		SCA	superior cerebellar artery
NPH	normal pressure hydrocephalus		SCSD	subacute combined systems degeneration
NSAID	nonsteroidal anti-inflammatory drug		SSRI	selective serotonin reuptake inhibitor
PCA	posterior cerebral artery		SUNCT	short-lasting, unilateral, neuralgiform headaches with conjunctival injection and tearing
PCA	patient-controlled analgesia			
PCom	posterior communicating artery		T	temperature
PCR	polymerase chain reaction		T1–T12	thoracic spinal cord levels 1–12
PD	Parkinson's disease		T$_4$	thyroxine
PE	physical exam		TCA	tricyclic antidepressant
PICA	posteriorinferior cerebellar artery		TSH	thyroid-stimulating hormone
PMHx	previous medical history		UMN	upper motor neuron
PNS	peripheral nervous system		V1–V3	ophthalmic, maxillary, and mandibular divisions of the trigeminal nerve
POMC	pro-opiomelanocortin			
PPRF	para-pontine reticular formation		V1–V5	also refers to visual cortex regions
PTSD	post-traumatic stress disorder		VMA	vanillylmandelic acid
REM	rapid eye movement		VOR	vestibulo-ocular reflex
RR	respiratory rate		VPL	ventral posterolateral nucleus (of thalamus)
Rx	medications		VS	vital signs

Normal Ranges of Laboratory Values

BLOOD, PLASMA, SERUM

Alanine aminotransferase (ALT, GPT at 30 C)	8–20 U/L
Amylase, serum	25–125 U/L
Aspartate aminotransferase (AST, GOT at 30 C)	8–20 U/L
Bilirubin, serum (adult) Total // Direct	0.1–1.0 mg/dL // 0.0–0.3 mg/dL
Calcium, serum (Ca^{2+})	8.4–10.2 mg/dL
Cholesterol, serum	Rec: < 200 mg/dL
Cortisol, serum	0800 h: 5–23 μg/dL // 1600 h: 3–15 μg/dL
	2000 h: ≤ 50% of 0800 h
Creatine kinase, serum	Male: 25–90 U/L
	Female: 10–70 U/L
Creatinine, serum	0.6–1.2 mg/dL
Electrolytes, serum	
Sodium (Na^+)	136–145 mEq/L
Chloride (Cl^-)	95–105 mEq/L
Potassium (K^+)	3.5–5.0 mEq/L
Bicarbonate (HCO_3^-)	22–28 mEq/L
Magnesium (Mg^{2+})	1.5–2.0 mEq/L
Ferritin, serum	Male: 15–200 ng/mL
	Female: 12–150 ng/mL
Follicle-stimulating hormone, serum/plasma	Male: 4–25 mIU/mL
	Female: premenopause 4–30 mIU/mL
	midcycle peak 10–90 mIU/mL
	postmenopause 40–250 mIU/mL
Gases, arterial blood (room air)	
pH	7.35–7.45
Pco_2	33–45 mm Hg
Po_2	75–105 mm Hg
Glucose, serum	Fasting: 70–110 mg/dL
	2-h postprandial: < 120 mg/dL
Growth hormone—arginine stimulation	Fasting: < 5 ng/mL
	provocative stimuli: > 7 ng/mL
Iron	50–70 μg/dL
Lactate dehydrogenase, serum	45–90 U/L
Luteinizing hormone, serum/plasma	Male: 6–23 mIU/mL
	Female: follicular phase 5–30 mIU/mL
	midcycle 75–150 mIU/mL
	postmenopause 30–200 mIU/mL
Osmolality, serum	275–295 mOsmol/kg
Parathyroid hormone, serum, N-terminal	230–630 pg/mL
Phosphate (alkaline), serum (p-NPP at 30 C)	20–70 U/L
Phosphorus (inorganic), serum	3.0–4.5 mg/dL
Prolactin, serum (hPRL)	< 20 ng/mL
Proteins, serum	
Total (recumbent)	6.0–7.8 g/dL
Albumin	3.5–5.5 g/dL
Globulin	2.3–3.5 g/dL
Thyroid-stimulating hormone, serum or plasma	0.5–5.0 μU/mL
Thyroidal iodine (^{123}I) uptake	8–30% of administered dose/24 h
Thyroxine (T_4), serum	5–12 μg/dL
Triglycerides, serum	35–160 mg/dL
Triiodothyronine (T_3), serum (RIA)	115–190 ng/dL
Triiodothyronine (T_3), resin uptake	25–35%
Urea nitrogen, serum (BUN)	7–18 mg/dL
Uric acid, serum	3.0–8.2 mg/dL

CEREBROSPINAL FLUID

Cell count	0–5 cells/mm^3
Chloride	118–132 mEq/L
Gamma globulin	3–12% total proteins
Glucose	40–70 mg/dL
Pressure	70–180 mm H$_2$O
Proteins, total	< 40 mg/dL

HEMATOLOGIC

Bleeding time (template)	2–7 minutes
Erythrocyte count	Male: 4.3–5.9 million/mm^3
	Female: 3.5–5.5 million/mm^3
Erythrocyte sedimentation rate (Westergren)	Male: 0–15 mm/h
	Female: 0–20 mm/h
Hematocrit	Male: 41–53%
	Female: 36–46%
Hemoglobin A$_{1C}$	≤ 6%
Hemoglobin, blood	Male: 13.5–17.5 g/dL
	Female: 12.0–16.0 g/dL
Leukocyte count and differential	
Leukocyte count	4500–11,000/mm^3
Segmented neutrophils	54–62%
Bands	3–5%
Eosinophils	1–3%
Basophils	0–0.75%
Lymphocytes	25–33%
Monocytes	3–7%
Mean corpuscular hemoglobin	25.4–34.6 pg/cell
Mean corpuscular hemoglobin concentration	31–36% Hb/cell
Mean corpuscular volume	80–100 μm^3
Partial thromboplastin time (activated)	25–40 seconds
Platelet count	150,000–400,000/mm^3
Prothrombin time	11–15 seconds
Reticulocyte count	0.5–1.5% of red cells
Thrombin time	< 2 seconds deviation from control
Volume	
Plasma	Male: 25–43 mL/kg
	Female: 28–45 mL/kg
Red cell	Male: 20–36 mL/kg
	Female: 19–31 mL/kg

SWEAT

Chloride	0–35 mmol/L

URINE

Calcium	100–300 mg/24 h
Chloride	Varies with intake
Creatine clearance	Male: 97–137 mL/min
	Female: 88–128 mL/min
Osmolality	50–1400 mOsmol/kg
Oxalate	8–40 μg/mL
Potassium	Varies with diet
Proteins, total	< 150 mg/24 h
Sodium	Varies with diet
Uric acid	Varies with diet

Part I

Brain Anatomy

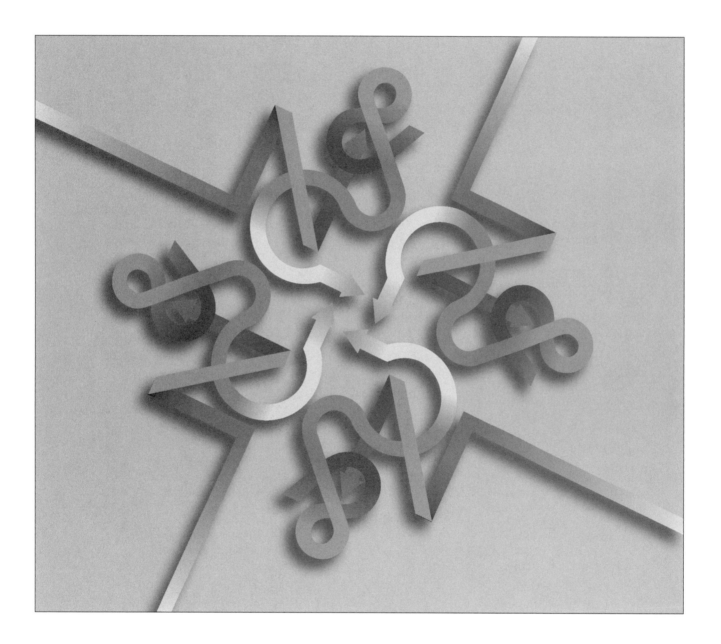

HPI: PT is a 67-year-old male who presents to the emergency department (ED) with altered level of consciousness and right hemiparesis. This morning at breakfast, he looked up with a puzzled expression, did not seem able to speak, and had twitching of the right side of the face. His right arm then became stiff and began to jerk, followed by his right leg. He fell out of his chair and began to jerk all over. The whole episode "seemed to last forever but probably was only a few minutes long." He has been lethargic ever since. His vital signs are stable. His wife is very upset, stating that "he is having another stroke." You determine that this patient presented in a similar manner 1 year ago. His wife says he was diagnosed as having a stroke and was ultimately treated with a blood thinner that required periodic laboratory tests. He did well but was left with residual mild right arm weakness. Language function was impaired initially, but this resolved.

Thought Questions

- What is the structural implication of hemiparesis?

- What is the structural implication of an inability to speak?

- What does the evolution of this patient's spell emphasize about cortical organization?

- Is this patient right handed or left handed?

- Where is the lesion?

Basic Science Review and Discussion

Frontal lobe dysfunction can be divided into rostral and caudal frontal lobe involvement. Rostral syndromes tend to disrupt higher order cognitive function. This category of disease is discussed within the context of the prefrontal cortex. Posterior frontal lobe syndromes are more likely to be associated with motor deficits. Language deficits can also be seen, particularly if the dominant hemisphere is involved. This case highlights several important concepts regarding the organization of the frontal lobes. The pattern of seizure spread in this case emphasizes the **somatotopic organization** of the frontal cortex. Adjacent cortical regions control adjacent body parts on the contralateral side. PT's seizure started in the cortical areas controlling the right side of the face and language (i.e., the **dominant hemisphere** in a right-handed individual). His seizure then spread to cortical areas controlling the arm and then the leg. This somatotopic propagation of seizure activity is called a **Jacksonian motor seizure.** PT did not loose consciousness, however, until the seizure spread to both hemispheres (both sides of the body became involved). This emphasizes that supratentorial (hemispheric) disease needs to be bilateral to cause loss of consciousness. Given the complex nature of cortical function, it is important to understand how the cerebral cortex is organized before undertaking a functional review.

Cortical Organization The **cerebrum** is divided into two hemispheres, each anatomically organized into **frontal,** **parietal, temporal,** and **occipital lobes.** The left hemisphere is dominant in most right-handed individuals and two thirds of left-handed individuals. Corresponding regions in the dominant and nondominant hemispheres often have different but complementary functions. The **cerebral cortex** is a sheet of gray matter, averaging 2 to 3 mm in thickness, covering the surface of the cerebral hemispheres. It is folded against itself, forming **gyri** separated by **sulci,** to accommodate its large surface area within the relatively small skull.

The **longitudinal fissure** separates the two hemispheres. The **lateral (sylvian) fissures** separate the frontal and temporal lobes on each side. The **insular cortex** is contained within the lateral fissure, forming a border between frontal, parietal, and temporal lobes. The central sulcus separates the frontal cortex from the parietal cortex, which contain the primary motor and sensory cortices, respectively.

The cerebral cortex is divided into layers on the basis of cellular morphology and axonal organization. It is also divided into three major types, based on the number of layers present. Phylogenetically, **neocortex,** which predominates in humans, is the newest type of cortex and has six layers. **Allocortex** is the oldest type of cortex and has three layers, and **mesocortex** has an intermediate structure. Allocortex and mesocortex are found predominantly in the temporal and limbic regions.

The cerebral cortex is further subdivided into **Brodmann's areas** on the basis of cellular organization within the cortical layers. There are 52 Brodmann's areas, although not all areas are present in all species. Only the most clinically relevant Brodmann areas are discussed here. Figure 1-1 illustrates the Brodmann areas of the human brain as seen from a lateral view.

Neocortical Layers

Organization of cortical layers Input to the cortex goes to **layers I, II, III,** and **IV.** Output from the cortex originates in **layers II, III, V,** and **VI.** Layer I has few neurons but serves as a venue for interaction of axons and dendrites originating in the other layers. Layers II and III are responsible for com-

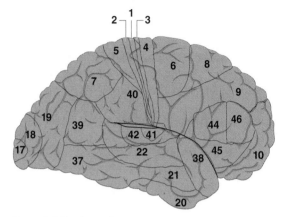

Figure 1-1 Brodmann's areas.

munication between different cortical areas, and the remaining layers mediate communication with subcortical structures.

Axons that mediate communication between adjacent cortical areas are called **U fibers** because of the shape of their path from one cortical area to the next. They originate from and project to cortical layers II and III. Groups of functionally related fibers are called *fasciculi.* For example, the **arcuate fasciculus** connects **Wernicke's area** for receptive language to **Broca's area** for expressive language. Fibers crossing the midline through the **corpus callosum** and the **anterior and posterior commissures** mediate communication between corresponding cortical regions in the two hemispheres.

Regions of the cerebral cortex can be divided functionally into primary cortical areas and associative cortical areas. **Primary cortical areas** are dedicated to a single modality (e.g., motor, somatosensory, visual, and auditory). **Associative cortical areas** are multimodal. They integrate information from a variety of cortical areas.

Cortical efferent fibers The main site of **motor output** from the cortex is **layer V.** The axons of large pyramidal neurons (of Betz) in this layer make up the **corticospinal (pyramidal) tract** and **corticobulbar tract.** Feedback to the thalamus is mediated by **corticothalamic fibers** originating in **layer VI.** As a general rule, fibers originating in layers V and VI leave the cerebrum and have subcortical targets.

Cortical afferent fibers Most sensory input pathways synapse in the thalamus on their way to the cortex (olfaction is the only sensory modality to reach its primary cortex without passing through the thalamus). Thalamic sensory pathway fibers exit the thalamus in a modality-specific manner and terminate in **layer IV** of their corresponding primary sensory cortex. Layer IV is histologically distinct in the primary visual cortex, where it is divided by the **line of Gennari.** This gives the primary visual cortex a striped

appearance in a cross section from which the name **striate cortex** is derived.

Several monoaminergic, cholinergic, and GABAergic (γ-aminobutyric acid) pathways that originate in the brainstem and basal forebrain project to different cortical layers and modulate cortical function. These systems are discussed separately.

Organization of the Frontal Lobe

Surface anatomy The **frontal lobe** extends posteriorly from the frontal pole to the **central sulcus.** It is bound medially by the longitudinal fissure and laterally by the lateral fissure. The **precentral gyrus** is immediately anterior to the central sulcus. This area contains the **primary motor cortex** (Brodmann's area 4). Three major gyri are arranged perpendicular to the precentral gyrus and extend anteriorly, toward the frontal pole. They are the **superior, middle,** and **inferior frontal gyri.** This region contains the **supplementary motor area** and **premotor area** (both in Brodmann's area 6), the **frontal eye fields** (Brodmann's area 8), **Broca's area** (Brodmann's areas 44 and 45), and the **prefrontal cortex** (Brodmann's areas 46, 9, 10, and 11). The frontal lobe is involved in the organization and control of **motor function, expressive language, cognitive function,** and **emotional behavior.** This case focuses on cortical motor systems. The remaining topics are covered in Cases 2 and 3.

Primary motor cortex The primary motor cortex in each hemisphere is organized somatotopically and controls motor function for the contralateral side of the body. **Somatotopic organization** means that adjacent cortical areas control adjacent regions of the body. A **motor homunculus** is a schematic representation of the human body as it would be drawn on the cortical surface. It is distorted because cortical areas devoted to fine motor function (e.g., the hand) are disproportionately large. The primary sensory cortex also can be depicted by a sensory homunculus.

Within the primary motor strip, areas controlling the face, tongue, and hand are located relatively lateral and those controlling the lower extremity are most medial (within the longitudinal fissure). A pathologic process that spreads across the surface of the primary cortex, like the **Jacksonian motor seizure** in the presented case, will progressively affect contiguous parts of the body on one side because of this organization.

Most of the primary motor cortex receives its blood supply from branches of the **middle cerebral artery.** The anterior cerebral artery supplies the medial primary motor cortex. This organization is clinically significant. A cortical infarction in the distribution of the middle cerebral artery may affect the face and upper extremity while sparing the lower extremity. The converse can be seen with infarction of the anterior cerebral artery. When both extremities and the face are involved, a subcortical lesion affecting fibers of the corticospinal tract should be suspected. Involvement of the extremities with sparing of the face is less commonly encountered in cerebral disease and may implicate a spinal cord process. A single **midsagittal lesion,** such as a meningioma or a sagittal sinus thrombosis, can cause bilateral lower extremity deficits while sparing upper extremity function.

Supplementary motor and premotor areas   The **supplementary motor area** is contained within the medial portion of Brodmann's area 6, anterior to the primary motor cortex. It is important for the **temporal organization of movements** and the coordination of complex movements. As would be expected, considerable communication between the supplementary motor areas of the two hemispheres is needed for this function. Each supplementary motor area has some bilateral motor function. This cortical area is also extensively interconnected with the primary motor, premotor, and somatosensory cortices, as well as with the basal ganglia, thalamus, and cerebellum.

The **premotor area** (Brodmann's area 6) is responsible for motor function that is dependent on sensory input. These motor behaviors can be relatively stereotyped. Examples include reaching for an object in the visual field and following commands or cues. This cortical area receives input from sensory and associative cortical areas.

Lesions in these motor-planning cortical areas are associated with apraxia. **Apraxia** is the inability to perform complex motor tasks despite retained motor strength, sensation, and coordination. It represents a disconnection between the frontal and the parietal lobes. Unlike frontal apraxias, parietal apraxias are associated with the inability to understand the meaning of gestures. The most commonly encountered apraxias are summarized later in this case (see Thumbnail: Frontal Cortex and Motor Function).

Frontal eye fields   **Saccades** are rapid eye movements (REMs) that shift the fixation of gaze from one point to another, skipping any intervening visual targets or distractions. **Voluntary saccades,** such as shifting your gaze from this sentence to another part of the page, are triggered by the **frontal eye fields** (Brodmann's area 8). The eye field in

each hemisphere drives gaze toward the contralateral side. Gaze is directed centrally when both frontal eye fields are equally active. Pathologic processes that cause an imbalance in this system lead to gaze deviation. For example, a frontal cerebral infarction would be associated with decreased activity on the affected side. The intact contralateral eye field would be relatively more active, driving gaze toward the affected side. Conversely, a focal frontal seizure would be associated with hyperactivity on the affected side driving the direction of gaze toward the intact, unaffected side. Focal frontal seizures associated with gaze deviation and/or head turning toward the unaffected side are called **versive seizures.**

The prefrontal cortex and inferior parietal cortex are involved in the planning and coordination of saccadic eye movements. The **supplementary eye fields** are located adjacent to the frontal eye fields and supplementary motor areas. They are involved in the coordination of voluntary saccades with complex motor behaviors. Eye fields in the inferior parieto-temporo-occipital association cortices (Brodmann's areas 19, 39, and 40) are responsible for reflexive **involuntary saccades.** These areas coordinate information from the field of vision with motor programs pertaining to eye movement and are involved in the coordination of **smooth pursuit** eye movements.

Clinical Correlation   Although a full medical history was not available in this case, PT's use of an anticoagulant requiring periodic blood tests (likely warfarin) suggests that an embolic etiology was either strongly suspected or proven at the time of his first stroke. Recurrence is an important consideration, but other etiologies also exist. It has been estimated that as many as 25% of patients with embolic strokes involving the cortex will ultimately develop epilepsy (a syndrome of recurrent seizures). Nearly half of all new-onset seizures occur in the elderly and previous infarction is believed to be one of the common causes in this patient population. These seizures are considered symptomatic because they are secondary to a known structural process (stroke, tumor, abscess, etc.). They are distinguished from idiopathic seizures, which are more common at younger ages. The most commonly encountered seizure types are summarized in Case 22 (see Thumbnail: Olfaction and Olfactory Nerve).

Case Conclusion   PT was evaluated through an acute stroke pathway but was not felt to be a thrombolysis candidate because of the recent use of warfarin and the apparent seizure at onset. A computed tomographic (CT) scan of the brain revealed a small wedge-shaped area of left frontal hypodensity extending to the cortex. This finding was unchanged relative to imaging performed at the time of his last admission. PT remained hemiparetic for several hours after his seizure but gradually improved. This is called **Todd's phenomenon,** or **postictal hemiparesis.** It is often seen in the setting of symptomatic frontal lobe epilepsy. An interictal electroencephalogram (EEG) confirmed the presence of left frontal epileptiform discharges, supporting the diagnosis of a symptomatic motor seizure with secondary generalization. PT was treated with phenytoin, which he tolerated without difficulty.

Thumbnail: Frontal Cortex and Motor Function

Apraxia

Syndrome	Clinical manifestation	Lesion localization
Limb apraxia	Disability of a single limb, often associated with fine motor function disturbance despite intact strength, sensation, and coordination	Supplementary motor and premotor areas
Orofacial apraxia	Normal strength but cannot whistle, blow out match, etc.	Supplementary motor and premotor areas
Ideomotor apraxia	Inability to follow motor commands or imitate movements that can otherwise be performed spontaneously	Dominant premotor cortex or dominant inferior parietal lobule or anterior corpus callosum
Ideational apraxia	Inability to carry out ideational plan or sort its motor components	Often bilateral frontal and/or parietal dysfunction
Constructional apraxia	Difficulty assembling components or drawing objects	Parietal cortex (usually nondominant)

Key Points

- ▶ Neocortex has six layers.
- ▶ Input to the cortex goes to layers I, II, III, and IV.
- ▶ Output from the cortex originates in layers II, III, V, and VI.
- ▶ Layers II and III are responsible for communication between different areas of cortex.

- ▶ Sensory input terminates in layer IV of the cortex and arrives via the thalamus.
- ▶ Cortical motor output originates in layer V of the primary motor cortex in the precentral gyrus and gives rise to the pyramidal tract.

Questions

1. You evaluate a right-handed patient with a suspected cortical infarction in the distribution of the left middle cerebral artery. Which of the following is most likely to be spared?
   A. Right-sided face motor function
   B. Right-sided arm motor function
   C. Right-sided leg motor function
   D. Language repetition
   E. Language fluency

2. A patient in the epilepsy monitoring unit is noted to turn her eyes and head to the left at the beginning of her seizures. She then becomes stiff all over. Finally she develops rhythmic jerking movements involving her whole body. Her seizures are probably originating from where?
   A. The right parietal cortex
   B. The right frontal cortex
   C. The left parietal cortex
   D. The left frontal cortex
   E. The right oculomotor nuclear group

3. A patient presents to the ED unresponsive and with a right-gaze preference. A hemorrhagic stroke is suspected in which of the following areas?
   A. The right parietal cortex
   B. The right frontal cortex
   C. The left parietal cortex
   D. The left frontal cortex
   E. The right oculomotor nuclear group

4. A patient is unable to demonstrate how he brushes his teeth. The nurse tells you she saw him brushing his teeth earlier that morning. The most likely explanation is which of the following?
   A. He is a difficult, uncooperative patient.
   B. He has an ideational apraxia.
   C. He has an ideomotor apraxia.
   D. He has a limb apraxia.
   E. He has an constructional apraxia.

> **HPI:** RS is a 66-year-old right-handed smoker who had sudden onset of right-hand clumsiness 2 hours ago. He initially thought nothing of this problem, but it has progressed to the point that he can barely move his right upper extremity. He presents for further evaluation.
>
> **PE:** He is awake and alert. His vital signs are stable. He is able to understand your instructions and follow commands but is frustrated by not being able to express himself adequately. He has a halting, stuttering speech pattern. He has trouble finding words. He is not able to repeat words or phrases. He cannot sustain his right arm against gravity and he has a weak grip on the right side. His strength is otherwise intact. His coordination is appropriate to his strength. Sensation and reflexes are normal.

Thought Questions

- What is the structural implication of impaired speech?
- What cortical areas mediate language?
- Is this patient right handed or left handed?
- Where is the lesion?

Basic Science Review and Discussion

When evaluating a patient with impaired speech, one must distinguish between dysarthria and the aphasias. Dysarthria implies a slurring speech quality. It is associated with disruption of motor control to the muscles of speech. Dysarthria is an important feature of lower cranial nerve dysfunction. Upper motor neuron lesions of the corticobulbar pathways innervating the cranial nerve nuclei also can be associated with dysarthria. The aphasias, on the other hand, represent disruption of the cortical language system that can be independent of motor function.

Perisylvian Language Areas The processing of language requires input of sensory information, processing of that information, integration of that information with previously acquired data, coordination of language output, and language expression. Disruptions of language function are called *aphasias.* The primary language areas involved in this series of functions are all located around the lateral (sylvian) sulcus, in the **dominant hemisphere. Perisylvian aphasias** are associated with disruption of these key structures and are all **characterized by an inability to repeat language.**

Wernicke's Area for Receptive Language Receptive aphasias involve Wernicke's area, which is located at the border of the temporal and parietal lobes (parts of Brodmann's areas 22 and 39). Patients with **Wernicke's aphasia** are unable to understand or repeat language but have fluent, albeit nonsensical, speech. They may make paraphasic errors, substituting words or syllables during relatively fluent speech.

Pure word deafness is a variant of Wernicke's aphasia limited to verbal language, with intact written language. The pathways connecting the auditory cortex to Wernicke's area is affected. **Alexia without agraphia** is a variant of Wernicke's aphasia limited to written language, with intact spoken language.

Broca's Area for Expressive Language Expressive aphasias involve Broca's area, which is located in the inferolateral frontal lobe (Brodmann's areas 44 and 45). Broca's area is involved in coordinating the motor programs needed to generate language. Like the current patient, patients with **Broca's aphasia** have a stuttering speech pattern. They may not be able to name objects. They are unable to repeat or produce fluent language, but they have intact comprehension of language. The **arcuate fasciculus** connects Wernicke's area to Broca's area. Patients with lesions of the arcuate fasciculus have a **conductive aphasia;** they can understand and produce language but cannot repeat. When all of these areas are affected, patients present with **global aphasia.** Comprehension, repetition, and fluent speech all are lost.

Transcortical Language Pathways The primary language areas must communicate with higher order associative cortical regions for language to be integrated into complex cognitive functions. Disruption of these connections results in **transcortical aphasias.** Transcortical aphasias are all **characterized by intact repetition** because Wernicke's area, the arcuate fasciculus, and Broca's area are all intact. Patients with **transcortical sensory aphasias** generally have lesions in the pathways connecting Wernicke's area to the higher order associative cortex. They have poor comprehension with intact repetition and fluent speech. Patients with **transcortical motor aphasias** generally have lesions of the pathways connecting associative cortical areas to Broca's area. They have intact comprehension and repetition with nonfluent speech. In **mixed transcortical aphasia,** repetition is the only language function left intact.

Nondominant Hemisphere The comparable cortical regions in the contralateral (nondominant) hemisphere mediate prosody. **Prosody** refers to the melodic emotional content of language. Patients with lesions of Brodmann's area 44 in the nondominant hemisphere have **aprosodic speech** (monotonic, unemotional). Patients with lesions of Brodmann's area 22 in the nondominant hemisphere are not able to detect speech inflection. For example, they cannot detect the difference between a statement of fact and a question, if both are similarly phrased (if you hold out an apple toward them and say "apple?" they may reply "Yes, it is"). As a general rule, one is more likely to see apraxia with nondominant hemispheric lesions and aphasia with dominant hemisphere lesions.

Case Conclusion   RS was evaluated through an acute stroke protocol that included routine laboratory studies and CT imaging on an emergent basis. He was determined to be a good candidate for thrombolytic therapy, which he tolerated without incident. His symptoms fluctuated over the following days but ultimately stabilized to a moderate right upper extremity hemiparesis. His speech became more fluent, although he continued to have some difficulty with naming. Magnetic resonance imaging (MRI) of the brain confirmed a small acute left frontal ischemic infarction. A definitive etiology could not be identified. He was started on an antiplatelet agent and was discharged with arrangements for out-patient therapies.

Thumbnail: Frontal Cortex and Language Function

Perisylvian Aphasias			
Syndrome	**Spontaneous speech**	**Comprehension**	**Repetition**
Broca's	Nonfluent	Good	Poor
Wernicke's	Fluent	Poor	Poor
Conduction	Fluent	Good	Poor
Global	Nonfluent	Poor	Poor

Transcortical Aphasias			
Syndrome	**Spontaneous speech**	**Comprehension**	**Repetition**
Transcortical motor	Nonfluent	Good	Good
Transcortical sensory	Fluent	Poor	Good
Mixed	Nonfluent	Poor	Good
Anomic	Fluent	Good	Good

Key Points

▶ Broca's area for expressive language is in Brodmann's areas 44 and 45.

▶ Wernicke's area for receptive language is in Brodmann's areas 22 and 39.

▶ Pure word deafness is a variant of Wernicke's aphasia limited to verbal language, with intact written language.

▶ Alexia without agraphia is a variant of Wernicke's aphasia limited to written language, with intact spoken language.

▶ **Prosody** refers to the melodic, emotional content of language.

Questions

1. You evaluate a right-handed patient who is brought by his family for evaluation of confusion. He has fluent speech but often uses "made-up" words or inappropriate words. When you try to speak to him, he repeats everything you say but does not interact. Where is his lesion?
   A. Right parietal lobe
   B. Left parietal lobe
   C. Wernicke's area
   D. Broca's area
   E. Left arcuate fasciculus

2. The family of the patient you have just evaluated would like to know the cause of his transcortical sensory aphasia. You explain that he has had a stroke. Compromise of which of the following vascular territories would lead to his deficit?
   A. Right middle cerebral artery (MCA)
   B. Left MCA
   C. Left MCA/anterior cerebral artery (ACA) border zone
   D. Left MCA/posterior cerebral artery (PCA) border zone
   E. Left PCA

3. You evaluate a 67-year-old right-handed gentleman who has had a stroke. He reports that he is having trouble reading. He took some notes while on the telephone but cannot read them even though they appear quite legible. Which of the following regions is likely to be affected?
   A. Left occipital cortex
   B. Right occipital cortex
   C. Left frontal cortex
   D. Right frontal cortex
   E. Left supplementary motor area

4. You are asked to evaluate a patient who was admitted for a cardiovascular evaluation following an episode of chest pain. The nurse tells you that the patient became aphasic about 20 minutes before your arrival. The patient is somewhat disoriented. He has normal speech rhythm but slurs his words as though intoxicated. He cooperates with your examination and is oriented to his name and the fact that he is in a hospital. He cannot state the year, month, or day of the week. Which of the following structures is implicated?
   A. Broca's area
   B. Wernicke's area
   C. Arcuate fasciculus
   D. Left parietal cortex
   E. None of the above

HPI: TR is a 65-year-old man who was in good health until approximately 9 months ago. His family reports that they did not notice any problems at the time, but in retrospect, they note that he became more withdrawn. When he does become involved, he seems confused and often interjects inappropriate comments. He also has become increasingly unsteady on his feet and has had several falls. Most recently, he has become incontinent of urine. This has prompted a referral to your office. His only remarkable medical history consists of an episode of meningitis several years ago. His family does not recall the details. Alcohol use is denied.

PE: You note that TR does appear confused at times. He knows the day but makes errors on naming the month and year. It is difficult to engage him in conversation during the examination. He has difficulty with naming, remote memory, and recall. His examination is unremarkable, except for a marked abnormality of gait. He walks with a wide base, seems very unsteady, and slides his feet across the floor as though being held down by magnets.

Thought Questions

- What is the nature of this patient's confusion?
- Does he have altered perception?
- What cognitive processes are affected?
- What brain regions might be implicated in this case?
- What brain regions are involved in cognition?

Basic Science Review and Discussion

TR presented with a chronic deterioration of cognition and gait with subsequent development of incontinence. This clinical triad (wacky, wobbly, and wet) is the hallmark of **normal-pressure hydrocephalus** (NPH). **Hydrocephalus** is a relative increase in the volume of cerebrospinal fluid (CSF) resulting in dilatation of the ventricles of the brain. Two major categories of hydrocephalus are recognized, either **communicating** or **noncommunicating.** The latter is generally associated with a structural process that obstructs the normal flow of CSF. Examples include tumors in the third or fourth ventricles. In communicating hydrocephalus, the normal flow of CSF is preserved, but most commonly, the reabsorption of CSF through the arachnoid granulations is slowed. This may be related to previous injury to the arachnoid granulations, as may be seen with meningitis or hemorrhage. Hydrocephalus can present either acutely or chronically, depending on the mechanics of flow disruption. Essentially, NPH is a chronic manifestation of communicating hydrocephalus in adults. Imaging confirms enlargement of the ventricular system out of proportion to any cerebral atrophy that may be present. Imaging is also important to exclude any other structural processes, such as previous extensive ischemia or tumor, which can present similarly. If all other reversible causes are excluded, then ventricular shunting has been reported to be helpful in some cases of

NPH. This intervention can be supported by a favorable response to large-volume lumbar puncture, suggesting that some of the deficits may be reversible.

The signs and symptoms illustrated in this patient can be localized to the frontal lobes in general and to the prefrontal cortex in particular. From a clinical standpoint, it is important to note that structural frontal lesions and more generalized processes such as hydrocephalus, metabolic encephalopathy, and dementia can all present similarly. This is related to the fact that the frontal lobes mediate those higher functions that define human behavior. The ventricular system is discussed in more detail separately. Here, we focus on the prefrontal cortex and to a lesser extent on the manifestations of dementia. Note that the dementias are not localized uniquely to the prefrontal cortex. However, the prefrontal manifestations of dementing disorders are particularly striking.

Organization of the Prefrontal Cortex From a clinical standpoint, the distinction between frontal and prefrontal lesions is somewhat blurred. The **prefrontal cortex** refers to the most anterior portion of the frontal lobe, including the frontal pole. It corresponds to Brodmann's areas 9, 10, 11, and 46. The prefrontal cortex is involved in higher order cerebral functions. It facilitates complex tasks that require **integration of information over time.** It is involved in **affective behavior, judgment, creativity,** and **planning of complex movements.**

Given the diverse nature of prefrontal cortical function, it is not surprising that this region is extensively interconnected with other brain areas. The prefrontal cortex receives input from and sends output to other associative cortical areas, the limbic system, the hypothalamus, the thalamus (mainly the dorsomedial nucleus), and the basal ganglia (mainly the head of the caudate nucleus). The prefrontal cortex also receives modulatory input from aminergic brainstem and basal forebrain nuclei. These latter pathways are discussed separately.

The complex nature of prefrontal cortical function makes it difficult to categorize different functional components on an anatomic basis. Much of what is known about the function of the prefrontal cortex is derived from animal studies or anecdotal reports of prefrontal lesions. One of the best known examples is the case of **Phineas Gage,** a 19th century railroad worker. An accidental explosion sent an iron rod through his skull, destroying most of his left prefrontal cortex. He survived and lived another 13 years but had dramatic personality changes. He was noted to have become moody, impulsive, and irresponsible.

Some gross generalizations can be made about prefrontal cortex function on the basis of these kinds of observations. Two major types of syndromes can be identified, although considerable overlap can be seen in the clinical setting. **Dorsolateral prefrontal lesions** tend to be associated with **behavioral apathy.** On the other hand, **orbitofrontal lesions** tend to be associated with **impulsive behavior** and **disruption of normal mood and affect.**

Dorsolateral Prefrontal Cortex   The **dorsolateral prefrontal cortex** seems to be important **for working memory.** This is a temporary storage area for information that is only needed in the moment, like keeping track of the location of other cars while driving. This area also seems to cooperate with the medial temporal in learning new facts. When this area is injured, patients are noted to have **psychomotor retardation,** difficulty with organization of complex tasks, and relative **indifference** to their environment. On examination, they may be noted to have **perseverative behavior,** difficulty generating word lists, and difficulty with repetitive or complex motor tasks. They may not be able to follow multistep commands. Performance of alternating or rhythmic tasks may be impaired. These last deficits also can be associated with extrapyramidal disorders, but remember that the prefrontal cortex is connected to the basal ganglia.

Patients whose lesions extend more medially may become **incontinent** of urine. Their **apathy** may be so profound that they are indifferent to their incontinence. The apathy associated with prefrontal lesions has been used to clinical advantage in the past. The prefrontal lobotomy was a surgical procedure that severed the connection between the prefrontal cortex and the **dorsomedial nucleus of the thalamus.** It was used to treat psychotic patients in the era before the introduction of neuroleptics. It also was used to treat patients with intractable pain. These patients did not experience less pain after the procedure, but they cared less about their pain.

Orbitofrontal Prefrontal Cortex   The **orbitofrontal cortex** is extensively interconnected with the **limbic system.** Patients with lesions in this area tend to have problems with **behavioral control.** They become disinhibited, impulsive, and distractible. They may be emotionally labile and euphoric, and they may have an inappropriate or jocular affect.

Clinical Manifestations of Prefrontal Disease   The clinical manifestations of frontal lobe disease can be quite varied. The features of orbitofrontal and dorsolateral syndromes often overlap. Other characteristic findings are difficult to localize to a specific anatomic location. Patients with prefrontal lesions may have difficulty with **abstract reasoning,** such as proverb interpretation. They may exhibit **poor judgment,** requiring close supervision. **Paratonia (gegenhalten)** may be found during the motor examination. This is a characteristic increase in tone that can seem as though the patient is intentionally resisting the examiner. Primitive reflexes, normally present only in infants, may reemerge. These **frontal release signs** include the grasp, suck, rooting, and snout reflexes. Finally, these patients often have a shuffling **magnetic gait** that can predispose to falls (gait apraxia).

Initial screening evaluations of patients with altered mental status are performed to identify potentially reversible causes. These studies include a careful examination to look for localizing clues and neuroimaging to identify structural disturbances or hydrocephalus. Routine laboratory studies include metabolic and hematology panels, thyroid function, and vitamin B_{12} level, as well as studies to identify infectious or inflammatory processes either systemically or localized to the central nervous system (CNS). EEG is used to identify nonconvulsive seizures and to confirm generalized encephalopathy.

Dementia and Delirium   Although the aforementioned features are commonly associated with frontal lobe lesions, it is important to note the broad range of generalized disorders that can present similarly. The cognitive changes in patients like TR are often seen in the setting of dementia. When assessing such patients, confusion often arises between the diagnosis of delirium and dementia. **Delirium** is an acute state of confusion associated with altered perception. **Dementia,** on the other hand, is a term used to describe chronic deterioration of cognitive function. The two conditions are not mutually exclusive. In fact, patients with dementia are often more susceptible to acute confusional states. Both conditions are commonly encountered as the consequence of general medical problems. Infections, metabolic disturbances, deficiency states, endocrine abnormalities, and toxin exposure (including alcohol and illicit drugs) can all be associated with altered mentation. Dementia, in particular, is often associated with clinical manifestations resembling the frontal lobe syndromes described earlier in this case. This does not mean that the frontal lobe is the primary site of pathology in dementing illnesses. The dementias generally lack specific neuroanatomic localization. The key features of some of the most common forms of dementia are discussed later in this case (see Thumbnail: Prefrontal Cortex).

Case Conclusion   TR was admitted to the hospital for evaluation of his deteriorating neurologic function. Initial screening laboratory studies were performed to exclude metabolic, endocrine, nutritional, and toxic causes for his symptoms. No evidence of systemic disease was found. An MRI of the brain did not reveal any structural causes. The ventricular system appeared to be enlarged. A large-volume lumbar puncture was performed and a normal opening pressure was documented. Several hours after the procedure, the family noted some improvement in TR's condition. His condition, however, deteriorated again over several days. Arrangements were made for ventricular shunt placement to treat his NPH.

Thumbnail: Prefrontal Cortex

Syndromes	Characteristics	Causes
Broad categories		
Cortical dementias	Memory problems, getting lost, aphasia, apraxia, agnosia, executive problems	Degenerative, vascular, infectious, inflammatory
Subcortical dementias	Bradyphrenia, poor attention and motivation apathy, irritability, depression	Degenerative, vascular, infectious, inflammatory, often reversible general medical conditions
Dementia plus	Dementia with associated pyramidal, extrapyramidal, or cerebellar signs	Dementia with Lewy bodies; Huntington's disease; Parkinson's disease; corticobasal degeneration; Creutzfeldt-Jakob disease
Specific syndromes		
Alzheimer's disease	Most common dementia; initially cortical dementia pattern with gradually broadening and worsening symptoms	Cerebral atrophy; neuronal loss; amyloid plaques; neurofibrillary tangles; both sporadic and hereditary forms are recognized
Vascular dementia	Second most common dementia; cause, stigmata of multiple infarctions such as hemiparesis, hemianesthesia, or visual field deficits may be seen	Multiple cerebral infarctions
Binswanger's syndrome	A vascular dementia syndrome; subcortical dementia features, prominent frontal lobe features	Extensive subcortical white matter ischemic disease
Dementia with Lewy bodies	Intermittent psychosis, parkinsonian features, second most common primary dementia	Intraneuronal Lewy body inclusions—more extensive than Parkinson's disease
Frontotemporal dementias	Prominent frontal lobe features	Anterior frontal and/or anterior temporal atrophy can be asymmetric
Pick's disease	A frontotemporal dementia; prominent frontal lobe features	Neuronal loss in cortical layers 1 through 3, Pick's bodies (neuronal inclusion bodies)
Creutzfeldt-Jakob disease and other spongiform encephalopathies	Rapidly progressive, aggressive dementing illnesses	Prion diseases; mostly sporadic, some hereditary Spongiform cerebral changes; may have elevated 14–3–3 protein in CSF (non-specific)
Pseudodementia	Variable features	Depression

Key Points

- The prefrontal cortex facilitates the integration of information over time.
- The prefrontal cortex is involved in affective behavior, judgment, and creativity.
- Dorsolateral prefrontal lesions are associated with behavioral apathy.
- Orbitofrontal prefrontal lesions are associated with impulsive behavior and disruption of normal mood and affect.
- Medial prefrontal lesions are associated with incontinence.

- Paratonia (gegenhalten) is a characteristic increase in tone associated with frontal lesions.
- Frontal release signs include the grasp, suck, rooting, and snout reflexes.
- Delirium is an acute state of confusion associated with altered perception.
- Dementia is a term used to describe chronic deterioration of cognitive function.

Questions

1. A 50-year-old man with a known history of meningioma is being evaluated for worsening leg weakness and new-onset urinary incontinence. Where is his tumor?
   A. Over the dorsolateral prefrontal cortex, on the left
   B. Over the dorsolateral prefrontal cortex, on the right
   C. Near the orbitofrontal prefrontal cortex, in the midline
   D. Along the falx cerebri, in the midline
   E. Near the pineal gland, in the midline

2. A 36-year-old woman has suffered a rupture of an aneurysm on the anterior communicating artery. She survives and the lesion is clipped. However, she sustains injury to the prefrontal cortex and has marked personality changes. She is noted to be profoundly apathetic to her condition. The connection between her prefrontal cortex and which thalamic nucleus has been affected?
   A. Anterior nucleus of the thalamus
   B. Dorsomedial nucleus of the thalamus
   C. Ventral posterior nucleus of the thalamus
   D. Ventral lateral nucleus of the thalamus
   E. Medial geniculate nucleus (MGN) of the thalamus

3. What are the cardinal manifestations of NPH?
   A. Gait disturbance, snout reflex, and confusion
   B. Incontinence, rooting reflex, and gegenhalten
   C. Incontinence, grasp reflex, and gait disturbance
   D. Gait disturbance, incontinence, and confusion
   E. Confusion, suck reflex, and incontinence

4. You evaluate a patient with an orbitofrontal lesion. Which of the following behaviors is most likely to be seen?
   A. Difficulty organizing complex tasks
   B. Impulsivity
   C. Poor working memory
   D. Apathy
   E. Perseveration

HPI: SD is a 45-year-old right-handed male who has been having headaches over the past 3 months. He does not have a history of headaches. He has attributed these headaches to stress at work and a recent downturn in the economy. His headaches seem to be at their worst in the morning and are exacerbated by lying down. He has been brought to the ED today by his wife, who reports he is no longer acting like himself. Earlier today he was complaining of an inability to write properly. He also was making prominent mathematical errors, which is unusual for him.

PE: His vital signs are stable and his general examination is unrevealing. He seems somewhat confused and somnolent but answers orienting questions. He does not appear able to write. He makes prominent calculation errors. He has difficulty naming objects and does not appear to recognize his own fingers on his right hand. Right-sided hemineglect is confirmed by simultaneous stimulation. Papilledema is noted on his funduscopic examination. His cranial nerves are intact. Power, coordination, and reflexes are normal.

Thought Questions

- What is the anatomic basis for object recognition?
- What is the implication of the hemineglect?
- What cognitive processes are affected?
- What brain regions might be implicated in this case?
- What is the significance of the positional headache?

Basic Science Review and Discussion

An important clue to the cause of his symptoms is the positional quality of the headache. Headaches that are worse when upright suggest low CSF pressure, as may be seen following a lumbar puncture. Headaches that are worse when lying down, as in this case, suggest increased intracranial pressure. This can be seen in the setting of mass lesions. Neoplasms in the CNS can be broadly divided into primary CNS neoplasms and metastatic lesions.

Supratentorial lesions are more common in adults, and infratentorial lesions are more common in children. Of the systemic neoplasms associated with spread to the CNS, the most common are carcinomas of the lung, breast, ovary, gastrointestinal (GI) tract, and melanoma. Of the primary CNS neoplasms, gliomas are the most common, followed by meningiomas. Among the gliomas, glioblastoma multiforme is both the most aggressive and the most common tumor type. Although any brain region can be affected, as was the parietal lobe in this case, these tumors are most commonly found in the frontal and temporal lobes. This case highlights the many functions attributed to the parietal lobes.

Organization of the Parietal Lobe   The anterior boundary of the parietal lobe is defined by the **central sulcus,** which separates the frontal and parietal lobes. The **postcentral gyrus** (Brodmann's areas 3, 1, and 2) contains the **primary somatosensory cortex.** Supplementary and associative somatosensory cortical areas are located along the dorsomedial aspect of the parietal lobe, in the **superior parietal lobule.** This region corresponds to Brodmann's areas 5 and 7. The **sylvian (lateral) fissure** defines the lateral border of the parietal lobe on the surface of the brain. The parietal cortex is adjacent to the temporal lobe and the insular cortex in this area. The portion of the parietal cortex between the somatosensory areas and the sylvian fissure is also known as the **inferior parietal lobule.** It is made up of two gyri, the **supramarginal gyrus** and the **angular gyrus.** This region contains the main **multimodal associative cortex** (integrating information from many different areas). It is made up of Brodmann's areas 40 and 39. Brodmann's area 39 is located at the posterior end of the sylvian fissure, where it borders Brodmann's area 22 of the temporal lobe. This region contains **Wernicke's area** for receptive language, which was discussed separately. The posterior boundary of the parietal lobe is the occipital lobe. The **parieto-occipital sulcus** that defines this junction can be seen only on the medial surface of the brain.

Primary Somatosensory Cortex   All sensory information, with the exception of olfactory information, reaches its modality-specific primary sensory cortex via the thalamus. The **somatosensory system** mediates tactile and kinesthetic information from the body and face. The ascending pathways that make up this system are discussed separately. Somatosensory information from the contralateral half of the body reaches the primary somatosensory cortex via the **ventral posterolateral nucleus of the thalamus.** Information from the face is relayed by the **ventral posteromedial nucleus of the thalamus.** As is the case with the primary motor cortex, the primary somatosensory cortex is organized somatotopically. This means that adjacent somatosensory cortical areas receive information from adjacent areas on the surface of the body. This organization can be depicted graphically as a **somatosensory homunculus** (Latin for *little man*), with the region representing the face being most lateral and the region representing the lower extremity being most medial.

The **primary somatosensory cortex** is contained within the postcentral gyrus (Brodmann's areas 3a, 3b, 1, and 2). Brodmann's area 3a is concerned primarily with information from **muscle spindles.** Brodmann's areas 3b and 1 are concerned primarily with information from **skin receptors.** Brodmann's area 2 is concerned primarily with information from **deep tissue receptors.** Within the cortical area responsible for a given region of the body, adjacent columns of cells are activated preferentially by either rapidly adapting or slowly adapting receptive fields.

Structural lesions involving the primary somatosensory cortex are often characterized by loss of sensation to all modalities in the early stages of injury. However, tests of **proprioception** and **discrimination** may be the most sensitive in identifying the deficits. Loss of proprioception can also occur with lesions anywhere along the dorsal column-medial lemniscus system and, therefore, is not specific to cortical lesions. Loss of sensory discrimination can be seen with lesions of the primary somatosensory areas, particularly if the lesions extend posteriorly into associative and supplementary sensory areas. This manifests as **cortical sensory loss,** in which primary sensory modalities are intact, but integrative sensory functions are impaired. Cortical sensory loss is best detected by tests of discrimination, as outlined in Table 4-1. In the subacute to the chronic phase, there may be some recovery of pain, temperature, and light touch.

Higher Order Somatosensory Cortical Areas

Parietal operculum The **secondary somatosensory cortex** is located at the inferolateral end of the postcentral gyrus,

Table 4-1 Tests of somatosensory discrimination

Test	Description
Stereognosis	Identifying an object by touch, with the eyes closed
Graphesthesia	Identifying a letter or symbol traced on the skin
Extinction	Tactile stimulus is perceived on either side of the body when tested individually but only on one side of the body when both sides are tested simultaneously. Also called double simultaneous stimulation.

in an area called the **parietal operculum.** It also has a degree of somatotopic organization. Both sides of the body are represented in this area, although the contralateral side of the body still predominates. This area receives input from the thalamus and from primary cortical areas in both hemispheres. Lesions in this area have been associated with dissociation between pain and its meaning. In the subacute to the chronic phase, a pseudothalamic pain syndrome may develop.

Superior parietal lobule The **supplementary and associative somatosensory cortical areas** (Brodmann's areas 5 and 7) are located in the superior parietal lobule, along the dorsomedial aspect of the parietal lobe. These cortical areas are responsible for the perception of texture, shape, and size. They receive input from primary and secondary somatosensory areas and project primarily to multimodal associative areas, such as the inferior parietal lobule. Lesions of these higher order sensory areas can manifest as **cortical sensory loss** (described earlier in this case) or may be associated with more profound deficits. Unilateral lesions may be associated with **hemineglect** of the contralateral side of the body. This deficit can be so profound that affected individuals may not recognize the affected limbs as their own. Bilateral parieto-occipital lesions are rarely encountered but are characterized by **Balint's syndrome** or optic ataxia (i.e., the inability to voluntarily direct gaze to a specified point). The parietal syndromes are summarized later in this case (see Thumbnail: Parietal Cortex).

Main Multimodal Associative Cortex

Inferior parietal lobule The inferior parietal lobule contains the **supramarginal gyrus** and the **angular gyrus** and roughly corresponds to Brodmann's areas 40 and 39. This is the main **association cortex,** where multimodal information from various cortical areas is integrated. All sensory cortical areas are interconnected with this region. This region of cortex also projects to motor cortex, prefrontal cortex, and other associative areas. In essence, this is the cortical region where sensory input is analyzed and implemented. Lesions of the major association cortex in the nondominant hemisphere can be associated with **constructional apraxia** and **contralateral hemineglect.** Comparable lesions in the dominant hemisphere are associated with **Gerstmann's syndrome** (right-to-left disorientation, agraphia, acalculia, and finger agnosia). The parietal syndromes are summarized later in this case (see Thumbnail: Parietal Cortex).

Case Conclusion   An emergent CT scan of the head confirmed a left parietal lesion consistent with the clinical presentation of Gerstmann's syndrome. This scan revealed no evidence of acute hemorrhage. It was most consistent with a mass lesion or old ischemia. There was evidence of mass effect and midline shift. An MRI of the brain confirmed an irregularly enhancing left parietal mass lesion with central hypodensity and surrounding edema. Glioblastoma multiforme, the most malignant and one of the most common glial cell tumors, was suspected. Steroids were initiated to help relieve the exacerbation of symptoms associated with cerebral edema and mass effect. The patient was referred to a specialized center where a comprehensive team approach including neurosurgery, neuro-oncology, neuroradiology, and radiation oncology could be applied to this patient's care.

Thumbnail: Parietal Cortex

Parieto-Occipital Syndromes

Syndrome	Manifestations	Location	Special notes
Hemineglect syndrome	Impaired response to stimuli and anosognosia (denial of deficits)	Contralateral parietal cortex	More prominent with nondominant hemisphere involvement
Anton's syndrome	Cortical blindness	Visual cortex	Anosognosia of blindness
Balint's syndrome	Optic ataxia	Bilateral parieto-occipital lesions	Inability to direct gaze to a given point
Gerstmann's syndrome	Right-to-left disorientation; acalculia; agraphia; finger agnosia	Dominant angular gyrus	
Callosal syndrome	Hemialexia; ideomotor apraxia; agraphia; tactile anomia; auditory extinction	Corpus callosum	Only perceptions by dominant hemisphere can be described
Dejerine's syndrome	Right homonymous hemianopia; amnesia; alexia without agraphia	Parieto-occipital cortex	PCA infarction

Key Points

▶ Proprioception and discrimination may be the most sensitive tests of early parietal deficits.

▶ Recovery of pain, temperature, and light touch can be seen in the subacute to the chronic phase of parietal injury.

▶ In cortical sensory loss, primary sensory modalities are intact but integrative sensory functions are not.

▶ Unilateral parietal lesions can result in contralateral hemineglect.

▶ The major association cortex is in the supramarginal and angular gyri, in the inferior parietal lobule.

▶ Nondominant major association cortex lesions are associated with constructional apraxia and contralateral hemineglect.

Questions

1. You evaluate a patient with hemineglect and constructional apraxia. You suspect a lesion in the contralateral major association cortex. Which of the following is most likely to be affected?
   A. Parietal operculum
   B. Superior parietal lobule
   C. Supramarginal gyrus
   D. Brodmann's areas 5 and 7
   E. Postcentral gyrus

2. A 66-year-old woman has cortical sensory loss following a stroke. Which of the following functions would be most affected in this patient?
   A. Stereognosis
   B. Sensation of pain and temperature
   C. Proprioception
   D. Muscle spindle function
   E. Function of deep tissue receptors

3. A right-handed patient that you have been asked to evaluate has a left-sided inferior parietal tumor. Which of the following manifestations is least likely to be found in this patient?
   A. Right-to-left disorientation
   B. Constructional apraxia
   C. Agraphia
   D. Acalculia
   E. Finger agnosia

4. You evaluate a man who has developed numbness involving the lower half of his left face shortly after having had a stroke. Which of the following structures may be involved?
   A. Facial nerve
   B. Ventral posterolateral thalamic nucleus
   C. Ventral posteromedial nucleus of the thalamus
   D. Trigeminal nerve
   E. Dorsomedial nucleus of the thalamus

HPI: BS is a 69-year-old right-handed male who presents to the ED with acute onset of vision loss and mental status changes 2 hours ago.

PE: His vital signs are stable. He has a history of atrial fibrillation, but only takes his medications intermittently. He is somewhat somnolent, but he is able to answer orienting questions and follows commands during examination. His cranial nerve examination reveals a left homonymous hemianopia. His cranial nerve function is otherwise spared. There are no abnormalities noted on testing of motor or sensory function. Coordination is appropriate to the remainder of his examination. He has symmetric reflexes and no long-tract signs.

Thought Questions

- What is the anatomic basis for visual processing?
- What structures are associated with hemianopia?
- What structures are associated with quadrantanopia?
- What other signs and symptoms might one expect in such a case?
- What clues do the acute manifestation and medical history give concerning etiology?

Basic Science Review and Discussion

The acute manifestation of neurologic deficits should always bring to mind the possibility of a vascular cause, particularly in the setting of cardiovascular disease. This patient's symptoms are localized to the occipital lobe. This area is supplied by the PCA, which branches from the posterior circulation of the CNS. Associated symptoms could include vertigo, cranial nerve deficits, motor and sensory deficits, thalamic dysfunction, and peduncular hallucinosis. The clinical manifestations of cerebral vascular disease are discussed in further detail separately. This case focuses on the functional implications of occipital lobe injury. The main function of the occipital lobe is the processing of visual information. Different regions within the occipital lobe process units of information of varying complexity.

Organization of the Occipital Lobe The **occipital lobe** extends anteriorly from the occipital pole. The anterior boundary of the occipital lobe on the lateral surface of the brain is poorly defined. In this region, the occipital lobe merges with the parietal and temporal lobes. On the medial surface of the brain, the **parieto-occipital sulcus** defines the anterior boundary of the occipital lobe. The **calcarine sulcus** is perpendicular to the parieto-occipital sulcus and extends posteriorly to the occipital pole. These two sulci, together, look like a capital letter *T*.

Visual Cortex and Visual Processing Remember that visual input to the cortex originates in the **lateral geniculate nucleus** of the thalamus and terminates in the fourth cortical layer of the primary visual cortex. The visual pathways leading from the retina to the cortex are discussed in more detail in Case 23. A key point, however, is that visual information processed in one hemisphere represents input from both eyes pertaining to the contralateral visual field. Thus, a cortical lesion involving the occipital lobe on one side, as in the current case, would be expected to result in a **contralateral homonymous hemianopia.** However, there is usually a degree of **macular sparing** in these lesions. This is related to an abundant collateral vascular supply of the primary visual cortex. The visual field defects associated with various visual pathway lesions are discussed further in Case 23.

The **primary visual cortex,** or calcarine cortex, is contained within and around the calcarine sulcus. It corresponds to **Brodmann's area 17.** It is also called the **striate cortex** because it has a striped histologic appearance. This is because the fourth cortical layer in the primary visual cortex is divided by a visible line of white matter, called the **line of Gennari.**

As we have seen in other sensory systems, the organization of the visual cortex is **retinotopic.** This means that adjacent retinal areas and adjacent regions in the visual field are processed in adjacent calcarine cortical areas. The cortical areas responsible for central vision are located most posteriorly in the calcarine cortex, near the **occipital pole.** The amount of cortical area devoted to central vision is disproportionately large, reflecting the importance of the information being received from the **macula.** The remaining retinal areas are represented by cortical areas extending anteriorly from the occipital pole like a collapsed spiderweb. Throughout this cortical system, the regions of cortex responsible for processing information from the upper retina (and lower visual field) are located superior to the calcarine sulcus, in an area called the **cuneus.** The regions of cortex responsible for processing information from the lower retina (and upper visual field), on the other hand, are located inferior to the calcarine sulcus, in an area called the **lingual gyrus.**

Primary Visual Cortex The processing of visual information has several layers of complexity. Visual processing in the primary visual cortex is concerned primarily with basic visual units that respond preferentially to specific stimuli. Electrical stimulation of the primary visual cortex results in the perception of flashes of light, rather than formed image. Neurons within the primary visual cortex have **receptive fields** that respond preferentially to specific linear visual stimuli (horizontal, vertical, etc.). Neurons that respond to a particular orientation in a particular region of the retina are grouped together within **simple units.** Within each unit, some neurons may respond preferentially to either onset or cessation of illumination. **Complex units** receive information from multiple simple units. Groups of units concerned with a particular stimulus type are called *columns.* **Ocular dominance columns** respond preferentially to input from a given eye. **Orientation columns** respond preferentially to stimuli in a particular orientation in space. Higher order visual cortex areas are involved in further processing of these basic components of visual input.

Secondary Visual Cortex   The primary visual cortex is generally designated as *V1.* Subsequently higher orders of visual processing occur in cortical areas designated *V2–V5.* The **main secondary visual cortical regions** are V2 and V3, which respectively correspond to **Brodmann's areas 18 and 19.** Like V1, V2 is organized retinotopically. Neurons in this area have more complex receptive fields. The remaining areas of visual cortex are more concerned with specific aspects of vision. V3 appears to be associated with the processing of more **complex forms.** The localization of V4 and V5 is less precise. Both areas are located in the border area between the occipital and temporal lobes. V4 appears to be associated with the processing of **color information.** V5 has been implicated in the processing of information regarding **the motion of objects in the visual field.** These cortical regions, in turn, project to higher order associative cortical areas where visual input is integrated with information from other sensory modalities.

Clinical Correlation   The disruption of cortical sensory function can manifest clinically as agnosia. **Agnosia** is a modality-specific inability to recognize sensory input, often localized near the junction of the parietal, occipital, and temporal lobes. The agnosias are summarized later in this case (see Thumbnail: Occipital Cortex and Visual Processing). Note that the visual system plays an important role in many of these clinical manifestations. Output from the visual association cortex to **Brodmann's area 7** in the posterior parietal cortex is thought to mediate the **perception of depth and movement.** Output to the associative parietal cortex in **Brodmann's areas 39 and 22** is implicated in the visual **recognition of objects and symbols.** Patients with lesions in these areas may not be able to identify objects **(visual agnosia)** and may not be able to read **(alexia).** Output to **Brodmann's area 37,** at the occipitotemporal border, is involved in the **recognition of faces.** The loss of this function is called **prosopagnosia.** Output to **Brodmann's areas 20 and 21** in the inferior and middle temporal gyri is thought to be associated with the **analysis of form and color.** Stimulation of these areas is associated with complex visual hallucinations.

Case Conclusion   BS was initially evaluated under an acute stroke pathway because of the nature and abrupt onset of his symptoms, as well as his cardiac risk factors. Stat routine laboratory studies, including a coagulation panel, were normal. A CT scan of the head revealed no evidence of hemorrhage or subacute changes. Thrombolytics were initiated and were tolerated without complications. An MRI of the brain confirmed the diagnosis of a right occipital lobe infarction in the distribution of the right PCA. The area of infarction was wedge shaped and consistent with an embolic cause. A cardiology consultation was obtained, and eventually, warfarin therapy was restarted. BS regained some vision in the left half of his visual fields, but it was incomplete. He was also troubled by visual illusions, suggesting a residual impairment of higher order visual processing.

Thumbnail: Occipital Cortex and Visual Processing

Agnosias		
Subtypes	**Manifestations**	**Localization**
Visual		
Apperceptive agnosia	Picture, object, or color not perceived	Parieto-occipital associative cortex
Simultanagnosia	Recognize the parts but not the whole	Parieto-occipital associative cortex
Associative agnosia	Objects perceived but devoid of meaning	Parieto-occipital associative cortex
Prosopagnosia	Inability to recognize faces	Occipitotemporal border
Alexia without agraphia	Pure word blindness; hemianopia; inability to read; writing is spared	Dominant primary visual cortex and splenium of corpus callosum; part of Dejerine's syndrome
Alexia with agraphia	Inability to read or write	Dominant angular gyrus
Acalculia	Inability to do math	Parieto-occipital associative cortex; part of Gerstmann's syndrome
Auditory		
Verbal agnosia	Pure word deafness	Disconnection of auditory cortex from Wernicke's area
Sound agnosia	Impaired recognition of nonverbal sounds	Associative auditory cortex
Sensory amusia	Inability to recognize music	Dominant temporal cortex in musicians Nondominant in nonmusicians
Tactile		
Astereognosia	Inability to recognize objects by touch	Contralateral parietal cortex
Asymbolia	Inability to associate objects to their meanings	Contralateral parietal cortex

Key Points

- The primary visual cortex is contained within and around the calcarine sulcus.
- Unilateral occipital injuries result in contralateral homonymous hemianopia.
- Neurons in the visual cortex have receptive fields that respond preferentially to specific linear visual stimuli.
- Neurons that respond to a particular orientation in a particular region of the retina are grouped together within simple units.
- Complex units receive information from multiple simple units.
- Ocular dominance columns respond preferentially to input from a given eye.
- Orientation columns respond preferentially to stimuli in a particular orientation in space.
- Agnosia is a modality-specific inability to recognize sensory input.

Questions

1. You evaluate a patient with a visual field deficit. You determine that she has a homonymous left superior quadrantanopia. Where is her lesion?
   A. Right occipital lobe
   B. Right parietal lobe
   C. Right temporal lobe
   D. Right optic tract
   E. Right lateral geniculate nucleus of the thalamus

2. You evaluate a patient with known epilepsy. His seizures are associated with vivid visual hallucinations, followed by secondary generalization. Which of the following is most likely to contain his seizure focus?
   A. Posterior parietal cortex
   B. Inferior temporal cortex
   C. Occipitotemporal junction
   D. Angular gyrus
   E. Calcarine cortex

3. You evaluate a woman who has lost color vision. Which region of visual cortex is most likely to be affected?
   A. V1
   B. V2
   C. V3
   D. V4
   E. V5

4. You evaluate a man who has developed visual illusions in the wake of an ischemic stroke. He states that as he is talking with you, your head appears to be floating away from your body. Which region of visual cortex is most likely to be affected?
   A. V1
   B. V2
   C. V3
   D. V4
   E. V5

HPI: HV is a 23-year-old man who comes to the ED with acute altered mental status. His girlfriend states that he was in his usual state of health until yesterday. He came home from work complaining of a headache. He subsequently developed a fever. This morning he awoke feeling ill and decided not to go to work. He has become progressively more confused throughout the day. His deteriorating mental status has prompted emergent evaluation.

PE: He is febrile but other vitals signs are stable. You find him to be stuporous and only minimally cooperative with your examination. However, he does not appear to have any clearly localizing or lateralizing neurologic findings. During your examination, the patient has a generalized tonic-clonic seizure.

Thought Questions

- What is the most likely cause of this patient's headache?

- What is the implication of his altered level of consciousness?

- What brain region is implicated by the seizure in this setting?

- What other functions are mediated by this brain region?

Basic Science Review and Discussion

The presentation of acute, severe headache in the setting of fever should always bring to mind the possibility of **meningitis.** Involvement of the cerebral cortex (encephalitis) is implicated when altered mentation is superimposed on these findings, as is the case with the present patient. Encephalitis or meningoencephalitis also can be associated with seizures, aphasia, and coma. Assessing for signs of meningismus (meningeal irritation) is important in this setting. **Nuchal rigidity** is stiffness of the neck that resists passive flexion. **Brudzinski's sign** describes involuntary flexion of the hips and knees in response to passive flexion of the neck. **Kernig's sign** describes resistance to passive extension of the knee in a seated patient.

A variety of bacterial, viral, and nonviral causes need to be considered. The most common **bacterial causes** include *Streptococcus pneumoniae, Neisseria meningitidis, Haemophilus influenzae,* and *Listeria monocytogenes.* The most common **viral causes** include herpes simplex viruses (HSV), arboviruses, and enteroviruses. HSV is particularly likely to involve medial temporal lobe structures, causing characteristic epileptiform abnormalities on EEG. CSF analysis must be performed to identify the cause of these conditions. However, empiric therapy should always be initiated, rather than waiting for laboratory results. Bacterial causes are usually associated with increased opening pressure, high protein level, low or normal glucose level, and polymorphonuclear (PMN) cell proliferation. Bacteria may be seen on Gram stain and should be cultured. Viral causes are usually associated with normal or increased opening pressure, high protein level, normal glucose level, and mononuclear cell proliferation. In the case of HSV, affected areas may be hemorrhagic and red blood cells (RBCs) may be found in the CSF.

Organization of the Temporal Lobe If the lateral view of the brain looks like a boxer's glove, then the temporal lobe is represented by the glove's thumb. This orientation emphasizes the C-shaped structure of the pathways connecting temporal and frontal areas. The temporal lobe extends anteriorly to the **temporal pole** and inferiorly to the base of the brain. The **sylvian fissure** defines the superior aspect of the temporal lobe. Posteriorly, the temporal lobe is continuous with the associative areas of the parietal and occipital lobes. The temporal lobe contains a number of important structures with diverse functional significance. The superior and posterior portions of the temporal cortex are concerned with the processing of auditory information and with associative functions. Several important subcortical white matter pathways are located within the temporal lobe. Among them, the **arcuate fasciculus** plays an important role in the language system by connecting Wernicke's area to Broca's area. The temporal lobe also contains a portion of the **optic radiations** connecting the lateral geniculate nucleus of the thalamus with the primary visual cortex. This fiber bundle, known as **Meyer's loop,** is discussed further within the context of the visual system. However, it is important to remember that temporal lobe lesions can be associated with a **homonymous superior quadrantanopia** related to compromise of Meyer's loop. The temporal lobe also contains important deep nuclear groups involved in memory and emotion. The **hippocampus** is, technically, a continuation of the cerebral cortex that has been largely internalized. It lies deep within the temporal lobe and gives rise to the **Papez circuit.** This system is critical for the formation of new memories. This circuit is reviewed later in this case (see Thumbnail: Temporal Lobe). The **amygdala** is located anterior to the hippocampal formation in the temporal lobe. It helps to mediate emotional experience. The hippocampus and amygdala are discussed further within the context of the **limbic system.** The inferior and medial regions of the temporal cortex are immediately superficial to these limbic structures. They are involved in limbic circuitry and mediate olfaction, which is discussed separately. In addition to mediating these important primary functions, the temporal lobes are often implicated in epilepsy.

Temporal Cortex Most of the cerebral cortex is made up of neocortex. The remaining types of cortex, **allocortex** and **mesocortex,** are found primarily in the inferomedial (mesial) temporal lobe. This area is susceptible to injury, leading to **mesial temporal sclerosis** (MTS). MTS is a structural abnormality commonly associated with intractable epilepsy. In these cases, early surgical resection of MTS can be curative.

Allocortex consists of three layers. It is found in the **hippocampal formation** (archicortex) and adjacent **piriform cortex** (paleocortex). **Mesocortex** has an intermediate structure and forms a transitional boundary between allocortex and the neocortex of the temporal lobe. Mesocortex forms the **entorhinal cortex** and **parahippocampal cortex** of the mesial temporal lobe. These cortical areas are involved in olfaction and limbic functions (Figure 6-1).

Auditory Cortex The superior and lateral temporal cortex can be divided into three gyri: the superior, middle, and inferior temporal gyri. The **superior temporal gyrus** extends into the inferior aspect of the sylvian fissure. This area includes the **transverse gyrus of Heschl** (Brodmann's areas 41 and 42), which contains the primary and secondary auditory cortex. The subcortical auditory pathways that ultimately terminate in this area are discussed separately.

Ascending auditory pathways project to the **MGN of the thalamus,** which subsequently projects to the primary auditory cortex (Brodmann's area 41). The auditory cortex is not involved in the determination of different frequencies. This occurs subcortically, beginning with the cochlea. In fact, the structure of the cochlea defines the **tonotopic organization** of the auditory system. In the cortex, lower frequencies are located more anteriorly within the transverse gyrus of Heschl.

The primary and secondary auditory cortical areas are responsible for the integration of different components of sound and for the integration of different sounds over time. These areas receive bilateral input and, therefore, are not expected to be associated with hearing loss when injured. Although unilateral lesions in the auditory cortex may be associated with a mild degree of contralateral hearing impairment, the most common finding in this setting is impaired **sound localization in space.**

Higher order **associative auditory cortex** (Brodmann's area 22) makes up the remainder of the superior temporal gyrus. This is the area where sounds are recognized and paired with particular images and memories. For example, when hearing a train whistle, one recognizes that this sound is associated with the concept of a train. This sound may also bring to mind the image of a train. The most posterior portion of this cortical region contains **Wernicke's area,** which mediates the comprehension of language. The systems involved in the processing of language are discussed separately. The middle and inferior temporal gyri are involved in higher order visual processing and are discussed within the context of the occipital cortex and visual system.

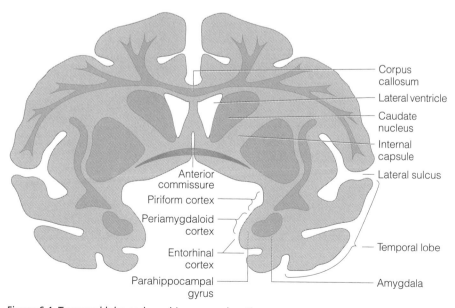

Figure 6-1 Temporal lobe and parahippocampal cortices.

Case Conclusion   HV's seizure activity was controlled with lorazepam. He was started on empiric ceftriaxone and acyclovir. A lumbar puncture was performed. The opening pressure was mildly elevated and the CSF was clear. Initial laboratory data confirmed an aseptic process consistent with viral meningoencephalitis. RBC counts were also elevated in the CSF. The suspicion of herpes simplex encephalitis was ultimately confirmed by polymerase chain reaction (PCR) analysis of the CSF. MRI scans of brain confirmed a right medial temporal inflammatory process, also consistent with the diagnosis. HV received high-dose intravenously (IV) administered acyclovir for 14 days. He gradually returned to his baseline. He subsequently did well but continued to have rare seizures, which ultimately resulted in the initiation of an antiepileptic medication.

Thumbnail: Temporal Lobe

Papez Circuit

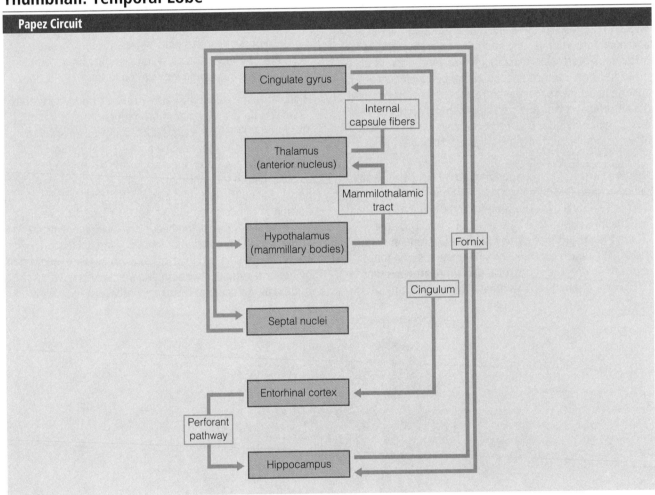

Key Points

- The arcuate fasciculus mediates language by connecting Wernicke's and Broca's areas.
- The optic radiations connect the lateral geniculate nucleus to the primary visual cortex.
- Lesions of Meyer's loop cause contralateral homonymous superior quadrantanopsias.
- Allocortex and mesocortex are found primarily in temporal and limbic regions.

- The primary auditory cortex is located in the transverse gyrus of Heschl.
- Auditory cortex damage may present as impaired sound localization in space.
- The middle and inferior temporal gyri are concerned with visual processing.
- The medial temporal lobe is concerned with memory and emotion.

Questions

1. A 35-year-old female undergoes right anterior temporal lobectomy to help control her seizures. Postoperatively, she reports impaired vision in the left upper quadrant of her visual field. Which structure is responsible?
   A. Uncus
   B. Amygdala
   C. Hippocampus
   D. Meyer's loop
   E. Transverse gyrus of Heschl

2. A 42-year-old male undergoes a selective surgical procedure on his right temporal lobe for treatment of his seizures. The goal of the procedure is to focus on the medial temporal lobe. Which of the following types of cortex is most likely to be relatively spared?
   A. Mesocortex
   B. Allocortex
   C. Piriform cortex
   D. Entorhinal cortex
   E. Neocortex

3. You evaluate a 67-year-old patient who can no longer localize sounds in space. Where might his lesion be located?
   A. Superior temporal gyrus
   B. Middle temporal gyrus
   C. Inferior temporal gyrus
   D. Medial temporal lobe
   E. MGN

4. You have determined that a 72-year-old gentleman has sustained an ischemic injury to his arcuate fasciculus. You know this because he has which of the following problems?
   A. He has a homonymous hemianopsia.
   B. He has a superior homonymous quadrantanopsia.
   C. He cannot repeat what you say.
   D. He cannot localize sounds in space.
   E. He seems unable to understand you.

HPI: AC is a 16-year-old boy who has been brought to the ED following a generalized convulsion. He was treated with lorazepam in the field and is no longer seizing at the time of your evaluation. He is very sleepy and cannot give a good history. His vital signs are stable. There are no focal findings on his neurologic examination. His mother reports that he has been having seizures frequently for several years. His spells are preceded by a sense that ongoing events have happened before and a rising sensation in the stomach. He sometimes smells burning rubber before his spells. His spells often resolve without generalized convulsions. He has tried several antiepileptic medications without success.

Thought Questions

- Which brain region is implicated by the symptoms preceding his spells?

- What other functions are mediated by this area?

- To what other brain regions is this area connected?

Basic Science Review and Discussion

Dysfunction of the limbic system manifests as altered mentation, memory, or behavior. Seizures, as in this patient, are a very commonly encountered clinical manifestation of limbic dysfunction. Although seizures can originate from any cortical area, seizures originating from medial temporal structures are a particularly important clinical entity. The clinical features associated with seizures arising from different cortical regions are summarized in Case 22 (see Thumbnail: Olfaction and Olfactory Nerve).

Seizures are the manifestation of excessively synchronized electrical activity involving the cortical surface of the brain. They can be either clinical or subclinical, in which case they are detected only by EEG. The new onset of seizures should always precipitate a search for possible causes. This search should include laboratory testing for possible metabolic or toxic processes, brain imaging to look for structural abnormalities, and evaluation for possible infectious processes. An EEG is indicated to evaluate for localizing epileptiform abnormalities and to exclude ongoing, nonconvulsive seizures in unresponsive patients.

Seizures are usually brief, lasting seconds to a few minutes. They are divided into several subtypes, depending on their clinical manifestations. Patients with recurrent seizures are diagnosed with **epilepsy** and need to be treated with antiepileptic medications. **Focal seizures** are associated with a localized disturbance of brain activity. For example, a focal motor seizure might be associated with abnormal movement of just one extremity. A **simple partial seizure** is a focal seizure during which consciousness is preserved. The electrical disturbance can then spread to adjacent brain areas. A **complex partial seizure** is a seizure in which cortical involvement is profound enough to alter consciousness or mentation. A **secondary generalized seizure** is one that starts as a partial seizure but spreads to involve the whole surface of the brain. **Primary generalized seizures** involve the entire surface of the brain from the beginning. They may be the cortical manifestation of subcortical processes. Because the entire surface is involved simultaneously, primary generalized seizures are not preceded by auras. When seizures become generalized, they most often manifest as **tonic-clonic seizures.** The tonic phase consists of whole-body stiffening. The patient may let out a cry as air is forced from the lungs. This is followed by the clonic phase, which consists of rhythmic jerking of the entire body. Although this is the most common manifestation, generalized seizures can also be associated with absence (blank staring), purely tonic, atonic, purely clonic, or myoclonic (rapid jerking) features. Combinations of these manifestations can also be seen.

Patients often describe an aura preceding their seizures. **Auras** are the focal manifestations of partial seizures before they spread. AC experienced an unpleasant odor preceding his seizure. This type of aura is commonly associated with seizures of temporal lobe origin. Other symptoms associated with auras of temporal lobe origin include fear, frequent feelings of déjà vu (a sense that what is being experienced has been experienced previously), and nausea or uneasiness of the stomach. These seizures can progress to unresponsive staring, a variety of orofacial automatisms (automatic movements), and other manifestations as other brain regions become involved. As we will see, many of these symptoms can be reproduced by stimulation of the **amygdala.** These seizures are sometimes called **uncinate seizures.** This is a reference to the uncus, which overlies the amygdala. When patients with temporal lobe epilepsy are treated with medications, they may report that their seizures have stopped, but they still have auras. This means that they are still having simple partial seizures, but their seizures are no longer spreading to other brain regions.

As a general rule, seizures that always begin in the same cortical areas may be associated with a structural abnormality in that area. In **younger patients,** one of the more commonly encountered underlying causes is MTS (hippocampal). These lesions may be related to insults to the temporal lobe early in life. Patients with these lesions may have seizures that are very difficult to control with medication. However, surgical resection of the abnormality can be curative in many cases. Thus, these patients must be identified early. In **older patients,** common causes for partial seizures include structural abnormalities related to previous **strokes** or to underlying neoplasms. These processes are discussed further within the context of other cases. This case focuses on limbic function and anatomy.

Limbic Function   The limbic lobe, as originally defined by early anatomists, included those structures on the inferior surface of the cerebrum that surround the brainstem. These included the inferior and medial aspects of the temporal lobes and associated structures (parahippocampal gyrus, uncus, isthmus, cingulated gyrus, and subcallosal gyrus). These areas were thought to mediate olfactory function, giving rise to the term **rhinencephalon.** We now recognize that olfaction, though closely associated with the limbic system, is a functionally separate process. The term **rhinencephalon** is still used to refer to the olfactory system, including the olfactory nerves, bulbs, tracts, striae, and primary olfactory cortex.

The **limbic system** and the **Papez circuit** are critical for **memory function,** particularly the acquisition of new memories. The limbic system and its adjacent structures have also been implicated in a wide variety of **emotional functions,** in **determining the importance of sensory information,** and in **coordinating somatic and visceral functions.** Behaviors that are associated with **self-preservation,** such as regulating nutrition, hydration, and self-defense, are partly mediated by these systems. Behaviors important to **survival of the species,** such as reproduction and social interaction, are also partly mediated by these areas.

Three major limbic emotion circuits have been proposed. Emotions related to self-preservation have been associated primarily with the amygdala and hippocampus. Emotions related to **pleasure** have been associated primarily with the cingulate gyrus and the septal nuclei of the basal forebrain, although the amygdala is also involved. Emotions related to **social cooperation** have been associated with the hypothalamus and the anterior thalamic nucleus. Of course, these are gross generalizations.

Memory   The association between the limbic system and memory is best demonstrated by the case of HM, a patient with intractable epilepsy who underwent bilateral temporal lobectomies. After these procedures, he was found to have severely impaired explicit memory and anterograde amnesia. His short-term memory and retrograde memory were not affected. **Short-term memory (working memory)** lasts seconds. This is the memory that helps one avoid bumping into others while walking through a crowd. It is localized to the frontal lobe. **Long-term memory** can last for years. It is subdivided into two types. **Explicit (declarative)** memory is concerned with learned facts. Episodic memory (of personal experience) and semantic memory (education) are both considered forms of explicit memory. The temporal lobes and septal nuclei have been implicated in forming explicit memories. **Implicit (procedural) memory** is concerned with learned skills. Structures implicated in mediating procedural memory include the dominant parietal cortex, cerebellum, basal ganglia, and frontal association cortex. Memory function is further subdivided based on cerebral dominance. The **left hippocampus** is needed to acquire new **verbal information.** The **right hippocampus** is needed to acquire new **nonverbal information.**

Organization of the Limbic System

Papez circuit   The concept of a "limbic system" has been in constant evolution over the past century. It arose from the combination of the limbic lobe with a circuit of several brain structures thought to mediate **emotional behavior and memory.** This circuit was defined by James Papez and still carries his name. The **Papez circuit** is illustrated in Case 6 (see Thumbnail: Temporal Lobe). It includes the **hippocampal formation, mammillary bodies, thalamus,** and **cingulated gyrus,** which then projects back to the hippocampus. Of course, the circuit also includes the fiber tracts that connect these different areas. The **fornix** connects the hippocampus to the mammillary bodies. The **mammillothalamic tract** connects the mammillary bodies to the anterior nucleus of the thalamus. Fibers from the anterior nucleus of the thalamus reach the cingulated gyrus via the **internal capsule.** The **cingulum** conveys fibers from the cingulated gyrus to the entorhinal cortex, in the parahippocampal gyrus. Finally, fibers from the entorhinal area reach the hippocampus via the **perforant path** and complete the circuit. As understanding of brain function has evolved, other structures have been included in this circuit. The **prefrontal cortex,** the **amygdala,** various **association cortical areas,** other **hypothalamic nuclei,** the **septal nuclei** of the basal forebrain, and the **nucleus accumbens** have all been postulated to subserve some limbic function. Some have even questioned whether the terms **Papez circuit** and **limbic system** have become obsolete, because they have grown to include so many structures.

Hippocampal Formation   The hippocampal formation is divided into three major areas whose main functions are input, processing, and output. The **dentate gyrus** is the main input area of the hippocampal formation. It is the darkly staining core at the center of most hippocampal cross sections. The **pes hippocampi,** or Ammon's horn, is the main area for hippocampal processing. It is the region immediately surrounding the dentate gyrus in hippocampal cross sections. The **subiculum** is the main output area of the hippocampal formation. It is also adjacent to the dentate gyrus but inferior to it in hippocampal cross sections. The subicu-

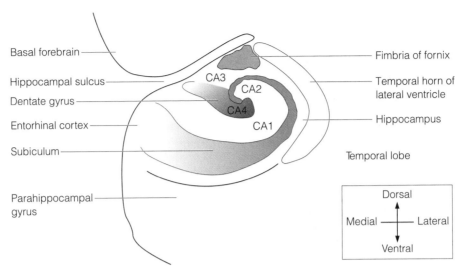

Figure 7-1 Hippocampal formation.

lum is continuous with the **entorhinal cortex** on the medial surface of the parahippocampal gyrus. This arrangement seems counterintuitive because the entorhinal cortex is a major source of input to the dentate gyrus, bypassing all of these other intervening structures (Figure 7-1).

The pes hippocampi itself is further divided into four fields, designated CA1 through CA4 (for cornu ammonis, or Ammon's horn). Region **CA4** corresponds to the border with the dentate gyrus. Regions **CA2** and **CA3** make up the body of the pes hippocampi. These areas are relatively resistant to anoxia. Region **CA1,** also called **Sommer's sector,** corresponds to the border of the pes hippocampi with the subiculum. This is also known as the **vulnerable zone,** because neurons in this area are particularly sensitive to anoxia. For this reason, the CA1 region is considered a **trigger zone** for seizures in **temporal lobe epilepsy.**

Hippocampal Neurons   Remember that the hippocampal formation is actually a cortical structure. It is made up of **allocortex,** which has only three layers. The **molecular layer** is the deepest within the hippocampal formation but is continuous with the molecular layer of the entorhinal cortex of the parahippocampal gyrus. This molecular layer, like the superficial molecular layer in other cortical areas, functions as a region of synaptic interaction. The intermediate layer of the hippocampal formation is the **pyramidal cell layer.** The pyramidal cell layer of the pes hippocampi is continuous with the granule cell layer of the dentate gyrus. The **granule cell layer** in the dentate gyrus is the main input site for information reaching the hippocampal formation.

Pyramidal neurons are the principle neurons of the hippocampus and are the only neurons in this area to project to other brain regions. The axons of these neurons in the

subiculum and the CA1 region project toward the ventricular surface of the hippocampal formation, forming the fimbriae of the fornix. The **fornix** is the main output fiber tract from the hippocampus. The third hippocampal layer is the **stratum oriens.** This layer contains various polymorphic cells that function as **inhibitory interneurons.**

The flow of hippocampal circuitry is summarized later in this case (see Thumbnail: Limbic System). Briefly, information from many brain regions reaches the hippocampal formation via the entorhinal cortex and the granule cells of the dentate gyrus. This information is processed within the layers of the pes hippocampi. The information is then projected to output targets via the pyramidal cells of the subiculum and the CA1 region.

Hippocampal Output   The **fornix** is the main pathway for hippocampal outflow. Feedback pathways also project back to hippocampal input sources via the entorhinal cortex. The fibers that make up the fornix arise from either the **subiculum** or the **hippocampal CA1** pyramidal neurons. The fibers from the subiculum project primarily to the mammillary bodies of the hypothalamus, the anterior subnucleus of the thalamus, and the amygdala. The hippocampal CA1 neurons project primarily to basal forebrain targets and the subiculum. The basal forebrain targets include the septal nuclei, inferomedial frontal cortex, anterior hypothalamic areas, and nucleus accumbens. (These structures are discussed further in this chapter and in subsequent chapters.)

Hypothalamus, Thalamus, and Cingulate Gyrus   These structures are covered in greater detail separately. The **mammillary bodies of the hypothalamus** are the main targets of hippocampal fibers in the fornix. They are strongly implicated in memory function. The mammillary bodies become atrophic in **Wernicke-Korsakoff syndrome.**

This is a syndrome of brain injury related to long-term thiamine deficiency, most often seen in the setting of alcoholism. These patients are encephalopathic, with features of psychosis. They often have anterograde amnesia and extraocular movement abnormalities. This syndrome can be induced iatrogenically when dextrose is given to alcoholic patients without thiamine supplementation.

The mammillary bodies are divided into medial and lateral nuclear groups. The medial nuclei project to the anterior nucleus of the thalamus. The lateral nuclei project to the midbrain and the pons. The **anterior nucleus of the thalamus** is the main target of fibers from the mammillary bodies via the **mammillothalamic tract.** This nucleus functions as a relay between the hypothalamus and the cingulate gyrus.

The **cingulate gyrus** is located on the medial surface of the cerebrum and is directly superior to the corpus callosum. This area coordinates the emotional content of limbic function with decision-making processes in the frontal lobes. Hyperactivity in this area has been implicated in **Tourette's syndrome.** Lesions in this area are associated with akinetic mutism.

Septal Nuclei and Amygdala   The **septal nuclei** are broadly divided into three groups (lateral, medial, and posterior groups). They are interconnected with the hippocampal formation, amygdala, and anterior hypothalamus. Functionally, the septal nuclei have been implicated in the modulation of **emotional, sexual,** and **maternal behaviors,** as well as in **memory functions.** Septal lesions have been associated with exaggerated behavioral responses.

The **amygdala** is broadly divided into three nuclei (central, corticomedial, and basolateral nuclei). It is extensively interconnected with many brain areas. Functionally, the amygdala helps to coordinate associations between stimuli and their importance to the organism. It also has been implicated in **autonomic homeostatic functions, emotional responses, control of appetite,** and **sexual behavior.** Electrical stimulation of the amygdala is associated with behavioral manifestations similar to those seen in mesial temporal lobe (uncinate) seizures.

Case Conclusion   The patient was admitted to the hospital for further evaluation. Seizure precautions were initiated for his safety. Laboratory studies confirmed therapeutic antiepileptic drug levels and failed to demonstrate any reversible metabolic or infectious causes for his spells. He was transferred to epilepsy monitoring for further clarification of his seizures. A high-resolution coronal MRI scan confirmed right-sided MTS. Several spells were captured during epilepsy monitoring. All appeared to originate from the right temporal area. Surgical resection of the lesion was performed without complication. At 2-year follow-up, the patient remained seizure free without medication.

Thumbnail: Limbic System

Hippocampal Circuit Flow

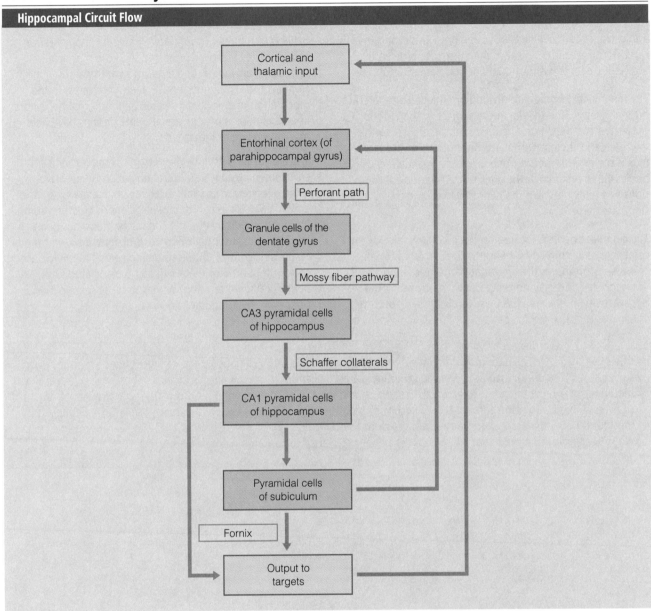

Key Points

▶ Explicit (declarative) memory is concerned with learned facts.

▶ Implicit (procedural) memory is concerned with learned skills.

▶ The dentate gyrus is the main input area of the hippocampal formation.

▶ The pes hippocampi, or Ammon's horn, is the main area for hippocampal processing.

▶ The subiculum is the main output area of the hippocampal formation.

▶ The hippocampal CA1 field, also called **Sommer's sector** or the **vulnerable zone**, is particularly sensitive to anoxia.

Questions

1. A 46-year-old man with a history of alcoholism presents with acute confusion, memory difficulties, and an apparent indifference to his condition. Which of the following structures is likely to have undergone significant atrophy?

   A. Hippocampus
   B. Nucleus basalis of Meynert
   C. Amygdala
   D. Mammillary bodies
   E. Cingulate gyrus

2. You evaluate a 12-year-old boy with intractable epilepsy. He has documented left-sided hippocampal sclerosis. In which area did his hippocampal atrophy most likely begin?

   A. Subiculum
   B. Sommer's sector
   C. Ammon's horn
   D. Dentate gyrus
   E. Entorhinal cortex

3. Following a temporal lobe injury, which of the following types of memory is least likely to be impaired?

   A. Long-term memory
   B. Semantic memory
   C. Explicit memory
   D. Declarative memory
   E. Short-term memory

4. You evaluate a 12-year-old boy with motor and vocal tics. Increased activity of which of the following regions has been implicated in this syndrome?

   A. Basal forebrain
   B. Amygdala
   C. Hypothalamus
   D. Cingulate gyrus
   E. Hippocampus

HPI: HR is an 8-month-old male infant who is being evaluated because of altered level of consciousness and poor feeding. He has had an upper respiratory tract infection and poor oral intake for a few days. He has also had an associated decrease in urine output and has become progressively lethargic. He was noted to be microcephalic at birth but has not been evaluated further for this. He has missed developmental milestones, but his medical history and family history are otherwise unremarkable.

PE: His vital signs are stable. He is sleepy, but easy to arouse, with a good cry. He is microcephalic but has no other prominent dysmorphic features. He is less interactive than his stated baseline. His tone and reflexes are somewhat increased, but he moves all extremities well.

Labs: He has a serum sodium level of 180 mEq/L with a serum osmolality of 350 mOsm/kg.

Thought Questions

- What type of brain disorders present with altered autoregulation?
- What other functions are mediated by this area?
- To what other brain regions is this area connected?
- What type of developmental problem might be implicated?

Basic Science Review and Discussion

The regulation of salt and water balance is mediated by a hormonal interaction between the hypothalamus, pituitary gland, and kidneys. This case highlights the important role of the hypothalamus in regulation of water balance. **Antidiuretic hormone (ADH) (arginine vasopressin [AVP] in humans)** is produced in the supraoptic and paraventricular nuclei of the **hypothalamus.** It is stored in the **posterior pituitary gland.** The hypothalamus is also involved in monitoring **serum osmolality.** The release of AVP from the posterior pituitary gland is normally triggered by increased serum osmolality, resulting of reabsorption of water in the distal convoluted tubule of the kidney. HR's dehydration from poor oral intake did not trigger an appropriate autoregulatory response. This failure of antidiuresis could be either central or renal. In this case, a **central diabetes insipidus** is suggested by the noted microcephaly and developmental delay. Central diabetes insipidus can be related to impaired osmoreceptor function or to impaired AVP production. However, both etiologies implicate the hypothalamus. This chapter focuses on the structure and function of the hypothalamus. The pituitary gland is discussed separately. Endocrine function and renal function are covered in other volumes in this series.

Organization of the Hypothalamus The **lamina terminalis** defines the anterior border of the hypothalamus. Structures rostral to this border include the septal nuclei and basal forebrain. The **mammillary bodies** are the most posterior nuclei of the hypothalamus and are rostral to the midbrain. The **internal capsule** forms the lateral border of the hypothalamus. Fibers of the internal capsule come together in this area to form the **cerebral peduncles.** The hypothalamus makes up the floor of the **third ventricle.** The **tuber cinereum is** the most ventral portion of the hypothalamus. The **median eminence** is the most central part of the tuber cinereum. The **infundibulum** (pituitary stalk) emerges from the median eminence.

Many different nuclei make up the hypothalamus. They can be broadly divided into anterior, tuberal, and posterior groups. Each group can be divided further into medial and lateral zones. The hypothalamic nuclei receive input from a wide variety of brain regions. The most important input sources include brainstem nuclei, the limbic system, intrinsic hypothalamic sensors for autoregulation, and feedback from hypothalamic target areas. Output from the hypothalamus can be divided into a neural division and an endocrine division. **Neural output** from the hypothalamus controls the function of the autonomic nervous system (ANS) and contributes to the limbic system and projects to many other brain regions. The **endocrine function** of the hypothalamus includes both the release of regulatory hormones that influence anterior pituitary gland function and the production of hormones that are transported to and released from the posterior pituitary gland. Pituitary gland function is discussed separately.

Anterior hypothalamic nuclei The anterior hypothalamus includes the anterior hypothalamic area and the supraoptic, suprachiasmatic, and paraventricular nuclei. The anterior hypothalamus monitors serum osmolality, produces the neuropeptides oxytocin and AVP, regulates autonomic function, and helps regulate sleep and circadian rhythms. The **anterior hypothalamic area** and the adjacent **lamina terminalis** contain the receptors that monitor serum osmolality. These **osmoreceptors** regulate the release of **ADH** (i.e., AVP) and help mediate **thirst.** In the present case, HR may have had osmoreceptor dysfunction. He was not able to dilute his serum by reabsorbing water and concentrating the urine (all mediated by AVP). He also did not seem to have increased thirst despite his high serum osmolality. Although this area regulates the release of AVP, it is not produced here. AVP is produced in the **supraoptic** and **paraventricular nuclei.** These nuclei are also located in the anterior hypothalamus. They produce oxytocin and AVP. Note that the hormones produced by these anterior hypothalamic nuclei are stored in and released from the **posterior pituitary gland.**

The anterior hypothalamus has two other important functions. Some neurons in the **paraventricular nuclei** project to autonomic nuclei in the brainstem and spinal cord where they help regulate **autonomic function.** In addition, the anterior hypothalamus is involved in regulation of sleep and circadian rhythms. The **suprachiasmatic nucleus** receives input from the retina. It projects to other hypothalamic nuclei, the pineal gland, and several other areas. This system is thought to mediate **circadian rhythms.** A role for the anterior hypothalamic area in the **regulation of sleep** has also been proposed.

Tuberal hypothalamic nuclei   The tuberal portion of the hypothalamus refers to the central portion of the hypothalamus directly superior to the tuber cinereum. This region includes the lateral, dorsomedial, ventromedial, and arcuate nuclei. The tuberal hypothalamus helps regulate feeding, emotional behavior, and endocrine function. The **lateral nuclei** are interconnected with the reticular formation and other brainstem nuclei. They have been implicated in **feeding behavior and arousal.** Lesions in the lateral hypothalamus are associated with **anorexia and weight loss.** The **dorsomedial** and **ventromedial nuclei** are closely related both anatomically and functionally. They are also involved in regulating **feeding (satiety center)** and **emotional behaviors.** Lesions in this area result in obesity and violent behavior. The ventromedial nuclei, in particular, receive considerable input from the amygdala.

The **arcuate nuclei** are located at the base of the hypothalamus, adjacent to the median eminence. The **median eminence** itself is located in the most proximal portion of the **infundibulum.** This is one of the few areas in the CNS where the **blood–brain barrier is compromised.** Humoral feedback on hypothalamic function is detected here. This is the area where all of the **releasing hormones** that act on the anterior pituitary gland are made. These endocrine interactions are covered in more detail separately. This is also an area where emotional experience can influence endocrine function.

Posterior hypothalamic nuclei   The posterior hypothalamus can be broadly divided into the posterior nuclei and the mammillary bodies. The posterior hypothalamus is involved in temperature regulation and participates in limbic and memory functions. The **posterior nuclei** are essentially continuous with the **periaqueductal gray matter of the midbrain.** Most neurons in this area project to brainstem nuclei. This area is thought to be important in **temperature regulation.** This area mediates reactions to cold ambient temperature, such as shivering and vasoconstriction. This area may also be involved in maintaining **arousal.**

The **mammillary bodies** have been discussed within the context of the limbic system. The nuclei of the mammillary bodies are the main target of axonal fibers in the **fornix.** Remember that the fornix is made up of fibers projecting from the **subiculum** and the **CA1 region of the hippocampal formation** to the hypothalamus. The mammillary nuclei are divided into medial and lateral groups, both of which receive input from the hippocampus. The medial **mammillary nuclei** subsequently project to the **anterior nucleus of the thalamus** along the **mammillothalamic tract.** This is a component of the main limbic circuitry. The lateral mammillary nuclei project to nuclei in the midbrain and the pons. This pathway may be involved in memory and autonomic systems.

Case Conclusion   The patient was admitted to the hospital for further evaluation. Supportive measures were initiated to treat the osmolality disturbance. The serum sodium level was stabilized with desmopressin (DDAVP). An MRI of the brain revealed holoprosencephaly, which is a failure of cerebral hemisphere separation. **Holoprosencephaly** is the most common developmental defect to involve the forebrain and midface, although the face may not be involved in all cases. This disorder is characterized by developmental delay, disruption of autoregulation, hydrocephalus, abnormal tone, and poor feeding. A variety of hypothalamic disturbances can be seen because the hypothalamus is a midline structure. These include dysautonomia, central diabetes insipidus, and other endocrine deficiencies. Nearly half of all cases have been linked to one of several genetic abnormalities. **Trisomy 13** is the most commonly encountered clinically. **Mutations of the Sonic hedgehog gene** are also an important association. Survival is correlated with cause. Few of these infants survive beyond the first year if a chromosomal abnormality is found. Survival at 1 year is as high as 50% in the absence of a documented chromosomal abnormality. HR ultimately returned to baseline and was discharge with arrangements for follow-up in the endocrinology and neurology clinics. Appropriate genetic testing was performed and counseling was provided to the family.

Thumbnail: Hypothalamus

Developmental Malformations of the CNS

A complete review of embryology and developmental disorders is beyond the scope of this text. However, several key elements from these disciplines should be emphasized. The manifestations of major CNS malformations can be divided on the basis of developmental stages. These categories are summarized in the following table.

Developmental period	Likely abnormality	Clinical manifestations
1–4 weeks of gestation	Failure of neural tube closure	Anencephaly Encephalocele Meningomyelocele
4–8 weeks of gestation	Midline malformations of prosencephalon	Holoprosencephaly Callosal agenesis Arrhinencephaly Septo-optic dysplasia Colpocephaly
8–20 weeks of gestation	Disruption of cortical organization	Lissencephalies Heterotopias
After 20 weeks of gestation	Predominantly secondary events (ischemia, etc.)	Schizencephaly

Key Points

- The hypothalamus has both neural and endocrine functions.
- Hypothalamic nuclei can be divided into anterior, tuberal, and posterior groups.
- The anterior hypothalamus monitors serum osmolality, regulates autonomic function, and helps regulate sleep and circadian rhythms.

- The anterior hypothalamus produces the neuropeptides oxytocin and vasopressin (AVP), which are stored in the posterior pituitary gland.
- The tuberal hypothalamus helps regulate feeding, emotional behavior, and endocrine function.
- The posterior hypothalamus is involved in temperature regulation and participates in limbic and memory functions.

Questions

1. A 52-year-old woman presents with acute confusion and memory difficulties. You suspect a nutritional deficiency may be related to her condition. Which of the following anatomic findings is most likely to be seen?
   A. Hypertrophy of the pituitary gland
   B. Atrophy of the paraventricular nuclei
   C. Atrophy of the mammillary bodies
   D. Hypertrophy of the mammillary bodies
   E. Arcuate nucleus degeneration

2. You evaluate a 12-year-old boy with intractable epilepsy. His seizures are characterized by episodes of uncontrollable laughter with retained consciousness. After the spells, he reports that he does not find anything particularly funny. He is rather scared during his spells. Which of the following regions is likely to be affected?
   A. Amygdala
   B. Hypothalamus
   C. Hippocampus
   D. Parahippocampal cortex
   E. Entorhinal cortex

3. You see a patient who is suspected of having a rare lesion involving his anterior hypothalamus. Which of the following is an unlikely manifestation of his lesion?
   A. Osmotic instability
   B. Disruption of circadian rhythm
   C. Dysautonomia
   D. Poor temperature regulation
   E. Trouble sleeping

4. You see another patient who is suspected of having a rare lesion. This one involves the posterior hypothalamus. Which of the following is an unlikely manifestation of his lesion?
   A. Disruption of appetite control
   B. Impaired arousal
   C. Poor memory performance
   D. Impaired vasoconstriction
   E. Poor temperature control

HPI: A 36-year-old woman presents to your gynecology practice complaining of amenorrhea for the past 8 months. With the exception of her one normal pregnancy at age 23, she reports having normal menses from age 13 until a year ago, when her periods became irregular and then ceased altogether. She has not lost any weight in this time but notes she has been having headaches with increasing frequency. Upon questioning, she notes a recent episode of galactorrhea, although she has not been pregnant or breast-feeding in more than 10 years. A pregnancy test in your office is negative.

Thought Questions

- Disease in what part of the CNS could produce this constellation of symptoms?

- What pathways does the brain use to affect endocrine function?

- What specific hormones are directly regulated by the brain, through which mechanisms?

Basic Science Review and Discussion

This patient describes symptoms of a **prolactinoma,** one type of tumor of the pituitary gland. To make this diagnosis and properly treat the tumor, one must understand the normal anatomy and function of the pituitary gland.

The pituitary gland lies at the **sella turcica,** inferior to the hypothalamus and just next to the optic chiasm. It is connected to the hypothalamus by the **pituitary stalk,** which allows for hypothalamic signals to directly regulate pituitary function. The pituitary gland has two parts: the anterior lobe (adenohypophysis) and the posterior lobe (neurohypophysis) (Figure 9-1).

The **anterior lobe** of the pituitary is the largest portion, making about three fourths of the mass of the pituitary. It receives hypothalamic input via a portal vascular system— vessels pass from the hypothalamus directly to the anterior lobe. Embryologically, the anterior lobe arises from Rathke's pouch and is connected to the brain by these blood vessels. Hypothalamic releasing hormones pass through the portal vessels to the anterior pituitary, where they stimulate the release of pituitary hormones. These include growth hormone **(GH),** adrenocorticotropic hormone **(ACTH),** melanocyte-stimulating hormone **(MSH),** thyroid-stimulating hormone **(TSH),** follicle-stimulating hormone **(FSH),** and luteinizing hormone **(LH).** Prolactin is the major exception to the positive effect of hypothalamic hormones; dopamine released by the hypothalamus *inhibits* prolactin secretion from the anterior pituitary. Some of these hormones have similar structures. For example, TSH, LH, and FSH share an α subunit and are only different in their β subunit. Likewise, ACTH

and MSH have similar precursors. Nonetheless, each of these hormones is made by specific cells with certain histologic characteristics. Acidophilic staining indicates somatotrophs, which make GH; or lactotrophs, which make prolactin. Basophilic staining indicates corticotrophs, which make ACTH; thyrotrophs, which make TSH; or gonadotrophs, which make FSH and LH. To further distinguish cell types, special antibody stains are used. Knowing the general staining patterns is useful in distinguishing which type of pituitary adenoma is present in a given histology sample from a pituitary biopsy (both clinically and on the USMLE).

The **posterior lobe** of the pituitary is the smaller portion, made of modified glial cells and direct axonal projections from the hypothalamus (as contrasted with the portal vascular system to the anterior pituitary). Embryologically, the posterior lobe arises from a budding of tissue from the floor of the third ventricle of the brain. Hypothalamic projections from the paraventricular nuclei to the posterior lobe release **oxytocin,** and those from the supraoptic nuclei release vasopressin (or **ADH).** Oxytocin is important in some smooth muscle contractions, particularly uterine contractions; whereas ADH acts on the collecting duct to allow the kidney to concentrate urine.

Clinical Correlation   The pituitary gland can cause disease either through hyperpituitarism or hypopituitarism. **Hyperpituitarism,** or too much hormone secretion, is usually the result of a hormone-secreting pituitary adenoma. **Prolactinomas** are the most common type of anterior pituitary adenoma, constituting 30% of these tumors. In advanced cases, pituitary adenomas can cause visual changes such as **bitemporal hemianopia.** In these instances, the enlarged pituitary compresses the optic chiasm, causing a loss of visual fields. Most typically this affects the vision in the lateral (temporal) fields of each eye. Before mass effects such as headaches or visual changes occur, pituitary adenomas will generally manifest through endocrine hyperfunction. For example, prolactin secretion is necessary in pregnancy for normal lactation. High prolactin levels also inhibit ovulation and normal menstruation. Therefore, a woman with a prolactinoma will present earliest with a loss of menses and sometimes galactorrhea caused by the end-organ effects of

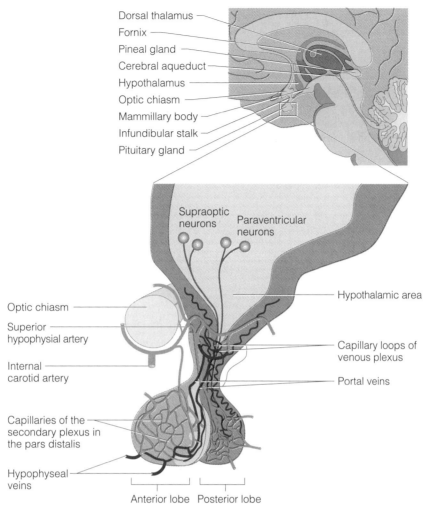

Figure 9-1 Anatomy of the pituitary gland. Note the location of the pituitary in relation to the hypothalamus, mammillary bodies, and optic chiasm. The anterior lobe of the pituitary is connected to the hypothalamus via a portal system of veins. These carry hormone signals to the anterior lobe. The posterior lobe receives signals through direct axonal inputs from the hypothalamus running through the infundibular stalk.

prolactin. Likewise, adenomas that secrete TSH can present with symptoms of hyperthyroidism, those that secrete ACTH can present with cushingoid features, and so on.

Hypopituitarism can be the result of ischemia in times of blood loss, radiation, inflammation, or tumors that do not actively secrete hormones but cause destruction of normal functioning tissue. In these cases, disease generally becomes apparent through the absence of hormone activity. As such, ischemic damage to the pituitary may not be immediately apparent but may manifest through chronic amenorrhea or hypothyroidism. Likewise, damage to the posterior pituitary may become apparent as **diabetes insipidus,** a problem of decreased ADH activity in the kidney. Patients with diabetes insipidus lose the ability to concentrate their urine; they present with symptoms of polyuria and polydipsia.

The **pituitary stalk** is a common site of injury in certain types of trauma, such as motor vehicle accidents. Shearing momentum of the brain against the skull in a jarring stop causes transection of the thin stalk, disrupting hypothalamic signaling to the pituitary. In these cases, panhypopituitarism may present acutely along with elevated prolactin levels. This is because most pituitary hormones have lost the stimulation of releasing factors from the hypothalamus, and prolactin has lost the inhibition of dopamine.

Pituitary disorders are often treated medically by supplementing hormone levels as needed. For example, glucocorticoids or thyroid hormone can be given to compensate for low levels of ACTH or TSH, respectively. Hyperpituitarism can be treated medically in the case of prolactinoma; bromocriptine is a dopamine agonist that can be taken to inhibit prolactin secretion. In other cases, surgery may be required to remove the adenoma. In these cases, trans-sphenoid surgery of the pituitary can remove the entire adenoma with minimal disruption of brain anatomy.

Case Conclusion   Given the patient's symptoms, you refer her for blood work and a CT to determine whether there might be a common cause of her headaches, galactorrhea, and amenorrhea. Indeed, CT reveals an enlarged pituitary gland, which corresponds with her elevated blood prolactin levels. You begin treatment with oral bromocriptine, which soon provides relief from her galactorrhea, and within months, normal menses return. Her adenoma is able to be well controlled by medical therapy alone at this time, but you plan regular follow-up to ensure no new symptoms arise and the adenoma does not grow further.

Thumbnail: Pituitary Gland

Characteristics of Pituitary Hormones				
Pituitary hormone	**Released by which lobe?**	**Produced by which cells?**	**Cell appearance**	**Hormone effects**
Prolactin	Anterior	Lactotrophs	Acidophilic	Lactation, inhibits menstruation
GH	Anterior	Somatotrophs	Acidophilic	Growth
TSH	Anterior	Thyrotrophs	Basophilic	Thyroid function
ACTH	Anterior	Corticotrophs	Basophilic	Cortisol release
FSH, LH	Anterior	Gonadotrophs	Basophilic	Ovulation, menstruation
Oxytocin	Posterior	Paraventricular hypothalamic projections	N/A	Uterine contraction
ADH	Posterior	Supraoptic hypothalamic projections	N/A	Urine concentration

Key Points

- The pituitary gland has two components: the anterior lobe and the posterior lobe.
- The anterior lobe is stimulated by releasing hormones from the hypothalamus, which are delivered via the portal vascular system.
- The anterior lobe releases prolactin, GH, ACTH, TSH, FSH, and LH.
- All anterior lobe hormone release is stimulated by hypothalamic releasing hormones. The only exception is prolactin, which is under inhibitory control by dopamine.
- The posterior lobe has direct axonal connections from the hypothalamus.
- The posterior lobe releases oxytocin and ADH.

Questions

1. A patient develops significant blood loss after childbirth, causing massive ischemic damage to the anterior pituitary. This condition, known as Sheehan's syndrome, would cause which of the following sets of hormone levels?

	Cortisol	FSH	Thyroxine (T$_4$)	Prolactin	ADH
A.	decreased	decreased	decreased	decreased	decreased
B.	decreased	decreased	decreased	increased	normal
C.	decreased	decreased	decreased	increased	decreased
D.	decreased	decreased	decreased	decreased	normal
E.	normal	normal	normal	increased	decreased

2. A 40-year-old patient presents with a hormone-secreting pituitary adenoma. Biopsy of the tumor shows proliferation of a single type of acidophilic cells. Which of the following signs and symptoms are most likely?
   A. Hypertension, obesity, diabetes
   B. Heat intolerance, weight loss, tachycardia
   C. Inability to breast-feed, menorrhagia, headache
   D. Enlarged jaw, diabetes, increased hand size
   E. Polyuria, increased thirst, low urine-specific gravity

3. A patient comes to her primary care provider complaining of fatigue, cold intolerance, weight gain, and hair loss. Suspecting possible hypothyroidism, the provider orders blood tests to assess her thyroid function. The assay for TSH must be specific for the β subunit, because TSH shares an α subunit with which of the following other hormones?
   A. FSH, LH
   B. FSH, ACTH
   C. ACTH, MSH
   D. MSH, LH
   E. FSH, MSH

4. A patient with central diabetes insipidus begins therapy with a vasopressin nasal spray. This medication replaces the hormone usually secreted by which set of pituitary cells?
   A. Acidophilic cells of the anterior lobe
   B. Basophilic cells of the anterior lobe
   C. Cells of the posterior lobe receiving projections from the paraventricular hypothalamus
   D. Cells of the posterior lobe receiving projections from the supraoptic hypothalamus
   E. Cells of the posterior lobe receiving signals through the hypothalamic portal vein

HPI: TD is a 68-year-old man who has been undergoing physical therapy for left shoulder pain over the past year. He has otherwise been in relatively good health despite a significant smoking history. He is being evaluated because of his persistent shoulder problems.

PE: On meeting him, you notice that his left pupil is somewhat smaller than the right one. His left eyelid also seems somewhat drooped. An extensive examination does not reveal any other deficits. Of incidental note, TD found his examination somewhat strenuous and had broken into a sweat. You notice that he seems to be sweating more on the right side of his face than on the left.

Thought Questions

- Which system regulates the identified abnormalities?
- Where in the brain does this system begin?
- What path does the system follow to its targets?
- What types of problems might be implicated?

Basic Science Review and Discussion

TD has the triad of **ptosis, miosis,** and **anhydrosis.** These are the classic features of **Horner's syndrome,** which results from disruption of sympathetic innervation to the face and eye. A lesion anywhere along the course of the sympathetic nervous system from the hypothalamus down to the upper thoracic spinal cord and back up along the carotid circulation can cause this syndrome. A CNS process can be excluded by the absence of any other neurologic deficits. The involvement of the face along with the eye on the left helps localize the lesion between the extra-axial thoracic spine and the carotid artery on the left. Combined with the smoking history and shoulder pain, the most likely explanation is a **Pancoast tumor** (involving the apex of the lung) with compression of the superior cervical ganglion.

Anatomy of the Autonomic Nervous System The ANS mediates control of **homeostasis,** influencing critical functions such as blood pressure (BP), heart rate (HR), and temperature regulation. The motor component of this system can be distinguished from the somatic motor system in several ways. Unlike somatic motor function (striated muscles), autonomic motor function is largely involuntary (smooth muscle and cardiac muscle). Somatic motor output from the CNS is monosynaptic (lower motor neuron projecting to target). Autonomic motor output is disynaptic (preganglionic neuron to postganglionic neuron to target). In the somatic system, motor output is always excitatory, and inhibition occurs centrally via interneurons. In the autonomic system, output to a given target can be either excitatory or inhibitory. The ANS is separated into **sympathetic** and **parasympathetic** divisions that often exert opposing influences on a given target. The varying effects of sympathetic

and parasympathetic function are summarized later in this case (see Thumbnail: Autonomic Nervous System).

Control of autonomic function occurs largely below the level of consciousness and is regulated by the **hypothalamus.** Changes in homeostasis are detected in the hypothalamus and appropriate responses are generated to help maintain homeostasis. Hypothalamic function is reviewed in Case 8. The hypothalamus influences the activity of **autonomic preganglionic neurons** (located in the brainstem or spinal cord). The axons of these neurons exit the CNS and make synaptic contact with postganglionic neurons located in **autonomic ganglia.** The location of the postganglionic neurons differs between the two divisions. Postganglionic neurons in the two divisions also use different neurotransmitters.

Sympathetic Nervous System **Sympathetic** control descends from the level of the hypothalamus to preganglionic neurons in the **intermediolateral cell columns** in the **thoracolumbar spinal cord.** Preganglionic axons, which are myelinated, leave the spinal cord and enter the adjacent sympathetic chain ganglia via the **white communicating rami (white** because the axons within are myelinated). Once in the sympathetic chain, these axons may ascend or descend briefly before making synaptic contact with **postganglionic neurons.** The postganglionic axons exit the sympathetic chain via the **gray communicating rami (gray** because the axons within are unmyelinated) and join peripheral nerves to get to their targets. For example, sympathetic innervation to the head originates in the **superior cervical (stellate) ganglion,** which is at the top of the **sympathetic chain.** These sympathetic nerves travel along the **carotid arteries,** their branches, and then join branches of various cranial nerves to reach their targets.

Outflow from the sympathetic chain to target organs is divergent. This means that many different target organs will be stimulated "in sympathy" (i.e., will all be influenced at the same time) by sympathetic activity. This ability to react in concert is important for those behaviors mediated by the sympathetic system **(fight or flight).** The sympathetic system mediates rapid responses to environmental stressors. Sympathetic effects include increased cardiac output, pupillary dilation, increased energy availability, and maintenance of temperature by shivering, piloerection, and vasoconstriction. Sympathetic innervation to the adrenal medulla is unique in that it is only preganglionic.

Parasympathetic Nervous System

Parasympathetic control descends from the level of the hypothalamus to preganglionic neurons in brainstem nuclei and sacral spinal cord. The parasympathetic system is also called the **craniosacral system,** based on the distribution of its preganglionic neurons. The preganglionic axons exit the CNS along cranial or peripheral nerves. They reach postganglionic neurons contained within peripheral parasympathetic ganglia, which are located close to the target organs. Postganglionic axons in the parasympathetic system then travel to their final target. The parasympathetic system is less divergent than the sympathetic system. The parasympathetic system is concerned with maintaining baseline conditions such as basal HR, respirations, and metabolic activity **(rest and digest). Cranial nerves III, VII, IX,** and **X** all have a parasympathetic component. Parasympathetic innervation to the eye is discussed further in Case 24. Cranial parasympathetic functions include pupillary constriction, lens accommodation, lacrimation, salivation, and control of cardiac function. The **sacral component** of the parasympathetic system innervates the urinary tract, bladder, distal large intestine, and reproductive organs. Autonomic functions in various organs are reviewed later in this case (see Thumbnail: Autonomic Nervous System).

Enteric Nervous System

Both the sympathetic and parasympathetic divisions of the ANS contribute to the innervation of the GI tract. The **enteric nervous system** is considered by many to be a third autonomic division. Sympathetic preganglionic fibers contributing to this system bypass the sympathetic chain ganglia and terminate in several **splanchnic ganglia** within the abdomen. Postganglionic sympathetic fibers from these ganglia then contribute to a meshwork of nerve fibers within the intestinal walls. The sympathetic contribution to the enteric nervous system inhibits motility and secretion.

Parasympathetic preganglionic fibers contributing to this system originate in both the cranial and the sacral portions of the parasympathetic system. They terminate in **enteric ganglia** located within the intestinal walls. The enteric ganglia, their postganglionic projections, and associated contributions from the sympathetic system make up the enteric nervous system. This system is further divided into a **submucosal (Meissner's) plexus** and a **myenteric (Auerbach's) plexus.** The parasympathetic contribution to the enteric nervous system promotes motility and secretion.

Autonomic Neurotransmitters

All autonomic preganglionic neurons use **acetylcholine (ACh)** as their primary neurotransmitter. A variety of **neuropeptides** can be co-secreted with ACh. The two divisions of the autonomic system differ in their postganglionic neurotransmitters.

Postganglionic parasympathetic neurons also use **ACh** as their primary neurotransmitter. Again, several neuropeptides also can be released as secondary neurotransmitters. **Postganglionic sympathetic neurons** use **norepinephrine (NE)** as their primary neurotransmitter and use neuropeptides as secondary neurotransmitters.

ACh acts through both nicotinic and muscarinic cholinergic receptors. The binding of ACh to **nicotinic receptors** triggers a fast excitatory postsynaptic potential (EPSP). This interaction often results in an **action potential.** It should be noted that autonomic nicotinic receptors are structurally different from the receptors found at the neuromuscular junction in striated muscle. The binding of ACh to **muscarinic receptors** may trigger either slow EPSPs or **slow inhibitory postsynaptic potentials (IPSPs).** The release of **neuropeptides** also can result in slow EPSPs. In addition, the release of neuropeptides can act through second-messenger systems to modify the efficiency of the co-secreted primary neurotransmitter. **NE** acts through several **different adrenoreceptors** (α_1, α_2, β_1, and β_2). Some of the major functions mediated by the different adrenoreceptors and muscarinic cholinergic receptors are summarized in Table 10-1.

Autonomic Dysfunction

Autonomic disorders are broadly divided into primary and secondary syndromes. The etiology

Table 10-1 Major functions mediated by adrenoreceptors and muscarinic receptors

	α_1-Receptors	α_2-Receptors	β_1-Receptors	β_2-Receptors	ACh$_{muscarinic}$
BP	Increased	—	Increased	—	Decreased
Cardiac output	—	—	Increased	—	Decreased
Heart rate	—	—	Increased	—	Decreased
Blood vessels	Vasoconstriction	—	—	Vasodilation in skeletal and cardiac muscle	—
Lungs	—	—	—	Bronchodilation	Bronchoconstriction
Pupils	Mydriasis	—	—	—	Miosis
Metabolism	—	Decreased insulin release	Increased lipid utilization	Increased glycogen utilization	Promotes glucose storage

of **primary dysautonomia** is often unclear. Both sympathetic and parasympathetic systems are usually involved. The most commonly encountered acute primary dysautonomia is vasovagal **syncope** (fainting), which is caused by increased parasympathetically mediated bradycardia in the setting of decreased sympathetic vasoconstrictor tone. The most commonly encountered chronic primary dysautonomia is **orthostatic hypotension** (in the absence of dehydration or other neurologic disease). Multiple system atrophy (MSA) describes a combination of dysautonomia, parkinsonism, and cerebellar dysfunction. Three forms of this disorder are recognized (parkinsonian, cerebellar, and mixed). The term Shy-Drager syndrome also has been used to describe dysautonomia in combination with other neurologic deficits.

The list of conditions resulting in **secondary dysautonomia** is extensive. As seen in TD's case, a structural lesion any-where along the course of the ANS can disrupt its function. Diseases of the brainstem and spinal cord such as infarction (as in **Wallenberg's syndrome**), demyelinating lesions, trauma, and tumors can all be associated with dysautonomia. Many conditions can also be associated with neuropathy causing peripheral dysautonomia. The most common of these include **diabetes mellitus** and the toxic effects of drugs or **alcohol.** Disorders of neuromuscular transmission can also result in impaired autonomic function. These conditions are discussed further in Case 43.

Synkinesis is another interesting manifestation of autonomic dysfunction in which functions not usually associated with each other become linked. This usually occurs as a result of aberrant reinnervation following injury to a nerve. For example, lacrimation may become linked to salivation **(crocodile tears)** following facial nerve injury.

Case Conclusion   TD was suspected of having a Pancoast tumor. A chest x-ray film was unrevealing. A CT scan of the chest confirmed a large left apical lung mass with extension into the adjacent soft tissues. Biopsy confirmed a non-small cell carcinoma. TD was referred for an oncology evaluation and further management of his carcinoma. Arrangements were made for presurgical irradiation and subsequent resection and chemotherapy.

Thumbnail: Autonomic Nervous System

	Sympathetic effects	**Parasympathetic effects**
Pupils	Mydriasis	Miosis
Ciliary muscle (lens shape)	—	Contraction (accommodation for near vision)
Lacrimation	—	Promotes tearing
Salivation	Thick secretions	Thin secretions
Cardiac output	Increased	Decreased
Blood vessels	Vasoconstriction and vasodilation	—
Lungs	Bronchodilation	Bronchoconstriction; increased secretions
GI tract	Decreased motility; decreased secretions	Increased motility; increased secretions
Urinary bladder	Relaxes detrusor (promotes retention)	Contracts detrusor (promotes excretion)
Sphincter muscles (bowel and urinary)	Contracts sphincters	Relaxes sphincters
Adrenal medulla	"Preganglionic" cholinergic fibers trigger epinephrine release	—
Sweat glands	"Preganglionic" cholinergic stimulation	—
Reproduction	Ejaculation; uterine relaxation	Erection
Metabolism	Promotes energy use	Promotes energy storage

Key Points

- Horner's syndrome is characterized by sympathetic dysfunction resulting in ptosis, miosis, and anhydrosis.
- Preganglionic sympathetic neurons are located in the intermediolateral cell columns of the thoracolumbar spinal cord.
- Sympathetic output is divergent, allowing target organs to react simultaneously to environmental stressors.
- The parasympathetic system is also called the **craniosacral system,** based on the distribution of its preganglionic neurons.

- The parasympathetic system is concerned with maintaining basal conditions.
- The most common acute primary dysautonomia is vasovagal syncope.
- The most common chronic primary dysautonomia is orthostatic hypotension.
- Neuropathy, as seen in diabetes mellitus, can be associated with peripheral dysautonomia.
- In synkinesis, functions not usually associated with each other become linked as a result of aberrant regeneration following nerve injury.

Questions

1. A 52-year-old woman presents with a left internal carotid artery dissection and associated right-sided hemiparesis. Which of the following might be an associated finding?

   A. Mydriasis on the left
   B. Mydriasis on the right
   C. Increased sweating on the left side of the face
   D. Miosis on the right
   E. Miosis on the left

2. A 63-year-old man has been diagnosed with a right-sided posterior communicating artery aneurysm. Which of the following might be an associated finding?

   A. Mydriasis on the left
   B. Mydriasis on the right
   C. Increased sweating on the left side of the face
   D. Miosis on the right
   E. Miosis on the left

3. You evaluate a newborn for excessive vomiting. He was born 48 hours ago and still has not passed any meconium. His abdomen is distended. You are able to appreciate colonic peristalsis and note a palpable fecal mass. You are able to determine that several family members have had similar problems. What neurons are affected?

   A. Preganglionic sympathetic neurons
   B. Postganglionic parasympathetic neurons
   C. Preganglionic parasympathetic neurons
   D. Postganglionic sympathetic neurons
   E. Neurons in the splanchnic ganglia

4. You evaluate a 34-year-old man who is recovering from a spinal cord injury sustained in a motorcycle accident. He confides in you that he has not been able to achieve an erection since his accident. Which of the following neurons is most likely to have been affected?

   A. Preganglionic sympathetic neurons
   B. Neurons in the splanchnic ganglia
   C. Cranial preganglionic parasympathetic neurons
   D. Postganglionic sympathetic neurons
   E. Sacral preganglionic parasympathetic neurons

HPI: A 47-year-old man comes to your neurology practice after noticing he has become "more and more forgetful" over the past 5 years. He has been having difficulty in his work as a salesman, forgetting certain tasks and making mistakes with accounts that he did not in the past. These changes have been noticed by his co-workers, who have suggested he's "not himself" anymore. He is more easily frustrated and angers easily. The patient also noticed that he has become more "clumsy" and finally decided to seek attention after spraining his ankle for a second time in 1 year falling on his front step. He has no known family history of any neurologic problems, but because his father left when he was young, he does not know about that side of his family.

PE: The patient has difficulty sitting still in his chair and makes many jerky and writhing movements with his fingers and lower extremities.

Thought Questions

- What parts of the brain are involved in motor control?

- How do they regulate one another?

- What disease can cause problems with motor control?

Basic Science Review and Discussion

This patient shows early signs of Huntington's disease (HD), a disease of motor dysfunction and dementia caused by progressive degeneration of the striatum in the basal ganglia. To recognize the disease and understand its transmission and prognosis requires a basic understanding of the circuits of the basal ganglia.

Basal Ganglia   The **basal ganglia** are groups of subcortical neurons, including the **caudate nucleus, putamen, globus pallidus,** and associated groups such as the **subthalamic nucleus** and the **substantia nigra,** all involved in motor control. Input about the environment and planned movements come from the cortex to the caudate and putamen. From here, the information is processed by the rest of the basal ganglia, before it is sent to the thalamus and relayed back to the cortex and finally to the corticospinal tracts. Although motor commands neither begin nor end in the basal ganglia, these nuclei are essential for their refinement.

The basal ganglia are often subdivided into a number of overlapping groups. Though somewhat confusing, it is essential to memorize these terms to understand discussions of motor processing. The **striatum** is the collective name for the caudate nucleus and the putamen, while the **lentiform nuclei** refer to the globus pallidus and the putamen. Less commonly, some texts refer to the striate body, which includes the caudate, putamen, and globus pallidus.

Once input arrives from the cortex, it is initially processed by the caudate and putamen. From there, information continues through the basal ganglia along two complementary pathways: the direct and indirect pathways. The direct pathway goes directly to the output nuclei (globus pallidus interna and substania nigra reticulata). The indirect pathway passes through the globus pallidus externa and subthalamic nucleus before reaching the output nuclei. Disruption of the balance between direct and indirect pathways leads to clinical disease. Although the precise details of these circuits are revised with ongoing research, Figure 11-1 provides a general overview.

Clinical Correlation   Lesions of the basal ganglia produce characteristic motor deficits. Among the best characterized is HD, a disease primarily affecting the caudate and putamen. HD is an autosomal dominant disease caused by an expanded trinucleotide repeat at a single gene. Although the disease is inherited in an autosomal dominant fashion, it also demonstrates anticipation; that is, symptoms tend to be worse and present earlier with each generation as the expanded region becomes longer.

In HD, the neurons of the caudate and putamen are progressively destroyed, decreasing GABAergic inhibition of the external segment of the globus pallidus. As a result, the globus pallidus is free to increase its own inhibitory input to the subthalamic nucleus. The subthalamic nucleus has too much inhibition and cannot regulate movement, resulting in **chorea** (Greek for dance), sudden jerky unintentional movements, and **athetosis,** writhing, snakelike movements. These motor problems are usually accompanied by progressive dementia. HD is always progressive and usually results in death within 15 years.

Other lesions of the basal ganglia cause equally characteristic deficits. Disease that affects the substantia nigra results in **parkinsonism,** slowness in movement along with rigidity and a resting tremor. Injury to the subthalamic nucleus causes **ballismus,** sudden flailing movements of the extremities. Injury to the striatum and globus pallidus, as in Wilson's disease, can cause either athetosis or difficulty in maintaining subconscious motor control such as posture.

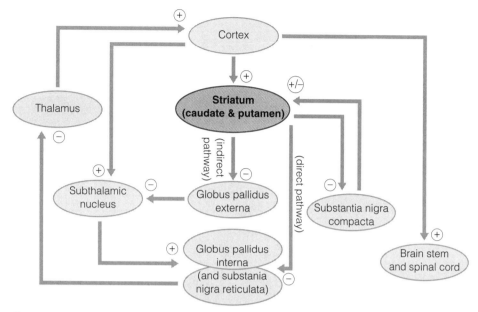

Figure 11-1 Interconnections of the basal ganglia and motor system. The striatum and subthalamic nucleus (STN) receive excitatory projections from the cortex. The striatum (caudate and putamen in humans) projects inhibitory inputs to the direct and indirect pathways, both of which project to the output nuclei. Because these pathways follow different paths, the indirect pathway is excitatory to the output nuclei whereas the direct pathway is inhibitory. Note also that most basal ganglia neurons are inhibitory GABA neurons. Exceptions include glutamate neurons in the subthalamic nucleus. Most of these neurons also co-express neuropeptides, which further complicates their interactions.

Case Conclusion   A more focused neurology examination reveals significant difficulty in motor tasks, such as sticking out the tongue for more than 10 seconds or reproducing a series of fine motor movements. Formal neuropsychological testing reveals marked deficits in frontal lobe function and some language function. Genetic testing confirms the presence of the CAG repeat on a single gene at chromosome 4. Although the patient still appears to be relatively early in his disease, he understands his long-term prognosis is poor.

Thumbnail: Basal Ganglia

Connections of the Basal Ganglia

Component of basal ganglia	Receives input from	Sends output to	Lesion results in
Caudate nucleus	Cortex, substantia nigra (compacta)	Globus pallidus, substantia nigra (reticulata)	Chorea, athetosis, dementia
Putamen	Cortex, substantia nigra (compacta)	Globus pallidus, substantia nigra (reticulata)	Chorea, athetosis
Globus pallidus (interna)*	Subthalamic nucleus	Thalamus	Athetosis, poor motor control
Globus pallidus (externa)	Caudate, putamen	Subthalamic nucleus	Athetosis, poor motor control
Subthalamic nucleus	Globus pallidus	Globus pallidus	Ballismus
Substantia nigra (compacta)	Claudate, putamen	Claudate, putamen	Parkinsonism
Substantia nigra (reticulata)*	Subthalamic nucleus	Thalamus	Parkinsonism

*Note that globus pallidus (interna) and substantia nigra (reticulata) are functionally equivalent.

Key Points

▸ The basal ganglia include the caudate, putamen, globus pallidus, substantia nigra, and subthalamic nucleus.

▸ The basal ganglia are required for motor control and refinement of movements.

▸ Input to the basal ganglia is from the cortex, and output is through the thalamus to the cortex and corticospinal tract.

▸ The caudate and putamen are the sites of input to the basal ganglia.

▸ The globus pallidus (interna) and substantia nigra (reticulata) are the output nuclei of the basal ganglia.

▸ Lesions to portions of the basal ganglia produce characteristic lesions; injury to the caudate and putamen causes chorea and athetosis.

Questions

1. After a stroke, a patient presents with new onset of flailing motions of the arms. The lesion that produces this problem has which of the following effects in the basal ganglia?
   A. Decreased inhibitory input to the globus pallidus
   B. Decreased excitatory input to the globus pallidus
   C. Decreased inhibitory input to the striatum
   D. Decreased excitatory input to the striatum
   E. Decreased excitatory input to the substantia nigra

2. In HD, the degeneration of striatal neurons has what direct downstream effect?
   A. Decreased inhibition to the globus pallidus
   B. Decreased excitation to the globus pallidus
   C. Decreased inhibition to the cortex
   D. Decreased inhibition to the spinal cord
   E. Decreased excitation to the spinal cord

3. Which of the following sends inputs directly to the cortex?
   A. Globus pallidus
   B. Thalamus
   C. Substantia nigra
   D. A and C
   E. All of the above

4. Considering a coronal section of the brain, which structure of the striatum is located most laterally?
   A. Caudate
   B. Putamen
   C. Globus pallidus
   D. Thalamus
   E. Cerebral cortex

HPI: A 76-year-old man notices at home that he has no feeling on his left side after getting up one morning. He is able to walk, although his coordination is impaired; he ignores the symptoms at the time because there is no pain or clear weakness. His daughter discovers his new problem and takes him to the ED, where he presents with nearly complete anesthesia of the face, arm, and leg of the left side.

PMHx: Hypertension, hypercholesterolemia, smokes one pack per day of cigarettes for the past 40 years. Rx: He takes no medications, although his doctor has written many prescriptions for him in the past.

PE: T 98.4°F   HR 84   BP 160/90   RR 14   SaO₂ 98% on room air

He has anesthesia of the left face, arm, trunk, and leg, which extends to the midline but does not affect the right side whatsoever. Strength is intact. He is able to walk, but movement of the left lower extremity is stiff and he takes smaller steps on the left side. He tends to ignore the left side of his body if he is not obliged to use it. He has a new burn on the left hand, which he had not noticed.

Thought Questions

■ Which neurologic structure is most likely to be the cause of the deficit?

■ What about the presentation is most characteristic of this type of lesion?

■ What is the essential organization of sensation in the nervous system?

Basic Science Review and Discussion

The thalamus, residing atop the brainstem at the epicenter of the subcortical structures, serves as the central relay station for almost all sensory input before it is relayed to the cortex. It plays an integral role in somatic sensation (touch and pain) of the entire body, but also relays visual and auditory input to the cortex. It also plays a role in processing language, and modulates motor movement.

The thalamus has been dissected into a collection of nuclei, some of which will be described here in some detail. Many of the nuclei of the thalamus do not have roles that are clinically significant, so they are listed only for the sake of completeness.

Anatomy   The thalamus is a bilateral, symmetric structure sitting at the internal core of the cerebrum, just superior to the midbrain. Its two halves are separated by the third ventricle, although they are joined by a small stalk that transverses the ventricle, the **interthalamic adhesion.** Each hemithalamus is roughly the shape of a small potato. Each half of the thalamus has a sagittally oriented **internal medullary lamina,** which separates the medial, anterior, and lateral nuclei of each hemithalamus. In addition, some nuclei are located within the internal medullary lamina itself, the most notable of which is the **centromedian nucleus.**

The Nuclei   More than a dozen nuclei of the thalamus have been named. Only a few of these have clinically significant roles that merit further explanation here.

Medial nuclei (are medial to the internal medullary lamina): **median, medial, medial dorsal** nuclei

Within the internal medullary lamina: centromedian, intralaminar nuclei

Lateral nuclei (lateral to internal medullary lamina): **lateral dorsal, lateral posterior, ventral anterior, ventral dorsal, ventral posterior** (includes **ventral posterolateral, posterointermediate,** and **posteromedial** nuclei), **pulvinar, lateral geniculate,** and **medial geniculate** nuclei

The ventral posterolateral nucleus   This nucleus serves as the relay station for all somatosensory information from the *body* to the postcentral gyrus of the parietal cortex. Contralateral vibration and simple touch arrives via the medial lemniscus after traveling in the dorsal columns of the spinal cord. Contralateral pain and temperature sensation arrives via the spinothalamic tract. This nucleus is therefore a crucial part of sensation, providing sensation of pain, temperature, vibration, touch, and conscious proprioception. Its neurons project directly onto the parietal cortex, where sensation becomes part of consciousness.

The ventral posteromedial nucleus   This nucleus serves as the relay station for all somatosensory information from the *face* to the postcentral gyrus. Its sensory input originates from the cranial nerves.

The lateral geniculate nucleus   The lateral geniculate nucleus (LGN) is the central relay station for visual information. The overwhelming majority (>99%) of optic fibers from the retina project directly to the LGN after passing through the optic chiasm. (The remaining optic fibers actually pass to the midbrain, where they regulate pupillary reflexes.) LGN neurons then project directly to the occipital cortex via the *optic radiations.* Though rare, LGN lesions may therefore result in homonymous hemianopsia.

The medial geniculate nucleus The medial geniculate nuclei receive all auditory input. Their neurons directly project ipsilaterally to the auditory cortex, located in the superior temporal gyrus. Hearing input originates in the cochlea of the inner ear, where it projects to the ipsilateral cochlear nuclei, which project to both the ipsilateral and the contralateral inferior colliculi of the midbrain. Neurons of the inferior colliculus relay directly to the ipsilateral medial geniculate nucleus (MGN). Because each MGN receives sensory input from both ears, loss of one MGN may not be clinically obvious.

Thalamic Lesions and Associated Syndromes The most common cause of thalamic injury is cerebrovascular, that is, stroke. Ischemic stroke is seen most often, but the thalamus is one of the areas of the brain most likely to be a site of spontaneous hemorrhage. Finally, tumors of the thalamus may also result in thalamic dysfunction. The more common presentations of thalamic lesions are described in the following sections.

Thalamic syndrome The "thalamic syndrome" refers to the symptoms seen in lesions involving only the thalamus. This is not always the case because of the proximity of the internal capsule and the basal ganglia, which may also be involved by the same disease. It describes **hemisensory loss affecting half of the entire body and face,** which may be followed by a **"thalamic pain syndrome"** of the affected side, as well as any other typical symptoms: changes in behavior, particularly inattention, thalamic aphasia, anterograde amnesia, or movement disorders such as chorea (the thalamus acts with the other basal ganglia to modulate movement). Parietal lobe infarcts cause similar loss of sensation but do not usually involve the leg, and they do not usually involve pain syndromes, amnesia, or movement disorders.

Thalamic pain syndrome Thalamic pain usually develops weeks to months after the injury and is usually described as

a persistent burning pain that is worsened by touching the affected side; it may respond to medical management.

Pure sensory A "clean" thalamic lesion that does not involve surrounding structures may result in hemisensory loss only, or **hemianesthesia.** There may be no motor involvement, aphasia, or behavioral changes. Paradoxically, pure thalamic injury may cause a transient hemiparesis, which usually resolves within hours (in contradistinction to hemisensory stroke, described later, where paresis may be permanent). Recovery of sensation varies according to the size of the lesion, and any sensory loss secondary to thalamic injury is at risk of developing a thalamic pain syndrome. Patients are prone to **neglect** the affected side, particularly with right-sided thalamic injury.

Sensorimotor Because of the proximity of the corticospinal motor fibers to the thalamus, ischemic, hemorrhagic, or neoplastic processes involving the thalamus may also cause loss of motor function. The adjacent motor fibers (the internal capsule is most likely to be the area involved) control the contralateral arm, leg, and face. Thus, the typical sensorimotor stroke involving the thalamus usually causes **hemiplegia and hemianesthesia of the contralateral side.**

Thalamic aphasia Thalamic lesions have been associated with receptive aphasias similar to Wernicke's aphasia, resulting in **fluent nonsensical speech** and impaired comprehension. Much as cortical aphasias are usually seen on the left side, thalamic aphasias **usually occur with left-sided thalamic injury.** However, the deficit is not usually as profound or as permanent as those seen in cortical aphasias. In addition, thalamic aphasias are **often dependent on the attentiveness** of the patient: alert patients may be able to overcome the aphasia with sufficient effort, only to relapse into noncoherent muttering when they are distracted or somnolent. Thalamic aphasias may be explained by considering the role of the thalamus in relaying language information.

Bilateral thalamic lesions Though rare, injury to both hemithalami may result in **impaired consciousness** or coma, because the sensory cortex is essentially deprived of sensory input.

Case Conclusion The patient was emergently taken for head CT scan, which showed a 2-cm (moderately sized) subacute infarct in the right thalamus, likely of several days' duration. The precise location appeared to be in the area of the ventral posterolateral and posteromedial nuclei, explaining the hemisensory loss and resulting hemineglect. He began to complain of a persistent burning sensation throughout his left side several months afterward, which made wearing clothes more difficult. Medications were somewhat effective in reducing his discomfort.

Thumbnail: Thalamus

Thalamic Nuclei and Functions

Nucleus	Input	Output	Function
Anterior	Mammillothalamic tract	Cingulate gyrus	Limbic and memory
Ventral anterior	Basal ganglia	Premotor cortex	Motor
Ventral lateral	Dentate nucleus	Motor and premotor cortices	Motor
Ventral posterior lateral	Dorsal column system	Postcentral gyrus	Somatosensory (body)
Ventral posterior medial	Trigeminal system	Postcentral gyrus	Somatosensory (face)
Lateral Geniculate	Retina	Visual cortex	Vision
Medial Geniculate	Inferior colliculus	Auditory cortex	Hearing
Dorsomedial	Amygdala	Prefrontal cortex	Limbic and memory
Pulvinar	Association cortices	Association cortices	Higher cognitive function
Centromedian	Reticular formation	Multiple cortical areas	Reticular activating system
Reticular	Thalamic nuclei	Thalamic nuclei	Thalamic feedback

Note: Thalamic subnuclei mentioned in other cases have also been included here.

Key Points

▶ The thalamus serves as a sensory relay station for all somatic, auditory, and visual input to the cortex.

▶ The thalamus also plays a role in arousing the cortex to language and modulating behavior.

▶ Thalamic lesions correspondingly may result in loss of somatic sensation, pain syndromes resulting from disruption of sensory input, thalamic aphasia, and changes in behavior.

Questions

1. A 76-year-old man in the hospital tells the story of the acute onset of right-sided weakness that occurred 2 days earlier. He describes losing feeling on his right face and arm as well, which has persisted; you notice he has a right lower facial droop and does not use his right arm. His leg was relatively unaffected. You notice that his speech is imprecise with incorrect word choice and he has some difficulty understanding your questions. What is the most likely cause?
   A. Right thalamic ischemic infarct with sensorimotor symptoms
   B. Left parietal lobe infarct
   C. Left thalamic ischemic infarct
   D. Left thalamic neoplasm
   E. Lesion likely outside of the thalamus

2. A 72-year-old woman experiences the inability to walk, consistently falling to the left side. While sitting, she does not notice anything unusual, although her left arm lies in an awkward position. She has no response to pain on the left arm or leg. With persistent requests, she will move the left side with full strength. What is the best explanation?
   A. Right parietal lobe infarct
   B. Right thalamic infarct with sensorimotor symptoms
   C. Right thalamic infarct with pure sensory symptoms
   D. Left thalamic infarct with pure sensory symptoms and apparent neglect
   E. Lesion likely outside of the thalamus

3. An 80-year-old woman is noted to have weakness of the right arm and a right lower facial droop upon waking up one morning. Sensation of the right arm and face is also significantly diminished. Her family member does not examine her lower extremity because she remains in bed. Based on the information given, which answers are possible?
   A. Left parietal lobe infarct
   B. Left middle cerebral artery infarct
   C. Left thalamic infarct
   D. Left frontal lobe infarct
   E. B and C are both possible

4. A 65-year-old right-handed man is noticed by his family to have developed bizarre speech several hours ago that is difficult to understand. Sensation and strength appear grossly normal. He complains of a new headache when carefully questioned. He also has difficulty understanding verbal commands, although he improves when he is compelled to give his full attention. What is the most likely diagnosis?
   A. Broca's aphasia
   B. Right thalamic infarct
   C. Left posterolateral frontal lobe infarct
   D. Left thalamic hemorrhage with thalamic aphasia
   E. Left parietal infarct

> **HPI:**   SM is a 15-year-old boy who has developed problems with his balance and coordination over the past few months. There has been a gradual progression of his symptoms. Recently, he has had several falls. He has also begun to speak less clearly. He has no other medical problems and has been doing well academically. His mother reports that she thinks there have been one or two other similar cases in other family members.
>
> **PE:**   SM has normal vital signs, although his heart rhythm is thought to be somewhat irregular at times. His general examination is otherwise unremarkable. On neurologic examination, his cranial nerves appear to be intact. Some gaze-evoked nystagmus is noted. He has nearly full strength, with some mild lower extremity weakness that is rated 4/5 bilaterally. His coordination is impaired on finger-to-nose testing. He also appears to have an unsteady and broad-based gait. He is not able to walk heel-to-toe. He has a positive Romberg's test. His deep tendon reflexes are absent in the lower extremities. He has diminished sensation to both pinprick and vibration in his feet. Babinski's sign is present bilaterally.

Thought Questions

- Which brain region is most likely affected?
- How is this structure organized?
- What other systems are affected in this case?
- What are some potential explanations for his symptoms?

Basic Science Review and Discussion

Prominent **ataxia** is most often seen with diseases of the cerebellum and its associated structures. Many different conditions and categories of disease can be associated with ataxia. One of the most common causes for cerebellar atrophy and dysfunction is exposure to any of a number of toxins, particularly **alcohol.** Several deficiency states are also associated with cerebellar dysfunction. A wide variety of vascular and structural processes can also result in ataxia. **Posterior fossa ischemia, neoplasms in the posterior fossa,** and **obstruction of CSF flow** can all manifest in this way. **Demyelinating disease** in the posterior fossa, **infectious diseases, hereditary disorders,** and **migraine** can all be associated with cerebellar dysfunction. **Paraneoplastic syndromes** can also present with ataxia as a principle feature. A complete review of the clinical syndromes associated with cerebellar dysfunction is beyond the scope of this text and should be reviewed in a clinical textbook. However, several important clinical points should be emphasized within the context of reviewing cerebellar function. Cerebellar dysfunction often occurs in the setting of other signs and symptoms. These associations can offer clues to the etiology of the disturbance. For example, the combination of cerebellar dysfunction and cranial nerve palsies would implicate brainstem involvement. Also, there are age-related differences in the onset of different cerebellar conditions. For example, alcohol-related causes and vascular causes of ataxia are more common in older patients. On the other hand, hereditary conditions, migraine, and posterior fossa tumors are more likely to be encountered in younger patients. SM's case is characterized by ataxia in the setting of bilateral corticospinal tract involvement and peripheral neuropathy. Given the involvement of multiple systems and the family history of similar symptoms, a **hereditary process** is likely in this case.

Cerebellar Anatomy   The organization of the cerebellum is summarized later in this case (see Thumbnail: Cerebellum). It is helpful to think of the cerebellum as being **organized in sets of three.** There are three lobes, three pairs of peduncles, three afferent fiber types, three cortical layers, three pairs of deep nuclei, and three functional divisions. These structures are reviewed within the context of information flow through the cerebellum. The vascular supply of the cerebellum is discussed separately.

Cerebellar lobes   The cerebellum can be broadly divided into an anterior lobe, a posterior lobe, and a flocculonodular lobe. The **primary fissure** separates the anterior and posterior lobes. The **anterior lobe** corresponds to roughly the anterior one third of the cerebellum and is primarily involved **in maintaining muscle tone.** The **posterior lobe** corresponds to roughly the posterior two thirds of the cerebellum. It is phylogenetically the newest part of the cerebellum and is mainly involved with **coordinating motor function.** The **flocculonodular lobe** looks like a mustache crossing the midline horizontally on the ventral surface of the cerebellum. It is made up of two parts: the **flocculus** (one on each side of the midline) and the **nodulus,** which is located on the midline. The flocculonodular lobe is phylogenetically the oldest part of the cerebellum. It is concerned with **vestibular function** and is interconnected with the vestibular nuclei. Several fissures on the cerebellar surface divide each of the lobes further, into several lobules. The most important of these to be able to recognize are the **cerebellar tonsils** (one on each side). They are located on the ventral surface of the cerebellum and are part of the posterior lobe. These are the structures that are pulled down through the foramen magnum in **herniation syndromes** and with **Chiari's malformations**. Chiari's malformations are herniation syndromes in which the cerebellar tonsils and caudal vermis are pulled down through the foramen magnum. Type I Chiari's malformations are relatively mild. Type II Chiari's malformations are more severe, with distortion of the medulla and the fourth ventricle. They are often associated with a syrinx of the cervical spinal cord. A similar condition, the Dandy-Walker malformation, is associated with enlargement of the fourth ventricle resulting from impaired outflow of CSF through the foramen of Magendie.

The cerebellum is also divided functionally into two **cerebellar hemispheres** and one midline portion, called the **cerebellar vermis**. This distinction ignores the differentiation of the cerebellum into lobes. For example, the nodulus (of the flocculonodular lobe) is just one part of the vermis on the inferior surface of the cerebellum. The distinction between the cerebellar vermis and the cerebellar hemispheres is clinically important. The **cerebellar vermis** helps coordinate movements of **muscles in the trunk and the proximal extremities**. It is particularly susceptible to injury from alcohol and other toxins. The **cerebellar hemispheres**, on the other hand, are more concerned with coordinating movements of **muscles in the distal extremities**. Note that a relatively larger and newer portion of the cerebellum is devoted to the coordination of fine motor movements.

Cerebellar cortex and white matter   The surface of the cerebellum has many in-foldings, similar to the gyri seen on the cerebral surface. In the cerebellum, these folds of cortex are called **folia** because they resemble leaves packed against each other. As with the gyri of the cerebral cortex, the effect of the folia is to greatly increase the amount of cerebellar surface area packed into a very small space. As in the cerebrum, the cerebellar cortical surface is made up of a layer of **gray matter** surrounding a **core of white matter** and several **deep gray nuclei**. The cerebellar white matter is made up of the fibers that bring information in to and out of the cerebellum. These fibers are organized into three pairs of **cerebellar peduncles**: the superior, middle, and inferior peduncles. The cerebellar peduncles connect the cerebellum to the brainstem at the level of the **pons**. The **fourth ventricle** separates the pons from the cerebellum. The inferior and middle peduncles convey information to the cerebellum. The middle peduncles are the largest and are continuous with the body of the pons. The superior peduncles convey information out from the cerebellum.

Cerebellar nuclei   The cerebellar cortex receives input from many sources. Output from the cerebellar cortex goes primarily to the deep nuclei of the cerebellum. The cerebellar nuclei are divided into three groups. The **fastigial nuclei** are closest to the midline. They receive input from the **cerebellar vermis**. They project out to the **vestibular nuclei** and the

reticular formation. The fastigial nuclei help regulate vestibular function. The output pathway originating in the fastigial nuclei is unique because it travels through the **inferior cerebellar peduncles**. All other cerebellar output goes through the superior cerebellar peduncles.

The **intermediate nuclei** receive input from the **paramedian cerebellar hemispheres**. They project out to the **red nucleus** and the **thalamus** via the **superior cerebellar peduncles**. The intermediate nuclei are further divided into globus nuclei and emboliform nuclei. These nuclei help regulate posture and balance. The **dentate nuclei** receive input from the **lateral portions of the cerebellar hemispheres**. They also project to the thalamus via the **superior cerebellar peduncles**. The dentate nuclei mediate coordination of the extremities.

Circuitry of the cerebellar cortex   The **cerebellar cortex** has three layers: the outer **molecular layer**, the middle **Purkinje's cell layer**, and the inner **granular layer**. The best way to review these layers is to consider their input and the organization of cerebellar circuitry. This circuitry is summarized in Figure 13-1.

Purkinje's cells are the main **output neurons** of the cerebellar cortex. They are all arranged next to each other, forming a layer of cells only one cell-width deep. The Purkinje's cells are inhibitory neurons that project primarily to the **deep cerebellar nuclei**. Their axons are all oriented downward toward the deep cerebellar nuclei. Purkinje's cell dendrites all project superficially into the **molecular layer**. This is the outermost layer of the cerebellar cortex. It is primarily a region of synaptic interaction (note that this is true of the molecular layer in all types of cortex). The dendrites of each Purkinje's cell form a two-dimensional array that is perpendicular to the long axis of the **cerebellar folia** within the molecular layer. These dendrites receive input from two different sources.

Climbing fibers are excitatory axons that originate in the **inferior olivary nuclei**. These nuclei receive input from both the **spinal cord** and the **cerebral cortex**. Climbing fibers exit the inferior olivary nuclei, cross to the contralateral side, and enter the cerebellum through the **contralateral inferior cerebellar peduncle** (also called the **restiform body**). They "climb up" along the descending Purkinje's cell axons. The terminal branches of the climbing fibers parallel the branches of the Purkinje's cell dendrites. Thus, each climbing fiber makes many synaptic contacts with its specific Purkinje's cell and exerts a strong influence on the function of that cell.

All other sources of input to the cerebellum enter the cerebellum as **mossy fibers**. The **pontine nuclei** are the most prominent source of cerebellar mossy fibers. The **corticopontine pathway** conveys information from the cerebral cortex to the pontine nuclei. Pontine neurons then give off

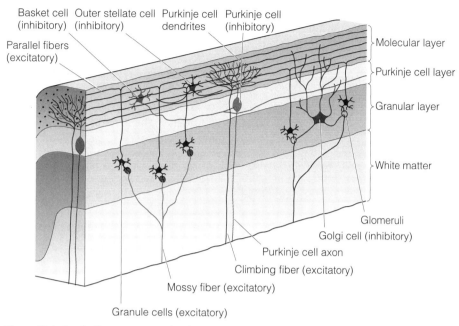

Figure 13-1 Cerebellar cortex organization.

mossy fibers, which **cross the midline** and enter the cerebellum through the **contralateral middle cerebellar peduncle.** Input conveyed to the cerebellum by the reticulocerebellar, vestibulocerebellar, cuneocerebellar, and spinocerebellar tracts also enter the cerebellum as mossy fibers. Most of these tracts enter the cerebellum through the inferior cerebellar peduncle. Note that the inferior and middle cerebellar peduncles primarily convey information to the cerebellum, and the superior cerebellar peduncles are output pathways.

Regardless of their origin, mossy fibers synapse on granule cells in the **granular layer** of the cerebellar cortex. Mossy fiber axons terminals interact with granule cell dendrites in clusters called **glomeruli.** Adjacent glomeruli are functionally linked by inhibitory interneurons called **Golgi's cells.** Granule cell axons extend superficially into the **molecular layer** of the cerebellar cortex. These axons are called **parallel fibers** because they are parallel to the long axis of the cerebellar folia and perpendicular to the plane of the Purkinje cell dendrites. Thus, each parallel fiber only contacts a Purkinje cell once but contacts multiple Purkinje's cells. This is in contrast to the arrangement of the climbing fibers (they make many contacts with just one Purkinje's cell). The function of groups of Purkinje's cells is coordinated by interneurons within the molecular layer (basket cells and stellate cells). These interactions are summarized in Figure 13-1.

Overview of Cerebellar Function   The cerebellum coordinates information regarding the planning and execution of movement on the **ipsilateral side of the body.** The cerebellum receives information from the **cerebral cortex** regarding the planning of movement and the execution of those plans. It also receives sensory information from the **spinal cord** and **vestibular system** regarding the execution of movements. Note that in most cases the cerebellum helps regulate the function of contralateral structures in the CNS. This means that fibers entering the cerebellum must first cross the midline. Fibers exiting the cerebellum also must cross the midline before getting to their targets.

The cerebellum has three functional systems. The circuit flow outlined in the preceding paragraphs applies to all three systems. These functional divisions can be confusing because they do not strictly adhere to the anatomic distinctions noted. The **vestibulocerebellum** includes the flocculonodular lobe, portions of the cerebellar vermis, and the fastigial nuclei. This system is concerned with **balance and eye movements.** It receives input primarily from and projects primarily to the vestibular nuclei. The cerebellum is important for visual **smooth pursuit** (tracking a moving object). Disruption of the vestibulocerebellum causes **nystagmus.**

The **spinocerebellum** is concerned with maintaining **muscle tone** and monitoring the **execution of movement.** This system receives input from the spinal cord and projects to the cerebral cortex via the thalamus. The spinocerebellum is further divided into two parallel systems. The **cerebellar vermis** helps regulate **medial motor systems** in the control of **axial and proximal muscles.** Disruption of this system causes ataxia of the trunk and postural imbalance. The **paramedian cerebellar hemispheres** help regulate **lateral motor systems** in the control of **distal limb muscles.** Disruption of this system causes limb ataxia.

The **cerebrocerebellum** mediates **feedback** to cerebral motor systems. It is made up primarily of the **lateral cerebellar hemispheres.** It receives input from the cerebrum via the pons and projects back to the cerebrum via the dentate nuclei and thalamus. It helps regulate **coordination** and the **initiation of movement.**

In essence, the cerebellum compares intended motor plans with the results of motor action. It then fine-tunes the function of descending motor systems to compensate for potential errors. The cerebellum may play a similar role in the fine-tuning of other, **nonmotor cerebral functions.** Finally, cerebellar circuits may be involved in **learning of motor skills.**

Clinical Correlation   Hundreds of diseases are associated with ataxia and dizziness. Some of the most common causes include vascular disease, peripheral vestibulopathies, demyelinating diseases, and structural processes involving the posterior fossa. In addition, many **hereditary diseases** are associated with cerebellar dysfunction. Many of these relatively rare disorders have been associated with **unstable trinucleotide repeats.** The first neurologic trinucleotide-repeat disease to have been well characterized is Huntington's disease (HD). The most commonly encountered ataxic disorders in this category are **Friedreich's ataxia** and **spinocerebellar ataxia** types 2, 3, and 6 (although 16 types have been identified, some only in individual families).

Trinucleotide-repeat diseases are often characterized by progressive neurodegeneration. The repeat expansions cause meitotic instability. The length of the expansion usually correlates with disease severity. **Anticipation,** disease onset at progressively younger ages in subsequent generations, is a common feature. These disorders often have an autosomal dominant inheritance pattern.

Case Conclusion   SM had an MRI to exclude any structural abnormalities of the posterior fossa or evidence of demyelinating disease. A lumbar puncture failed to reveal any abnormalities suggestive of infectious or inflammatory disorders. Electrical studies were performed to exclude neuropathy. Vitamin E deficiency and other metabolic abnormalities were also excluded. His clinical picture was most consistent with Friedreich's ataxia or one of the other rare spinocerebellar ataxias. An electrocardiogram (ECG) was obtained. No arrhythmias were seen but T-wave inversions, consistent with Friedreich's ataxia, were seen. Genetic testing confirmed the diagnosis. He was referred to a neuromuscular center where comprehensive supportive services could be arranged. Unfortunately, treatment options for hereditary ataxias are limited.

Thumbnail: Cerebellum

Cerebellum is Organized in Groups of Three	
Three lobes	Flocculonodular lobe—phylogenetically oldest Anterior lobe Posterior lobe—phylogenetically newest
Three cortical layers	Molecular layer—venue for synaptic interaction Purkinje's cell layer—output to deep nuclei Granular layer—sight of mossy fiber input
Three Purkinje's cells afferent paths	Mossy fibers—all other sources of input Climbing fibers—from inferior olivary nuclei Aminergic fibers—from the brainstem
Three pairs of deep nuclei	Fastigial Interposed (globose and emboliform) Dentate
Three pairs of peduncles	Superior—primarily output Middle—primarily input Inferior—primarily input
Three functional divisions	Vestibulocerebellum—balance and eye movements Spinocerebellum—muscle tone and movement Cerebrocerebellum—coordination and movement

Key Points

▶ The cerebellum coordinates information regarding the planning and execution of movement on the ipsilateral side of the body.

▶ The flocculonodular lobe is mainly concerned with vestibular function.

▶ The posterior lobe is mainly involved with coordinating motor function.

▶ The anterior lobe is primarily involved with maintaining muscle tone.

▶ The cerebellar vermis helps coordinate movements of the trunk and proximal extremities.

▶ The cerebellar hemispheres help coordinate movements of the distal extremities.

▶ Climbing fibers originate in the inferior olivary nuclei and synapse directly onto Purkinje's cells.

▶ All other sources of input to the cerebellum enter the cerebellum as mossy fibers.

▶ Purkinje's cells are the main output neurons of the cerebellar cortex and project to the deep nuclei of the cerebellum.

▶ The cerebellar nuclei project out to brainstem and thalamic targets via the superior cerebellar peduncles.

Questions

1. A 52-year-old man presents with progressive ataxia that has developed over several months. He has a long-standing history of alcoholism. Which of the following structures is most likely to be abnormal on imaging studies of his brain?
   A. Fastigial nuclei
   B. Flocculus
   C. Dentate nucleus
   D. Interposed nuclei
   E. Vermis

2. You evaluate a patient with suspected cerebellar disease. You note that the patient has prominent gaze-evoked nystagmus. Which of the following structures is implicated?
   A. Fastigial nuclei
   B. Globose nuclei
   C. Dentate nuclei
   D. Interposed nuclei
   E. Emboliform nuclei

3. You evaluate a patient who has had a stroke involving a large portion of the ventral cerebellum on the right. Which of the following vessels is most likely to have been occluded?
   A. Anteriorinferior cerebellar artery (AICA)
   B. Posteriorinferior cerebellar artery (PICA)
   C. Basilar artery
   D. Superior cerebellar artery (SCA)
   E. Vertebral artery

4. You evaluate a patient who complains of positional headache. An imaging study revealed low-riding cerebellar tonsils and a possible syrinx in the cervical spinal cord. What type of malformation does this patient have?
   A. Chiari's type I
   B. Chiari's type II
   C. Dandy-Walker malformation
   D. Spinal stenosis
   E. Magendie's malformation

Case 1

1. C
2. B
3. B
4. C

Case 2

1. B
2. D
3. A
4. E

Case 3

1. D
2. B
3. D
4. B

Case 4

1. C
2. A
3. B
4. C

Case 5

1. C
2. B
3. D
4. E

Case 6

1. D
2. E
3. A
4. C

Case 7

1. D
2. B
3. E
4. D

Case 8

1. C
2. B
3. D
4. A

Case 9

1. D
2. D
3. A
4. D

Case 10

1. E
2. B
3. B
4. E

Case 11

1. B
2. A
3. B
4. B

Case 12

1. E
2. C
3. E
4. D

Case 13

1. E
2. A
3. B
4. B

Part II

Spinal Cord and Peripheral Nerves

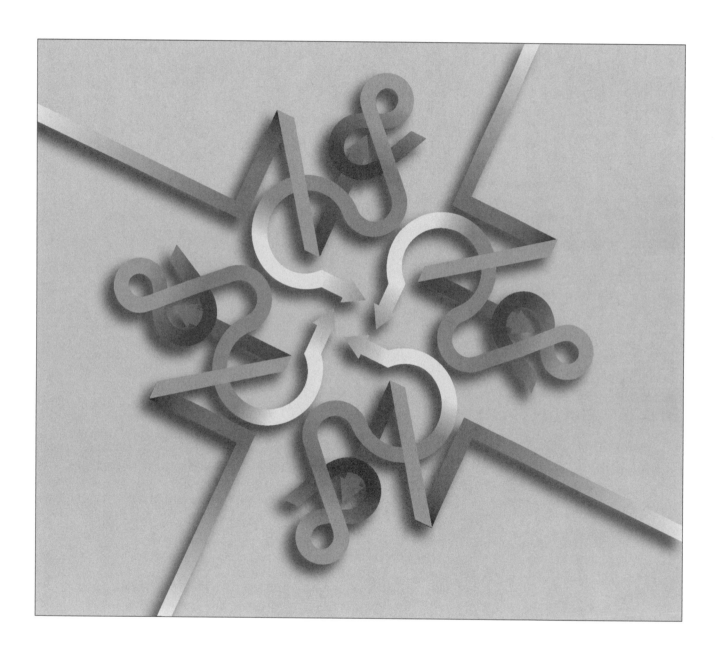

HPI: A 25-year-old man is brought to the hospital after being shot in the back. He is conscious and shouts that he is unable to walk and cannot feel his left leg. He is taken to the neurosurgical suite where the bullet and bone fragments are removed. You are able to examine him after he has been stabilized and the anesthesia has worn off. He is now able to tell you that he still cannot feel his left leg and cannot move it, but he does note that his left toes feel cold. **PMHx:** The patient had an appendectomy 14 years ago. **Rx:** He did not take any medications before this incident.

PE: T 100.4°F   HR 105   BP 155/85   RR 14   SaO$_2$ 94% on room air

Sensation to pressure and light touch is absent on the left side up to and including the T10 dermatome. Surprisingly, sensation to temperature and pain is absent on the *right side* up to the T10 dermatome. He cannot feel pain or temperature bilaterally in the T10 dermatome itself. Strength is absent in the left leg and hip muscles, but upper extremity strength is intact bilaterally. He has a clean and dry dressing over the surgical site in the lower thoracic region of the back.

Thought Questions

- How can this constellation of symptoms be explained?
- Where is the likely lesion?
- What is the prognosis?

Basic Science Review and Discussion

The Somatosensory System: From Nerve Endings to Cortex

Nerve endings, types of sensation   Somatic sensation, using the skin, muscles, and joints as sensory organs, begins at the level of the receptor, usually located within or just deep to the dermis. The viscera also have receptors, which are not discussed here. Each different receptor type allows for a slightly different type of sensation. A few major types are highlighted here, although there are many other types of receptors.

Pacinian corpuscles: the largest receptors, "onion-skin" structure, detect deep pressure

Muscle spindle and Golgi's tendon organ: provide proprioceptive information by recognizing stretch on muscles and tendons, respectively

Nociceptors: simple free nerve endings that detect pain

Meissner's corpuscles: smaller receptors that detect light touch

Peripheral sensory nerves   Once an action potential has been generated with the appropriate stimulus at a nerve ending, it is transduced to the spinal cord via the afferent peripheral nerves, which come in various nerve fibers. Pain fibers are either **unmyelinated** or **thin myelinated** fibers. On the other hand, fine touch may be transmitted via thick myelinated fibers.

Spinal cord tracts   Afferent input from the somatosensory system arrives at the spinal cord via the **dorsal nerve root** (Figure 14-1). Action potentials transverse the **dorsal root ganglion** along this pathway, as peripheral sensory nerves are **pseudounipolar** neurons (there is no synapse at the ganglion, merely the transition from dendrite to axons). The dorsal root transmits action potentials to the **dorsal horn** of the spinal cord.

There are three major somatic sensory systems, each of which is discussed separately. The **dorsal columns system** governs sensation of fine touch, conscious proprioception, and vibratory sense. The **spinothalamic system** governs sensation of pain and temperature, as well as crude touch. The **spinocerebellar system** governs sensation of unconscious proprioception.

Dorsal columns system   Afferent fibers from the periphery arrive via the dorsal nerve root and enter the dorsal columns of the spinal cord (hence the name). Axons from the sacral and lumbar nerve roots run directly into and up (without synapsing) the **medial** dorsal column of the spinal cord, more specifically named the **fasciculus gracilis.** Thoracic and cervical dorsal root axons run up the other (more lateral) dorsal column, the **fasciculus cuneatus.** These fascicular axons synapse on the **nucleus gracilis and nucleus cuneatus,** respectively, in the ipsilateral medulla. Second-order neurons located in these nuclei collectively project fibers that cross the midline to form the **medial lemniscus,** which projects onto the **ventral posterolateral nucleus of the thalamus.** Finally, third-order neurons located in the thalamus project to the **postcentral gyrus** of the cortex, where all sensation is brought to consciousness.

Spinothalamic system   The spinothalamic system crosses at the level of the dorsal root, unlike the dorsal column system. Multiple modulatory factors are in place throughout the spinothalamic system, which explains why the same

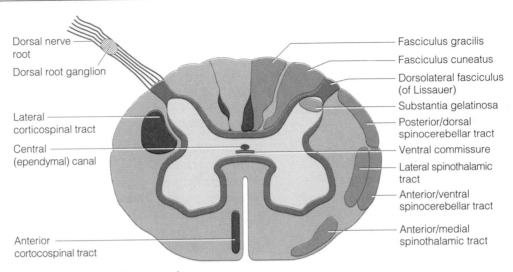

Figure 14-1 Spinal cord in cross section.

stimulus may be mild or excruciating, depending on the context.

The initial stimulus must excite a receptor in the periphery, be it for temperature, crude touch, or free nerve endings (nociceptors) for pain. Free nerve endings are stimulated by the local release of bradykinins, prostaglandins, histamine, and particularly **substance P** (a polypeptide that is one of the major neurotransmitters and stimulants in the pain pathway) secondary to inflammation or tissue damage.

The afferent impulse arrives via the dorsal nerve root. These axons first run up or down several spinal levels in **Lissauer's tract** of the dorsal horn before synapsing in the **substantia gelatinosa** (also of the dorsal horn). Second-order neurons then cross the midline in the **ventral commissure** to form the **medial** (crude touch) and **lateral** (pain, temperature) **spinothalamic tracts,** which run superiorly to synapse (again) in the ventral posterolateral nucleus of the thalamus. The spinothalamic tracts run contralateral to the afferent nerve ending due to decussation at the ventral commissure, unlike the dorsal columns system. Third-order neurons again project to the postcentral gyrus of the cortex, bringing pain, temperature, and crude touch to consciousness.

Spinocerebellar tract   The spinocerebellar tracts, dorsal and ventral, receive unconscious proprioceptive input via the dorsal horn and transmit it to the ipsilateral anterior lobe of the cerebellum. The **dorsal** tract remains ipsilateral and travels via the inferior cerebellar peduncle, whereas the **ventral** tract crosses the midline at the level of the dorsal root and crosses back again in the pons to arrive at the anterior lobe of the cerebellum via the superior cerebellar peduncle. This system allows the cerebellum to modulate balance and fine motor activity by recognizing limb placement. Because these tracts do not run to the cerebral cortex, they are not brought to consciousness.

Modulation of Pain Sensation and the Gate-Control Theory
As experience tells us, a stimulus that may seem painful while lying in bed at night may not even be recognized when sufficiently distracted. The perception of pain at the level of the postcentral gyrus may be modified at almost every step in the sensory system, including the receptor, the sensory nerve, and in particular, within the spinal cord and brain. Medications and the environment play a role in affecting pain perception, as described later in this case.

Peripheral nociceptors, which are stimulated by the release of prostaglandins and substance P, may be modulated by **nonsteroidal anti-inflammatory drugs (NSAIDs),** which decrease local prostaglandin production. **Capsaicin** (the active ingredient in hot pepper spray) may deplete stores of substance P to deaden the sensation of pain.

Peripheral nerves, which rely on sodium channels to propagate action potentials, may be deadened by using sodium channel blockers such as **lidocaine.**

The **spinal cord** modifies pain input at the level of the dorsal horn in the **substantia gelatinosa.** Second-order spinothalamic neurons are excited by input from nociceptive peripheral nerves. At the same time, they are inhibited by input from certain non-nociceptive peripheral nerves (specifically thick myelinated fibers). This inhibition explains why rubbing or massaging a tender area may decrease the sensation of pain via the competitive interaction of pain fibers versus dorsal column fibers. Finally, feedback interneurons from the brain also project onto the substantia gelatinosa to modify neuronal activity in accordance with emotional state, anxiety, and so on. This complex "gating" function of the substantia gelatinosa is referred to as the **gate-control theory.**

The **brain** also has numerous sites that modify the perception of pain, including the periaqueductal gray matter, the thalamus, and the reticular formation and limbic system. Opioid receptors in these locations, stimulated by endogenous opiates (called **endorphins** or **enkephalins**), as well as prescribed **opiates** (such as morphine or methadone), act to decrease the sensation of pain.

Pathologic States of the Somatosensory System The list of diseases that affect the sensory system is far too long to go over in detail. A few important conditions that are specific or particularly significant to the sensory system are described in the following sections.

Brown-Séquard's syndrome *Brown-Séquard's syndrome* refers to the constellation of symptoms seen with hemisection of the spinal cord: **ipsilateral paresis, ipsilateral dorsal column** sensory loss, and **contralateral spinothalamic** sensory loss. Patients will present with loss of fine touch ipsilateral to the lesion but will lose sensation to pain and temperature contralateral to the lesion. They may lose pain and temperature bilaterally at the site of the lesion because entering pain fibers may be obliterated within the dorsal root. The most common causes of Brown-Séquard's syndrome are trauma and compression secondary to tumor. As with all spinal cord lesions, recovery is usually minimal, unless decompression is an option.

Tabes dorsalis *Tabes dorsalis* ("dorsal softening") refers to the syndrome seen in neurosyphilis of sensory loss due to selective destruction of the dorsal roots and dorsal columns of the spinal cord. The spirochete *Treponema pallidum* disproportionately involves the dorsal columns system, which results in **sensory ataxia** (a "staggering gait" may be seen), loss of proprioception (positive Romberg's sign), and potential loss of reflexes. Dysesthesias may also present, often described as "lightning pains." The autonomic fibers may be involved and may cause urinary incontinence, impotence, and constipation. Penicillin will cure the infection, but the symptoms may persist because of permanent spinal cord damage.

Subacute combined systems degeneration Subacute combined systems degeneration refers to the subacute involvement of multiple neurologic systems seen in **vitamin B$_{12}$ (cobalamine) deficiency**. Vitamin B$_{12}$ is a cofactor used by methyltransferases, which in turn play a role in fatty acid metabolism and myelin synthesis. Vitamin B$_{12}$ deficiency leads to inadequate myelin production and the accumulation of abnormal fatty acids, causing demyelination and axonal degeneration in the peripheral nerves, dorsal columns, and spinocerebellar and corticospinal tracts. This initially presents **with distal paresthesias,** followed by distal numbness, then a **sensory ataxia** with gait difficulty, and finally **distal weakness** as the corticospinal tracts become

involved. As is the case with most peripheral neuropathies, long nerves are most susceptible, resulting in hand and foot involvement initially in a "glove and stocking" distribution. Vitamin B$_{12}$ repletion is curative if started within a few months of symptom onset, otherwise, some of the CNS effects may be permanent.

Syringomyelia The spontaneous formation of a "syrinx" (tube) within the spinal cord (an enlargement of the central canal) is known as **syringomyelia.** Cause is not entirely clear; patients with anatomic abnormalities such as the **Arnold-Chiari malformation** (elongated brainstem with downward displacement of the cerebellar tonsils into the foramen magnum) are at greater risk. A syrinx is most often found in the **low cervical cord.** Central cord fibers are initially affected, with the decussating spinothalamic fibers in the ventral commissure being most vulnerable, initially causing **pain** and discomfort in the **hands/upper extremities** bilaterally. This may progress to a **"capelike" distribution** of insensitivity to pain and temperature of the upper extremities and torso (the legs are not involved because their spinothalamic fibers are crossed in the lumbosacral cord, well inferior to the syrinx). Treatment usually involves medical pain management, with severe cases leading to surgical drainage of the syrinx, which has limited benefit in arresting syrinx progression.

Multiple sclerosis Multiple sclerosis (MS) is a disease of unclear origin, which causes spotty demyelination in apparently random areas of the CNS white matter, both brain and spinal cord. It may result in **patchy** areas of **anesthesia/ dysesthesia,** as well as **weakness.** Symptoms usually flare at varying intervals, although they predictably flare in warmer weather. Medical treatment is employed with varying success.

Peripheral neuropathy Various diseases cause peripheral neuropathies. As a general rule, nerve fibers are more susceptible to any ischemic, inflammatory, or demyelinating process in proportion to their length. Sensory fibers are generally smaller and more susceptible than motor fibers. Peripheral neuropathies thus selectively involve the hands and feet and progress proximally as the disease progresses in what is often referred to as a **glove-and-stocking distribution. Diabetes** causes an ischemic neuropathy that usually presents with **distal sensory loss. Vitamin B deficiency** (in addition to vitamin B$_{12}$ **deficiency**) and **folic acid deficiency** cause a demyelinating neuropathy with similar symptoms. **Alcohol abuse** (possibly secondary to nutritional deficiencies) and lead poisoning may cause sensory loss. Human immunodeficiency virus **(HIV)** neuropathy may cause bilateral foot pain on the soles of the feet. Finally, familial peripheral neuropathies have also been reported.

Case Conclusion   An operative report from this patient's surgery indicates that the bullet transected the left half of the spinal cord before lodging in the T10 vertebral body. Destruction of the left half of the spinal cord at the level of the T10 spinal nerves was essentially complete, but the right side was relatively unaffected. The functional consequence is hemisection of the spinal cord on the left side, resulting in **Brown-Séquard's syndrome.** Regrettably, the prognosis for spinal cord lesions is poor, and it is anticipated that he will not regain motor function of the left lower extremity, which will require him to use a wheelchair.

Thumbnail: Sensory Systems

Sensory Systems and Pathologic States

Anatomic location	Disease	Function or symptoms
Dorsal columns		Fine touch, vibration, proprioception
	Tabes dorsalis	Sensory ataxia, staggering gait
	Subacute combined systems degeneration	Distal paresthesias/sensory loss, distal numbness, distal weakness
Spinothalamic		Contralateral pain/temperature/crude touch
	Syringomyelia	"Capelike" loss of pain sensation in arms/torso
Spinocerebellar		Unconscious proprioception
Peripheral nerves		Peripheral sensation or motor function
	Peripheral neuropathy	Distal glove and stocking loss of fine touch, may progress to involve proximal areas or pain sensation
Other		
	Brown-Séquard's syndrome (cord hemisection)	Ipsilateral plegia and loss of fine touch with contralateral pain and temperature loss
	Multiple sclerosis	Patchy areas of weakness and sensory loss

Key Points

▶ The somatosensory system is divided into three major systems based on spinal cord tracts: the dorsal columns (fine touch and proprioception), spinothalamic (crude touch, pain, and temperature), and spinocerebellar (unconscious proprioception).

▶ Sensation of pain is affected by various factors including medications and neuronal feedback, as shown in the gate-control theory. Substance P is the major transmitter of pain.

▶ A number of diseases affect sensation by interfering with nerves and sensory tracts, including trauma (Brown-Séquard's syndrome), neurosyphilis, alcohol abuse, nutritional deficiencies (particularly vitamin B_{12}, folic acid), multiple sclerosis, and syringomyelia.

Questions

1. A patient has a spinal cord tumor that has affected the dorsal horn only on the right side at the C7 level. Which of the following symptoms should be seen on examination?
   A. Right-sided pain and temperature loss of the right C7 dermatome only
   B. Right-sided fine touch/vibratory loss of the right C7 dermatome only
   C. Right-sided fine touch/vibratory loss, left-sided pain/temperature loss of the C7 dermatome
   D. Right-sided fine touch/vibratory loss, right-sided pain/temperature loss of the C7 dermatome
   E. Left-sided pain/temperature loss of the C7 dermatome only

2. A 45-year-old male is brought to the hospital for difficulty walking and appearing confused. He does not have any significant medical history. He has diminished sensation to light touch bilaterally involving the upper and lower extremities and looks at his feet while walking. Proprioception is markedly diminished, with a positive Romberg's sign. Reflexes are almost completely absent, including no pupillary reflex to light. What is the most likely diagnosis?
   A. Peripheral neuropathy
   B. Syringomyelia
   C. Neurosyphilis
   D. Subacute combined systems degeneration
   E. Brown-Séquard's syndrome

3. A 32-year-old woman develops diffuse burning pain in her right arm that is now beginning to affect the left arm as well. On examination, sensation to pinprick and pain is markedly diminished across her upper torso and arms but is intact beneath the shoulder blades and around the neck. She is otherwise intact. What might an MRI of the brain and spinal cord be expected to show?
   A. Bilateral foraminal stenosis of cervical spine
   B. Downward displacement of cerebellar tonsils into foramen magnum, central syrinx in low cervical/upper thoracic cord
   C. Diffuse patchy demyelination bilaterally throughout brain white matter
   D. Normal
   E. Low cervical disk herniation with cord compression

4. A homeless patient visits the clinic for the first time for a routine physical. He does not have any complaints and is not aware of previous medical history. On examination, you note numerous cuts on his feet and markedly reduced sensation to pain and light touch up to the ankles and wrists bilaterally. The scent of alcohol is noticeable on his breath. His neurologic examination is otherwise intact. What is the most likely diagnosis?
   A. Peripheral neuropathy
   B. Subacute combined systems degeneration
   C. Syringomyelia
   D. Tabes dorsalis
   E. Multiple sclerosis

HPI: RK is a 33-year-old woman who has been in good health until 5 days ago when she developed tingling in her feet. A sensation of numbness then gradually ascended up her legs. She has also noted worsening back pain. There is no history of trauma. She did not seek medical attention initially but has now developed bilateral leg weakness. She reports that the weakness came on gradually and was subtle yesterday. This morning she awoke to find she could not stand or even get out of bed. She has been unable to urinate. She denies any other medical problems. She had the flu a few weeks earlier. She has never had anything like this before.

PE: Her vitals signs are all within normal parameters. Her neurologic examination reveals marked paraparesis. Reflexes are somewhat brisk in the lower extremities only. Toes are up-going bilaterally. She appears to have a T8 sensory level to all modalities. She is neurologically intact above the T8 level and her general examination is unremarkable.

Thought Questions

- Does this patient have a peripheral or a central lesion?

- What structure(s) is/are affected?

- What pathways are affected?

- What is the significance of the brisk reflexes?

Basic Science Review and Discussion

If this patient had presented earlier in the course of her syndrome, consideration might have been given to the possibility of a peripheral process. At this point, however, her syndrome represents central dysfunction. **Upper motor neuron (UMN) signs** including **brisk reflexes** and **extensor plantar (Babinski's)** responses accompany her leg weakness. She also has a **sensory level,** which helps to localize her lesion to the midthoracic spinal cord. This is further supported by her inability to void, evidence of **autonomic dysfunction.**

This **acute myelopathy** most likely represents an inflammatory, infectious, or parainfectious process (given her recent viral syndrome). Spinal cord ischemia, spinal vascular malformations, and spinal tumors would be important differential considerations. However, vascular processes manifest more acutely with maximum deficits reached within the first few hours. Tumors, on the other hand, tend to present more insidiously. Trauma is an important consideration but is excluded by history.

This chapter focuses on the **motor pathways.** Sensory systems, the autonomic system, spinal anatomy, and spinal nerves are all discussed separately. Cortical motor function is also discussed in more detail in Case 1. Other structures are also critically involved in motor function. The basal ganglia and cerebellum are also integral to normal motor function. Lesions in these areas result in various movement disorders. These regions are also discussed further in other chapters.

Motor System Organization The execution of movement begins in the **frontal cortex. Premotor** and **supplementary motor** areas contribute to the preparation of movement. The **primary motor cortex (Brodmann's area 4)** initiates movement. Cortical output is carried by the axons of pyramidal neurons in cortical layer V, which make up the pyramidal tract. The **pyramidal tract** is a more generic term that reflects all of the **corticofugal pathways.** The **corticospinal tract** is the main motor output pathway and is part of the pyramidal tract. However, the majority of pyramidal axons actually end at targets within the brainstem. These latter pathways include the **corticopontocerebellar pathway** and several **corticobulbar pathways.** Each of these systems is also part of the pyramidal tract. The motor cortex of each hemisphere controls movement of the contralateral side of the body via the corticospinal system. To reach contralateral targets, these fibers cross the midline at the **pyramidal decussation** in the caudal medulla.

Corticospinal Tract The main motor output pathway is a two-neuron system, consisting of an **upper motor neuron** (UMN) and a **lower motor neuron** (LMN). The large **pyramidal neurons** of **cortical layer V** in the **primary motor cortex** are the UMNs of this system. The **corticospinal tract** primarily contains the axons of these pyramidal neurons. However, this pathway also contains some axons originating in premotor, supplementary motor, and primary sensory cortical areas. Together, these fibers make up the **corona radiata** of the subcortical white matter. This name reflects the cone-shaped appearance of these fibers as they funnel together to pass between the **deep gray nuclei** and through the **diencephalon.** Of course, the corona radiata also contains ascending sensory fibers. Within the corona radiata, fibers mediating motor function of the face, arm, and leg are relatively separated from each other. Thus, focal lesions in this area are not likely to cause complete hemiparesis of the face, arm, and leg. However, as these fibers pass between the basal ganglia and the thalamus, they become more densely packed within the **internal capsule.** Lesions of the internal capsule (such as from **lentic-**

ulostriate ischemia) are more likely to manifest as hemiparesis involving the face, arm, and leg contralateral to the lesion.

The corticospinal tract remains tightly packed together as it passes though the **cerebral peduncles** of the **midbrain.** As these fibers reach the **pons,** they become more dispersed, passing between clusters of **pontine nuclei.** Fibers making up the **corticopontocerebellar pathway** end here while the corticospinal fibers continue caudally. The corticospinal tracts are visible on the ventral surface of the **medulla,** where they are called the **pyramids.** The **pyramidal decussation** is also visible in the caudal medulla. This is where the majority of corticospinal fibers cross the midline.

Throughout the brainstem, **corticobulbar fibers** that innervate various **cranial nerve nuclei** also branch of from the pyramidal tract and terminate at their corresponding brainstem levels.

Most of the corticospinal fibers (about 80%) cross the midline at the pyramidal decussation and descend through the spinal cord as the **lateral corticospinal tract** within the contralateral **lateral funiculus** of the spinal cord. The remaining fibers descend ipsilaterally through the **ventromedial corticospinal** tract in the **anterior funiculus** of the spinal cord. Most of these fibers ultimately cross the midline when they reach their terminal spinal cord level. A very small percentage of these fibers terminate on ipsilateral targets. Lesions of UMNs can occur anywhere from the cortical surface to the spinal cord. They usually manifest as weakness at first. UMN lesions are subsequently characterized by **pathologic reflexes** (such as **Babinski's sign**), **hyper-reflexia, clonus,** and ultimately by **spasticity** and **increased tone.**

Alpha Motor Neurons   The primary targets of the descending UMN fibers include both **LMNs (alpha motor neurons)** and **interneurons** located in the **ventral horns** of the spinal cord. The **somatotopic organization** found at higher levels is maintained within the spinal cord. LMNs innervating axial and proximal muscles are located more medially in the spinal cord gray matter. LMNs' innervating distal muscles, on the other hand, are located more laterally with the spinal cord gray matter of the ventral horns. Alpha motor neurons that innervate muscles in the **upper extremities** are clustered together at several cervical spinal levels where the spinal cord becomes enlarged. This is called the **cervical enlargement.** Alpha motor neurons that innervate muscles in the **lower extremities** are similarly arranged in the **lumbosacral enlargement.** Axons of the alpha motor neurons exit the spinal cord through the ventral roots to join peripheral nerves. Most muscles are innervated by neurons from multiple spinal levels. However, some muscles receive their innervation predominantly from one prominent spinal level. Weakness in these muscles can aid in the localization of

lesions. These muscles are summarized later in this case (see Thumbnail: Motor Systems).

Spinal nerve anatomy is discussed further in Case 16. Gamma motor neurons are similar to alpha motor neurons but innervate muscle spindles, which are involved in mediating spinal reflexes. Spinal reflex mechanisms are discussed within the context of sensory systems. **LMN lesions,** such as peripheral nerve compressions and radiculopathies, manifest as **weakness** with **diminished reflexes. Muscle wasting** and **fasciculations** ultimately develop.

Corticopontocerebellar and Corticobulbar Tracts   Many of the axons contained within the pyramidal tract terminate on brainstem targets. The most prominent example of this is the **corticopontocerebellar tract.** The axons in this tract outnumber the axons in the corticospinal tract by nearly 20:1. They terminate on **pontine neurons** in the **pontine nuclei.** Axons from the pontine neurons cross the midline to enter the **contralateral middle cerebellar peduncle.** These pontocerebellar fibers are a major source of **mossy fibers** to the cerebellum. Cerebellar circuitry is discussed further in Case 13.

Remember that the function of the cranial nerve nuclei in motor and sensory systems of the head is analogous to that of the spinal cord for the rest of the body. Similarly, the function of the **corticobulbar tract** is analogous to that of the **corticospinal tract.** Although some corticobulbar fibers project directly onto their associated **brainstem LMN,** most influence their targets via **reticular interneurons.** One important difference between the corticobulbar system and the corticospinal system is that many of the cranial nerve nuclei receive **bilateral cortical input** via corticobulbar fibers. However, these two systems essentially mediate the same motor functions albeit for different muscle groups.

Bulbospinal Tracts   Some brainstem nuclear groups act as regions of intermediate processing for the motor system or provide feedback information to the motor system through various modalities. These brainstem regions give rise to several **bulbospinal pathways** that influence the interaction between UMNs and LMNs. Four major tracts are reviewed. The locations of the major motor pathways within the spinal cord are summarized in Figure 15-1.

Rubrospinal tract   The **red nucleus** is a venue for integration of information coming from the **cerebral cortex** and information coming from the **cerebellum.** Lesions in this area result in **tremor.** Two major red nucleus output pathways are recognized. The first pathway projects to the **inferior olivary nucleus** on the same side. This is the major pathway in humans. It provides feedback to the **contralateral cerebellum.** The second is the **rubrospinal tract.** The rubrospinal tract is, in essence, an indirect corticospinal pathway. Axons of neurons in the red nucleus cross the

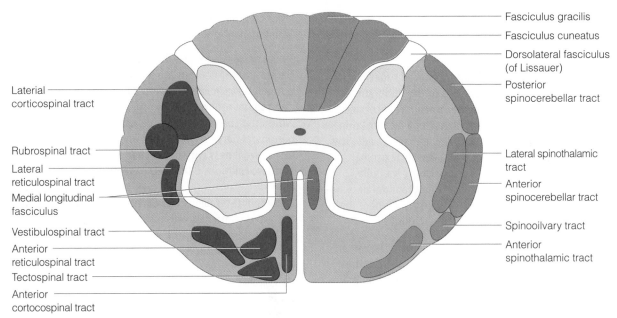

Figure 15-1 Principal fiber tracts of spinal cord.

Labels (clockwise from top right): Fasciculus gracilis; Fasciculus cuneatus; Dorsolateral fasciculus (of Lissauer); Posterior spinocerebellar tract; Lateral spinothalamic tract; Anterior spinocerebellar tract; Spinoolivary tract; Anterior spinothalamic tract; Anterior cortocospinal tract; Tectospinal tract; Anterior reticulospinal tract; Vestibulospinal tract; Medial longitudinal fasciculus; Lateral reticulospinal tract; Rubrospinal tract; Lateral corticospinal tract.

midline in the **ventral tegmentum,** course through the central tegmental tract, then through the lateral funiculus of the spinal cord to their target level.

Tectospinal tract   The **tectospinal tract** originates in the **superior colliculi.** These fibers cross the midline within the midbrain and descend medially through the brainstem to the spinal cord. In the medulla, it joins with the **medial longitudinal fasciculus.** The function of this system in humans is not clear. However, given the visual function of the superior colliculi and the vestibular function of the medial longitudinal fasciculus, this system may be involved in orienting movements of the head and body to visual cues.

Reticulospinal tract   The *reticular formation* makes up a central core through much of the brainstem. It contains many different nuclear groups. Many of these nuclei use monoamine neurotransmitters. These systems are discussed further in subsequent chapters. As a general rule, the *rostral reticular formation* is concerned with *consciousness and vigilance.* More *caudal reticular formation* regions are involved in regulating *cardiovascular and respiratory tract mechanisms.* Several *pontine and medullary reticular nuclei* project to the spinal cord and *influence motor function* (voluntary and reflexive movements, muscle tone).

Vestibulospinal tract   The **vestibular system** detects motion in several planes. This information is conveyed to brainstem vestibular nuclei by the **vestibulocochlear nerve** (cranial nerve [CN] VIII). The vestibular nuclei (superior, lateral, medial, and inferior) are interconnected with medial cerebellar structures, the oculomotor nuclei, and the cervical spinal cord. The **lateral** and **medial vestibular nuclei** give rise to descending fibers that project to the spinal cord as

the **vestibulospinal tract.** This complex system helps coordinate eye, head, and neck movements. The vestibular system is discussed in detail in Case 29.

Clinical Correlation   **Acute transverse myelitis** (ATM) is focal inflammation of the spinal cord. The inflammation is evident on MRI studies and in the spinal fluid. Prompt diagnosis is very important. The first goal of therapy is to minimize further injury. **Intravenous steroids** are the standard of care. Plasma exchange, intravenous immunoglobulin (IVIG), and immunosuppressive agents also have been used. Primary ATM is the result of an autoimmune process. Secondary ATM can be seen in the setting of acute infection, during the postinfectious period, and after immunizations. **Molecular mimicry,** a similarity between an extrinsic antigen and a self-antigen, may be involved in these cases. ATM can also be encountered within the context of the connective tissue diseases.

ATM affects people of all ages but is most often seen in the second and fourth decades. Its clinical manifestation is characterized by sensory, motor, and autonomic symptoms. The sensory symptoms are usually associated with a distinct spinal sensory level. As a general rule, about one third of patients will recover with little or no residual deficit. One third will be left with more moderate disability. One third will be left with severe disability.

ATM can represent the first clinical manifestation of what will ultimately become **multiple sclerosis** (MS). Patients who have white matter lesions on their MRI scan of the brain at the time of their ATM are much more likely to develop MS than those who have normal brain MRI studies. Of course, a history of demyelinating disease in another CNS region supports the diagnosis of MS.

Case Conclusion   RK was admitted to the hospital. An MRI of the thoracic spinal cord confirmed a focal inflammatory lesion involving the T7 and T8 spinal levels. MRI scans of the brain, cervical spine, and lumbosacral spine did not reveal any other areas of abnormality. A lumbar puncture revealed mild inflammatory changes with no evidence of infection. The patient received a 5-day course of high-dose IV steroids followed by an oral tapering dose. She was ultimately transferred to the rehabilitation service where she gradually regained most of her function. In follow-up at 1 year, she was self-ambulatory with only mild residual weakness.

Thumbnail: Motor Systems

Spinal Segments and Their Major Muscles

Roots	Muscles
C3, C4	Levator scapulae
C5 + C6	Deltoid, supraspinatus, infraspinatus, rhomboids, biceps, brachioradialis, supinator
C6 + C7	Flexor carpi radialis, pronator teres, extensor carpi radialis
Mostly C7	Triceps, extensor digitorum, anconeus
Mostly C8	Extensor indicis proprius, most other forearm extensors and flexors
C8 + T1	Intrinsic hand muscles
L2 + L3	Iliopsoas, rectus femoris
L3	Adductor longus
L3 + L4	Gracilis, vastus medialis and lateralis
L4 + L5	Tibialis anterior
Mostly L5	Extensor hallucis longus, extensor digitorum longus and brevis, peroneus longus and brevis, posterior tibial, flexor digitorum longus, medial hamstrings, gluteus medius
Mostly S1	Abductor hallucis, abductor digiti quinti, soleus, gastrocnemius, lateral hamstrings, gluteus maximus
S2, S3	Sphincter ani

Key Points

▶ Many of the axons contained within the pyramidal tract terminate on brainstem targets.

▶ The corticospinal tract is the main motor output pathway and is part of the pyramidal system.

▶ Corticospinal fibers cross the midline at the pyramidal decussation in the caudal medulla.

▶ Approximately 80% of corticospinal fibers cross the midline at the pyramidal decussation and descend as the lateral corticospinal tract.

▶ The remaining fibers descend ipsilaterally through the ventromedial corticospinal tract.

▶ UMN lesions are characterized by pathologic reflexes (such as Babinski's sign), hyper-reflexia, clonus, and spasticity.

▶ LMN lesions manifest as weakness with diminished reflexes and eventual muscle wasting and fasciculations.

Questions

1. You evaluate a patient whose right arm is markedly weak. Reflexes in the arm are diminished. However, you note that reflexes are rather brisk in the right leg and the patient has an up-going toe on the right. Reflexes are normal on the left. What structure is involved?

   A. Peripheral nerves
   B. Ventral roots
   C. Spinal cord
   D. Brainstem
   E. Alpha motor neurons

2. You evaluate a 63-year-old patient who has developed progressive muscle weakness and wasting over several months. Muscle fasciculations are diffusely evident on examination. Reflexes are rather brisk. Which structure is most likely affected?

   A. Peripheral nerves
   B. Ventral roots
   C. Muscles
   D. Neuromuscular junction
   E. Alpha motor neurons

3. You evaluate a 38-year-old acutely myelopathic female. She has previously been treated for optic neuritis. Which of the following tissues is most likely affected in her spinal cord?

   A. White matter only
   B. Gray matter only
   C. Both gray and white matter
   D. Small caliber vasculature
   E. All of the above

4. You evaluate a patient who has a spinal cord injury and note very brisk reflexes in the lower extremities. Which of the following is responsible?

   A. Increased sensory input to alpha motor neurons
   B. Increased corticospinal axon function
   C. Decreased alpha motor neuron function
   D. Decreased corticospinal axon function
   E. Increased alpha motor neuron function

HPI: An elderly 78-year-old female is brought to your attention for recurrent arm and neck pain. She recalls no trauma or inciting event, but for the past 6 months, she has noted a recurrent sharp pain originating in the back of her neck, which shoots down her right arm to her thumb. This is often brought about when she coughs or turns her head and is minimized when she lies down. She has a history of hypertension and has had bilateral hip replacements. She takes Tylenol and occasional Motrin for joint pains, and hydrochlorothiazide for high BP.

PE: T 36.7°C   HR 72   BP 135/85
On neurologic exam, she has diminished sensation to pinprick on her right lateral arm and forearm, as well as the thumb. Right biceps strength and reflex is diminished, though still present. She has some neck pain on palpation throughout. On turning her head, the shooting pain from her neck to her right arm is reproduced.

Labs: White blood cell (WBC) 7, hematocrit (Hct) 35, sodium (Na) 136, potassium (K) 3.6

Thought Questions

- What nervous structure is the likely source of the problem?
- What adjacent anatomic structures are contributing?
- What about this patient has likely placed her at risk?

Basic Science Review and Discussion

The spinal cord gives off a tetrad of nerve roots (left and right, ventral and dorsal) at each spinal level. The motor nerve root (ventral) and sensory nerve root (dorsal) come together to form a unified **spinal nerve.** The spinal nerves are grouped into basic categories by the vertebrae they accompany, namely cervical, thoracic, lumbar, and sacral. Each spinal nerve is named for the vertebrae that it runs adjacent to (C5, T1, etc.). Cervical spinal nerves are named for the vertebrae that they run superior to (i.e., C5 nerve root runs just superior to the C5 vertebral body), whereas all other nerve roots are named for the vertebrae they run inferior to (the T6 nerve root runs inferior to the T6 vertebral body, in the T6–T7 intervertebral space).

As the nerve roots emerge from the spinal cord, the dorsal and ventral roots coalesce and the single nerve runs laterally toward the "neural foramina," the intervertebral openings through which the spinal nerve passes out of the bony spine. It is in the foramina, surrounded by bone (namely, the bony pedicle of the vertebra), that the nerve is most vulnerable to compression. Once outside of the foramina, spinal nerves either intertwine to form the cervical, brachial, and lumbosacral plexuses, or run solitary as the intercostal nerves.

Compression of these nerve roots or spinal nerves is referred to as a **radiculopathy** (*radiculo-* refers to a root).

Cervical Spinal Nerves   The cervical spinal nerves are of particular note for a variety of reasons. For one, because there are in fact eight cervical nerves and seven cervical vertebrae, the C8 nerve root deserves special mention as running in the C7-T1 intervertebral space. They are of particular importance because they innervate the upper extremities. Finally, because the cervical vertebrae are relatively small with relatively small neural foramina to match, the stage is set for nerve root compression (radiculopathy).

Cervical radiculopathy   As the spinal nerves run toward neural foramina, they run tangentially and adjacent to the intervertebral disks. Lateral protrusion or **herniation** of the disks will in turn compress the nerve root against the bony pedicle, resulting in radiculopathy. It is worth noting that posterior herniation of the disk (the notorious "slipped disk") will potentially compress the cord itself, resulting in spinal cord compression, or **myelopathy.**

Radiculopathy may also be caused by alterations in the bony architecture of the neural foramen, as is seen with degenerative joint disease, that is, osteoarthritis. In this case, hypertrophy and/or degeneration of the bony facet joints will contort the foramina. This is referred to as **foraminal encroachment,** and it causes the majority of cervical radiculopathy. In rarer cases, a mass, fracture, localized infection, or other process may also compress a spinal nerve root.

Foraminal encroachment occurs most often in the joints that receive the most wear and tear, namely the C4–C7 vertebral joints (they have greater rotational and flexional mobility). As a result, C5, C6, and C7 cervical radiculopathies are the most common.

Cervical radiculopathy is often manifested by particular symptoms, namely a sharp, shooting pain running from the neck along the dermatomal distribution of the affected nerve root, which is usually along the arm. Paresthesias and numbness may also often occur. Weakness and loss of reflexes may occur in muscle groups that are innervated by the affected nerve root. Movements that promote further impingement or movement of the nerve in the restrictive foramen tend to make this worse: coughing, straining, and turning the head. Conversely, lying down with the neck in a neutral position often affords relief. Management is usually conservative, involving relative immobilization of the neck and decreased use of the involved extremity, which is generally effective.

Lumbar radiculopathy The lumbar region deserves special mention because it is a region of particular strain, as it supports the weight of the spinal column and is thus most prone to disk herniation. Disk herniation, or **lumbar disk prolapse,** usually occurs laterally and thus leads to radiculopathy (posterior herniation, on the other hand, poses a risk for cord compression or cauda equina compression). Lumbar radiculopathy is symptomatically similar to cervical radiculopathy. It often presents with sharp pain radiating down the leg, paresthesias, numbness, and potential weakness and loss of reflexes in the segmental distribution pertaining to the affected nerve root. The L4, L5, and S1 nerve roots are most often affected.

Case Conclusion   On account of thumb paresthesias, biceps weakness, and reduced biceps reflex, this patient's C6 radiculopathy became apparent. She was started on conservative management with a soft neck collar to minimize turning of her head for 3 days, which reduces her symptoms. NSAIDs such as ibuprofen may also be used for pain. She is able to use her arm with only occasional twinges thereafter. Should her symptoms recur and cervical immobilization or traction prove ineffective, she may become a candidate for **foraminectomy,** or surgical enlargement of the offending neural foramen.

Thumbnail: Spinal Nerves

Selected Spinal Nerves: Key Functions and Resulting Deficits

Note: It is important to recognize that the functions stated in the following table are by no means all inclusive. They merely reflect key functions to aid memorization; more specific details have been omitted.

Nerve	Function	Presentation with injury
C5	Biceps strength and reflex; sensation lateral arm	Biceps weakness; paresthesias/ pain lateral arm; pain referred to scapula
C6	Biceps strength and reflex; sensation lateral forearm, thumb	Biceps weakness; paresthesias/pain in forearm/thumb
C7	Triceps strength and reflex; sensation second, third digits (lateral fingers)	Triceps weakness; paresthesias/pain to lateral fingers
L4	Quadriceps strength and reflex; gluteal strength; sensation kneecap, medial calf	Quads weakness, decreased knee jerk; pain/paresthesias kneecap, medial calf
L5	Extensor hallucis longus (EHL)/foot dorsiflexor strength; gluteal and hamstring strength; sensation lateral calf, dorsal foot	EHL, foot dorsiflexor weakness; moderate gluteal/hamstring weakness; pain/paresthesias lateral calf, dorsal foot
S1	Gastrocnemius strength, ankle jerk; gluteal and hamstring strength; sensation lateral foot and sole	Gastrocnemius weakness, reduced ankle jerk; moderate gluteal/hamstring weakness; pain/paresthesias
Myelopathy	Unilateral/bilateral strength and sensation at and below compression; autonomic functions (bowel/bladder)	Weakness or paralysis at or below lesion; pain/paresthesia/anesthesia; bowel/bladder incontinence

Key Points

▶ The spinal nerve roots emerge from the spinal cord in segmental tetrads, with the dorsal and ventral roots coalescing to form pairs of spinal nerves (left and right).

▶ Spinal nerves and nerve roots are vulnerable to compression, resulting in partial or complete dysfunction. The dysfunction is specific to the myotome (motor function) and dermatome (sensation) of the affected nerve or nerve root.

▶ Compression usually occurs as a result of bony deformation of the spine and neural foramina but may also result from disk prolapse and/or herniation; other processes are also possible.

▶ Treatment usually involves rest and immobilization, although surgical decompression may be warranted in severe cases.

Questions

1. On a radiology rotation, you are given a cervical spine x-ray film of a 35-year-old man. You can detect only mild congenital narrowing of the cervical spinal canal. The only clinical information available is that the patient has been experiencing neck pain worsened by movement, radiating along the left arm to "some of his fingers." Triceps reflex is reduced on the left. What is the most likely diagnosis?
   A. Radial nerve injury
   B. C7 radiculopathy
   C. Musculocutaneous nerve injury
   D. C6 radiculopathy
   E. Cervical cord compression

2. On examining an older male patient, you discover complete anesthesia on the sole of the left foot. The patient tells you that this has been the case since sustaining a grenade blast in Vietnam, with shrapnel hitting his back in multiple locations. He has healed since surgical removal of the shrapnel and is not bothered by this lack of sensation. What might explain this finding?
   A. Sciatic nerve injury
   B. Left dorsal L4 nerve root transection
   C. Left ventral S1 nerve root transection
   D. Left dorsal L5 nerve root transection
   E. Left dorsal S1 nerve root transection

3. Routine examination of a 69-year-old man demonstrates relative weakness of the left EHL muscle (big toe extension is weakened). Ankle jerk and plantar flexion are intact. He appears to have decreased sensation on the dorsum of the left foot and mentions a history of low back pain with occasional "shooting pain" down the side of the left leg. What is the most likely diagnosis?
   A. Left L4 radiculopathy
   B. Left L5 radiculopathy
   C. Left S1 radiculopathy
   D. Left S2 radiculopathy
   E. Lumbar myelopathy

4. After an automobile accident, a 35-year-old man is placed on a backboard and transported to the hospital. Although he remains conscious, you note that sensation to pinprick is reduced but present bilaterally over the kneecaps and below. As the ambulance goes over bumps, you note that he transiently loses continence of stool. What is the best explanation?
   A. Bilateral L4 radiculopathy secondary to acute nerve root compression
   B. Bilateral L4 spinal nerve transection
   C. High cervical cord transection
   D. Diffuse lumbar radiculopathies bilaterally secondary to lumbar vertebral fractures
   E. Lumbar cord compression causing myelopathy

HPI: A 40-year-old male construction worker visits the ED with a new paralysis of the left hand. He describes using his left arm over his head and vigorously attempting to pull down a sliding lever when he felt a tearing sensation in the shoulder the previous day. Although some of the shoulder pain has resolved, he also notes lack of sensation along the medial arm. He is able to clench his fingers, but otherwise the fingers are paralyzed. His symptoms have not improved since the day before. His medical history is unremarkable.

PE: T 37.8°C   HR 75   BP 145/85
He has a claw hand and lack of sensation in the medial arm and hand corresponding to the C8 and T1 dermatomes, all on the left side. Finger flexion is relatively intact, but he has reduced extension and cannot use intrinsic muscles of the hand (finger abduction and adduction). Neurologic exam is otherwise unremarkable.

Thought Questions

- Damage to which structure is the most likely cause of this deficit?

- What about the adjacent anatomy is most likely to have caused the problem?

- What is the prognosis?

Basic Science Review and Discussion

The peripheral nerves of the upper extremity are derived from five spinal nerve roots that intertwine to form the **brachial plexus** (Figure 17-1). These roots are the C5, C6, C7, C8, and T1 segments, which are interwoven into three **trunks,** which again are interwoven to form three **cords,** which finally again are interwoven to form its five terminal

branches, the **five major peripheral nerves** of the upper extremity.

The plexus lies in the posterior neck where it runs just over the first rib and under the clavicle into the deep axilla. It evolves into the terminal branches within the axilla, which continue into the upper extremity.

In the process of ultimately forming these five major peripheral nerves of the upper extremity, the brachial plexus gives off a number of smaller peripheral nerves, which will be discussed here.

The brachial plexus specifically includes the C5–T1 spinal nerve roots, the trunks, the cords, and its own smaller branches; the five major terminal branches are not considered part of the brachial plexus. These terminal branches, namely the axillary, radial, musculocutaneous, median, and ulnar nerves, are discussed in Case 18 in more detail.

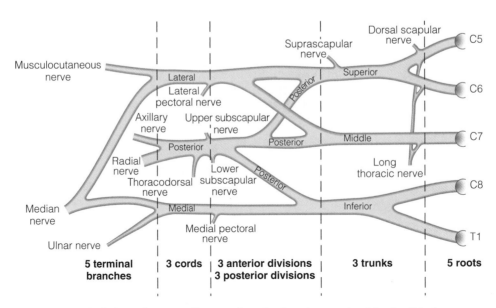

Figure 17-1 Brachial plexus. (Note: Smaller nerve branches have been omitted for simplicity.)

The function of the brachial plexus, as the name implies, is **to provide motor and sensory innervation to the entire upper extremity,** either through its own smaller nerve branches or through the five major terminal branches. All of the muscles located within the upper extremity are supplied by the brachial plexus, although some truncal muscles that move the upper extremity or shoulder girdle (e.g., trapezius) may have other nerve supplies. The great majority of cutaneous sensation of the upper extremity is also supplied by the brachial plexus. (The exception is a small medial segment of the proximal arm, whose cutaneous sensation is supplied by the **intercostobrachial nerve,** which is derived from the T2 root.)

Specific Structures

Nerve roots   The proximal brachial plexus includes the spinal nerve roots C5–T1. Roots C5, C6, and C7 immediately drop fibers to form the **long thoracic nerve,** which innervates the serratus anterior muscle. C5 also sends fibers to the **dorsal scapular nerve** (rhomboid muscle), as well as to the **phrenic nerve.** C5 fuses with C6 and C8 with T1, with C7 standing alone, to form the three **trunks.**

Trunks   Predictably, the C5 and C6 trunk is the superior trunk, the C7 trunk the middle trunk, and C8 and T1 the inferior trunk. The superior trunk sends off the **suprascapular nerve,** which innervates the supraspinatus and infraspinatus muscles. Each trunk then divides into an **anterior and posterior division.**

Anterior and posterior divisions   There are three anterior divisions and three posterior divisions, totaling six structures, none of which give any side branches. The divisions then merge to form the **cords** of the brachial plexus. All of the posterior divisions merge to form the **posterior cord.** Of the anterior divisions, the superior and middle form the **lateral cord,** and the inferior simply becomes the **medial cord.**

Cords   The lateral cord, now composed of C5–C7 segments, gives off the **lateral pectoral nerve** (pectoralis major muscle). The medial cord gives off the **medial pectoral nerve** (pectoralis major and minor muscles). The posterior cord gives off the **thoracodorsal nerve** (latissimus dorsi muscle), the **upper subscapular nerve** (subscapularis muscle), and the **lower subscapular nerve** (teres major and subscapularis muscles). The cords then simply divide into the **terminal branches** (or major peripheral nerves). There is no intermingling of the cords, with the exception of the medial and lateral cords, which combine in part to form the **median nerve.**

Terminal branches   Each terminal branch includes divisions of the cords as follows:

Musculocutaneous nerve: derived from the lateral cord (C5, C6, C7)

Axillary nerve: from the posterior cord, but only includes the C5, C6 contributions

Radial nerve: from the posterior cord, includes all C5–T1 nerve roots

Median nerve: from both lateral and medial cords, includes all C5–T1 nerve roots

Ulnar nerve: from medial cord, C8 and T1

Brachial Plexopathies and Associated Neuropathies

Upper plexus lesion (Erb-Duchenne palsy)   An upper plexus lesion is usually seen in the context of birth or shoulder trauma, usually resulting from tearing of the superior trunk or C5 and C6 nerve roots resulting from excessive traction on the arm. This results in C5–C6 dysfunction, causing deltoid, biceps, and supraspinatus plus infraspinatus palsy. The patient may be unable to abduct the shoulder or flex the elbow. Recovery is often minimal or incomplete.

Lower plexus lesion (Klumpke's palsy)   A lower plexus lesion, usually resulting from forced abduction of the arm due to trauma or during birth, results in intrinsic hand muscle weakness and C8–T1 sensory loss. Lower plexus lesions have been seen from falling asleep after drinking with an arm slumped over a chair or table resulting in prolonged abduction.

Thoracic outlet syndrome   Thoracic outlet syndrome refers to the constellation of venous with or without arterial insufficiency, combined with brachial plexus dysfunction secondary to compression of the plexus and subclavian artery and vein. All three of these structures run over the first rib, rendering them vulnerable to compression by anomalous structures such as a cervical rib or congenital fibrous band.

The syndrome may present with neck and/or shoulder pain, forearm paresthesias, intrinsic hand muscle weakness, subclavian venous thrombosis, or possibly arterial insufficiency. Downward tension on the affected arm places greater traction on the neurovascular bundle, exacerbates compression against the first rib, and generally makes symptoms worse. Neurologic symptoms are most notable in the T1 distribution because the inferiorly located T1 root, lying closest the rib, is compressed most of all. Treatment is surgical decompression.

Brachial neuritis   Brachial neuritis is a debilitating inflammatory condition of the brachial plexus that results in shoulder pain and **proximal upper extremity weakness.** Cause is usually idiopathic but may often occur in the setting of a viral infection or after vaccination; it may also occur after IV heroin use. Patients present with shoulder pain, proximal more than distal arm weakness, and possible muscle wasting of the proximal arm muscles after about 4 weeks. Sensory loss of the shoulder may also occur. Both arms may be involved. No curative treatment is available, but the symptoms usually resolve with time.

Long thoracic nerve palsy (C5, C6, C7)   Long thoracic nerve palsy occurs in the setting of placing significant weight on the shoulder or lifting heavy objects with the arm, or spontaneously secondary to diabetes. The resulting **serratus anterior palsy** results in **winging of the scapula** (protrudes posteriorly from the back) when the arm is raised anteriorly.

Patients have difficulty raising the arm above the head because the scapula, which anchors these abducting arm muscles, is no longer stabilized by the serratus anterior. A common complaint is the inability to comb the hair with the affected arm. The effects are often permanent.

Suprascapular nerve palsy (C5, C6)   The suprascapular nerve may also be compromised by placing a large amount of weight on the shoulder, or from an ischemic neuropathy secondary to diabetes. The supraspinatus muscle weakness leads to difficulty abducting the arm, whereas infraspinatus muscle weakness compromises external rotation of the arm. Wasting of the spinati muscles is made clearer by abnormal prominence of the scapular spine.

Case Conclusion   The history of injury during forced abduction is suggestive of a lower plexus lesion, which is also suggested by the paresthesia and weakness in a C8–T1 distribution. Regrettably, such traumatic injuries are very slow to heal, and in many cases, traumatic brachial plexus lesions may improve very little.

Thumbnail: Brachial Plexus

Syndromes of Brachial Plexus and Associated Nerves			
Syndrome	**Structure**	**Symptoms**	**Nerve roots**
Upper plexus lesion	C5, C6 roots	Weakness of shoulder abduction, elbow flexion, ± C5, C6 sensory loss	C5, C6, ± C7
Lower plexus lesion	C8, T1 roots	Intrinsic hand muscle weakness, ± C8, T1 sensory loss	C8, T1, ± C7
Thoracic outlet syndrome	T1 root, subclavian artery and vein	Neck pain, intrinsic hand weakness, subclavian venous thrombosis	T1, ± C8 depending on severity
Brachial neuritis	Brachial plexus	Shoulder pain, proximal arm weakness, occasional shoulder anesthesia	C5–T1 with variable degrees of involvement
Long thoracic nerve palsy	Long thoracic nerve, serratus anterior muscle	Winging of scapula, difficulty combing hair	C5, C6, C7
Suprascapular nerve palsy	Suprascapular nerve, spinati muscles (supraspinatus and infraspinatus)	Weakness of shoulder abduction, prominent spine of scapula	C5, C6

Key Points

▶ The brachial plexus supplies virtually all of the sensory and motor function of the upper extremity, which is derived from the C5–T1 nerve roots.

▶ The most common neuropathies specific to the brachial plexus include upper and lower plexus lesions, thoracic outlet syndrome, and long thoracic nerve palsy. Traumatic lesions generally may not recover, whereas spontaneous palsies are more likely to recover fully.

▶ The brachial plexus supplies several independent nerves and then ultimately gives rise to the five major nerves of the upper extremity: the axillary, radial, musculocutaneous, median, and ulnar nerves.

Questions

1. After undergoing right mastectomy with axillary node dissection for breast cancer, a 35-year-old woman notes a small area of anesthesia in her medial right upper arm. The surgeon assures her that he did not approach the brachial plexus during the operation. She has no discernible weakness or other neurologic findings. What is the most likely explanation?

   A. Right T1 nerve root injury secondary to excessive abduction during the operation
   B. Development of thoracic outlet syndrome secondary to wound closure
   C. Right lower plexus injury secondary to excessive abduction during the operation
   D. Right upper plexus injury resulting from excessive traction during the operation
   E. The lesion is outside the brachial plexus

2. A 69-year-old female patient describes difficulty combing her hair using her dominant right hand. She has learned to accommodate this by using her left hand but is puzzled by this problem, which began 2 weeks ago. She is able to abduct her right arm to 90 degrees, but not above the shoulder. There is no sensory loss. What is the most likely problem?

   A. C5 nerve root injury
   B. Long thoracic nerve palsy
   C. Thoracodorsal nerve palsy
   D. Suprascapular nerve palsy
   E. Upper plexus lesion

3. A 75-year-old woman visiting her doctor complains of difficulty abducting her left arm, which she has noticed for several months. On exam, sensation is intact, but she has weakness initiating left shoulder abduction; she is able to raise her arm above her head. Elbow flexion and extension is unaffected. Her left shoulder blade appears to be more prominent than her right. What is the most likely cause?

   A. Upper plexus injury
   B. Lower plexus injury
   C. Suprascapular nerve injury
   D. Long thoracic nerve injury
   E. C7 radiculopathy

4. A newborn infant is noted to have decreased movement of the right arm after a traumatic birth involving significant traction on the right arm. The infant does not appear to abduct the shoulder or flex the elbow and has decreased sensation to pinprick on the lateral arm. What is a likely cause?

   A. Lower brachial plexus injury
   B. Axillary nerve injury
   C. C5 radiculopathy
   D. Upper brachial plexus injury
   E. Brachial neuritis

HPI: A 65-year-old woman with a history of recent weight gain (15 pounds over 3 months) comes to your office complaining of tingling sensation in her palms on both sides, usually worse after she types or uses her hands for a prolonged period. She has been noticing this for several weeks and feels that it seems to be getting worse. She also notices more fatigue over the past few months. Otherwise, she feels well. She has no previous illnesses and takes no medications.

PE: T 35.5°C   HR 55   BP 112/62

On neurologic exam, she has diminished sensation to pinprick on the palmar surface of both hands, and notes pain radiating into the palms when her ventral wrist is struck with a reflex hammer. Biceps and triceps reflexes are normal, and strength in the forearm is preserved. She appears to have subtle weakness in opposition of both thumbs.

Labs: WBC 6, Hct 38, TSH 25 (normal TSH 0.5–5.0)

Thought Questions

- Which nerve is affected?

- Where in the nerve's course is the lesion?

- What other conditions are likely contributing to the neurologic problem?

Basic Science Review and Discussion

As discussed previously, the brachial plexus gives rise to the five major nerves of the upper extremity, whose function may be summarized into broad categories (with some minor exceptions). Keeping these generalizations in mind is helpful in determining which nerve is affected for many patient presentations.

The **axillary** nerve supplies the deltoid and teres minor muscles, as well as sensation of the shoulder. The **radial** nerve supplies motor function to the extensor (dorsal) compartments of the arm and forearm, as well as sensation of the dorsal hand. The **musculocutaneous** nerve supplies motor function to the flexor (ventral) compartment of the arm, as well as sensation of the ventral arm and part of ventral forearm. The **ulnar** nerve supplies motor function to the bulk of the intrinsic hand muscles (except the thumb), as well as sensation of the ulnar aspect of the hand (fifth and medial fourth digits). The **median** nerve supplies motor function to the flexor (ventral) compartment of the forearm and the thumb, as well as sensation of the ventral (or palmar) hand.

Each of these nerves run different anatomic courses, generally running close to the muscles and cutaneous regions that they innervate. In remembering which areas each nerve serves, and thus where they are likely to be found, it becomes clearer which injuries may affect a given nerve. Injuries involving the ulnar and median nerves are most common because they have the longest courses and have anatomically vulnerable spots.

The **axillary** nerve runs adjacent to the shoulder (glenohumeral) joint en route to the deltoid muscle. It is thus sometimes injured with **shoulder dislocation.**

The **radial** nerve runs around the humerus (in the **radial** or **spiral groove**) as it innervates the triceps, then forms the posterior interosseous nerve of the forearm. It is the most likely nerve to be injured by **humerus fracture.** Injury to the radial nerve results in unopposed wrist flexion, sometimes described as the characteristic **waiter's tip.**

The **musculocutaneous** nerve runs anteromedially to the humerus. It is sometimes injured by **humerus fracture.**

The **ulnar** nerve runs posterior to the humerus prior to passing in the **ulnar canal** of the medial epicondyle (here the nerve is colloquially called the *funny bone*), then runs in the anterior compartment of the forearm to the hand. It is thus injured by **elbow dislocation,** or **entrapment** in the ulnar canal. This results in an **ulnar neuropathy,** which results in denervation of the hand musculature, particularly the muscles of the fourth and fifth digits, resulting in **hypothenar atrophy** and the characteristic **ulnar claw.** The ulnar claw is caused by denervation of the lumbricals of the fourth and fifth digits, preventing extension of the phalanges against the preserved flexor tension of the flexor digitorum (median nerve).

The **median** nerve runs in the anterior compartment of the arm en route to forming **the anterior interosseous nerve** of the forearm, where it innervates the majority of the muscles in the anterior forearm compartment. It sends its most distal branch through the flexor compartment of the wrist, the **carpal tunnel.** The carpal tunnel is the narrow channel defined by the carpal bones and the ventral fibrous band known as the **flexor retinaculum,** or **transverse carpal ligament.** It contains the flexor tendons of the hand and the median nerve, with little room to spare. As a result, the majority of median neuropathies occur by compression in this tunnel causing **carpal tunnel syndrome.**

Carpal Tunnel Syndrome Carpal tunnel syndrome results from median nerve dysfunction secondary to mechanical compression in the carpal tunnel. Only the fibers in the median nerve present in the carpal tunnel will be affected; all branches that diverged from the median nerve proximally are spared.

Physical findings are focused on exacerbating the compression of the median nerve in the carpal tunnel, thus causing wrist pain. These include **Tinel's sign,** eliciting wrist pain by striking the midline anterior wrist with a reflex hammer on the irritated median nerve. Another is **Phalen's maneuver,** which also elicits wrist pain by holding the wrist in 90-degree palmar flexion for 60 seconds.

By the time the median nerve has reached the carpal tunnel, it has already innervated the anterior forearm compartment, and it has already given off the **recurrent median nerve,** which passes outside of the carpal tunnel to provide sensation for the thumb. It then follows that only sensation of the palmar second, third, and lateral fourth digits are generally affected by carpal tunnel syndrome. The motor innervation of the thumb (specifically, the opponens pollicis, abductor pollicis brevis, and flexor pollicis brevis) may also be affected. As these muscles begin to atrophy from the relative denervation, **thenar atrophy** develops.

Medical causes of carpal tunnel syndrome All causes of carpal tunnel cause mechanical compression of the median nerve by enlargement of the structures in the carpal tunnel, or compressing the tunnel itself. It is most often found in women and is often associated with **repetitive motions** that involve pressure on the ventral surface of the wrist, with **typing** being a common offender. Various medical conditions also may contribute by causing swelling of the nerve, connective tissue, or tendons within the carpal tunnel. Hypothyroidism should be mentioned because it is a relatively common and correctable ailment that is often associated with carpal tunnel syndrome (presumably through water retention).

Case Conclusion This older female's clinical hypothyroidism (manifested by recent weight gain, relative hypothermia, and significantly elevated TSH level) was identified and treated with thyroid hormone replacement. Over the next few weeks, she noted return of her weight to previous levels, and the tingling sensation in her palms left her. If it should return and is unresponsive to conventional modes of therapy such as wrist splints or weight loss, surgical transection of the flexor retinaculum may be considered.

Thumbnail: Nerves of Upper Extremity

Structure	Function	Characteristics of injury
Axillary nerve	Shoulder sensation and innervation	Deltoid weakness, shoulder anesthesia
Radial nerve	Extension and posterior sensation of upper extremity	**Waiter's tip,** loss of triceps reflex, posterior anesthesia
Musculocutaneous nerve	Flexion of arm, anterior arm sensation	Biceps weakness, loss of biceps reflex
Ulnar nerve	Innervation of hand, sensation of ulnar hand	**Ulnar claw**
Median nerve	Flexion of wrist and fingers, thumb innervation, sensation of palm	Thenar wasting, palmar anesthesia (**carpal tunnel syndrome**)
Cervical nerve root	Myotomal innervation, dermatomal sensation	Weakness of one nerve root (which usually affects multiple nerves), dermatomal anesthesia, may lose reflexes
Spinal cord injury	Motor function and sensation at and below level of injury	Hyperreflexia, clonus, possible loss of bowel/bladder function, may lose strength/sensation at and below level of lesion

Key Points

- There are five major nerves of the upper extremity, all derived from the brachial plexus. They are the axillary, radial, musculocutaneous, ulnar, and median nerves. Each nerve's function may be generalized into sensation and motor function of a part of the upper extremity.

- The more common injury syndromes include ulnar neuropathy (usually due to entrapment at the ulnar canal) and carpal tunnel syndrome.

- Carpal tunnel syndrome often may be improved by treatment with rest or treating the underlying cause, but if not, surgical transection of the flexor retinaculum is usually curative.

Questions

1. You are asked to see a 72-year-old woman with several weeks of spontaneous neck pain and pain in the area of the right scapula. She has no history of trauma or arm/shoulder injury. She describes occasional numbness running down her right arm anterolaterally, which stops proximal to the wrist. On examination, you appreciate slight biceps weakness and deltoid weakness on the right. X-ray film of right shoulder and humerus shows no evidence of fracture or bony deformity other than degenerative changes in the cervical spine. What is the most likely diagnosis?

   A. Median nerve injury
   B. C5 radiculopathy
   C. Axillary nerve injury
   D. Musculocutaneous nerve injury
   E. Upper brachial plexus injury

2. A 55-year-old man is found to have new difficulty moving his left arm hours after a car accident in which both the left humerus is fractured in the diaphysis (midshaft) and the left elbow is dislocated. On examination, he has inability to extend the wrist or fingers, anesthesia in the posterior forearm and dorsal hand, and wasting of the thenar eminence, all on the left. His fourth and fifth fingers are flexed more so than the others. He tells you that he has had tingling in his left fingers before. What is the most likely constellation of injury?

   A. Acute radial nerve injury, acute median nerve injury (carpal tunnel syndrome)
   B. Acute ulnar nerve injury
   C. Acute radial and ulnar nerve injury, chronic median nerve injury (carpal tunnel syndrome)
   D. Acute median nerve injury, chronic ulnar and radial nerve injury
   E. Acute axillary and ulnar nerve injury

3. A 60-year-old man describes chronic weakness in abducting the left shoulder and left shoulder numbness. He does not have shoulder pain or back pain. The left deltoid appears wasted on examination, and sensation to pinprick of the left shoulder is diminished. He thinks that these problems began after he dislocated his shoulder 4 years ago. What is the most likely cause?

   A. Left C6 radiculopathy
   B. Left C4 radiculopathy
   C. Left axillary nerve injury
   D. Left musculocutaneous nerve injury
   E. Left radial nerve injury

4. A trauma surgeon is repairing an open fracture of the humerus. While reducing the humeral fracture, she notes that the large nerve running within a groove around the humerus has been torn. What deficit is the patient expected to have?

   A. Inability to extend fingers with posterior forearm anesthesia
   B. Inability to flex fingers with anteromedial forearm anesthesia
   C. Ulnar claw with intrinsic hand weakness, dorsal hand anesthesia
   D. Inability to adduct thumb with palmar anesthesia
   E. Inability to flex elbow with lateral forearm anesthesia

HPI: A 36-year-old man is seen in the ED for leg weakness. He describes being unable to stand on his toes and having difficulty when he walks. This has gradually worsened over the past 2 weeks. On further questioning, he says that he has begun intermittently dribbling urine since yesterday and had one episode of fecal incontinence. He was diagnosed with HIV several months ago and is not taking antiretroviral therapy.

PE: T 99.6°F   HR 96   BP 120/65   RR 16 SaO_2 97% on room air
He appears thin and somewhat emaciated. Neurologic examination is notable for absent ankle jerks and two-fifths strength of plantar flexors and intrinsic foot muscles bilaterally. In addition, he has anesthesia on the back of both legs and the perianal region. Rectal tone is relatively absent. Hamstring and quadriceps strength is relatively preserved. There is no tenderness along the spine. He has fullness in the suprapubic area and voids a small amount of urine when this is compressed.

Thought Questions

- Which single location could best explain his symptoms?

- Which types of processes are more likely given the gradual onset?

- Which findings are most important to demonstrate the location?

Basic Science Review and Discussion

The spinal cord runs from the motor decussation of the lower medulla at the level of the foramen magnum to the conus medullaris around vertebral level L1–L2. It serves to relay sensory and motor information between the brain and peripheral nerves. In addition to serving as a relay instrument, it coordinates reflexes via spinal interneurons, thus expediting the reaction without having to wait for impulses to be transmitted to and from the brain. Essentially all sympathetic and parasympathetic bowel and bladder functions (non-vagal parasympathetic functions) are conducted through the cord as well.

Anatomy of the Cord The spinal cord is divided into four parts corresponding to their adjacent vertebrae. Each of these parts is divided into multiple **spinal levels,** or segments that have a tetrad of **spinal roots:** dorsal and ventral, right and left.

The **cervical** segment, contained within the cervical vertebrae, has spinal nerves that run **superior** to their corresponding vertebrae; for example, C1 runs superior to the C1 vertebra (also known as the atlas), and C7 runs superior to the C7 vertebra. C8 runs between the C7 and T1 vertebrae; there is no C8 vertebra. The cervical cord is wider than most other parts of the cord because many of its spinal roots are involved in the brachial plexus.

The **thoracic** segment, contained within the thoracic vertebrae, has spinal nerves that run inferior to the corresponding vertebra, as is the case for the rest of the spinal cord. The thoracic cord gives off the majority of **efferent sympathetic** fibers, the **white rami,** which innervate the **sympathetic trunk.**

The **lumbar** segment is involved in the lumbosacral plexus and is thus also wider than other parts of the cord.

The **sacral** cord also is involved in the lumbosacral plexus and gives rise to efferent parasympathetic fibers to bowel and bladder, the **sacral nerves.** The caudal end of the sacral cord forms a cone, referred to as the **conus medullaris.** The array of sacral spinal roots that fan out from the conus is the **cauda equina** ("horse's tail").

Finally, the paired **coccygeal nerves** descend from the tip of the conus. A filamentous anchor of pia and arachnoid mater, the **filum terminale,** also extends from the tip of the conus to anchor it to the caudal dura.

The Cord in Cross Section The spinal cord has a characteristic "butterfly" appearance of internal gray matter surrounded by the myelinated tracts of white matter (see Figure 14-1). At the center lies **the ependymal canal,** straddling the midline defined in part by the **dorsal** and **ventral fissures.**

The **ventral horns,** containing the lower motor nuclei of motor tracts (largely the **corticospinal** tracts), give rise to the ventral nerve roots at each spinal level.

The **dorsal horns,** containing sensory neurons of sensory tracts (largely the **spinothalamic** and **dorsal column** tracts), receive incoming axons from sensory peripheral nerves via the dorsal nerve roots.

The **lateral** horn, located only at levels T1–L2, projects efferent white rami to the sympathetic trunk.

Running between the dorsal and ventral horns are the **internuncial** neurons, which serve the crucial bridge in **spinal reflexes.** They link noxious sensations arriving in the dorsal horn to LMN nuclei located in the ventral horn, causing an immediate muscle contraction designed for self-preservation. This can cause withdrawal of the affected extremity before the noxious stimulus is fully recognized by the cortex.

Adjacent Neuroanatomy

The sympathetic trunks   All sympathetic activity is ultimately conducted through the **sympathetic trunks,** the paraspinal chains of sympathetic ganglia. The sympathetic center of command is the hypothalamus, which projects via the hypothalamospinal tract to the **lateral horn** of the spinal cord. The lateral horn is seen on **spinal levels T1–L2,** from which emerge the **white rami,** which innervate the entire sympathetic trunk. All sympathetic nerves then come from the sympathetic trunk, supplying blood vessels of the head and throughout the body, sweat glands, and so on. In addition, the sympathetic trunk gives off **gray rami** (appears more gray because it is not myelinated) at all spinal levels that supply sympathetic innervation to the spinal cord itself.

Diseases of the Spinal Cord and Paraspinal Processes

Cord compression   Various processes may result in compression of the spinal cord, most notably neoplasm, slipped disk, trauma, and epidural abscess. Bilateral weakness and/or sensory loss at or inferior to a given spinal level generally localizes a lesion to the spinal cord.

Because the spinal cord contains both UMNs within the corticospinal tracts and LMNs in the ventral horns, elements of both UMN and LMN lesions may occur with cord compression. Sensory loss may also occur. In addition, parasympathetic fibers that serve the parasympathetic sacral nerves may also be affected (these are usually the last to be affected with gradual compression), resulting in urinary or fecal **incontinence,** loss of **rectal tone,** and/or **impotence.**

As a rule, **cord compression causes UMN signs (hyperreflexia, clonus, spasticity) inferior to the lesion and may cause LMN signs (flaccid weakness, atrophy, and areflexia) at the level of the compression.**

An important exception applies in rapid or immediate compression, in which a condition known as spinal shock occurs. **Spinal shock** refers to the transient complete loss of function of the cord, including loss of spinal reflexes and LMN dysfunction, inferior to the site of an abrupt lesion. The cord regains its intrinsic function over days to weeks, restoring spinal reflexes and allowing UMN signs to return.

Patients who initially present with flaccid weakness and areflexia will develop spasticity and hyperreflexia if the lower motor neurons remain intact.

All cord compression syndromes must be treated by immediately removing or diminishing the size of the compressing mass, whether through surgery, radiation therapy, or chemotherapy/steroids.

Cauda equina syndrome   The cauda equina, consisting solely of sacral spinal nerves (LMNs), will present with **flaccid weakness,** sensory loss, **areflexia,** and possible bowel/bladder symptoms when compressed. Cauda equina syndrome is often seen with neoplasms, although lumbar disk prolapse at the L2–L3 level will put the cauda at risk. One or both sides may be affected, depending on whether the lesion is midline or parasagittal. Sacral motor dysfunction causes a **footdrop** and **loss of intrinsic foot muscles.** The pattern of sacral nerve root anesthesia seen in cauda equina syndrome is referred to as **saddle anesthesia,** because the S1–S5 dermatomes innervate the perianal area and posterior thighs and legs, including the parts of the skin that sit on a saddle. Compression of the pain fibers may also result in intense **pain.** The loss of parasympathetic bladder innervation results in **overflow incontinence** due to detrusor muscle paralysis (parasympathetic) with relative preservation of the sympathetic sphincter, as well as impotence and/or fecal incontinence.

Conus medullaris lesions   Lesions at the conus medullaris may affect UMNs within the cord itself or LMNs within the cauda, depending on their size. The presence of hyperreflexia or spasticity thus helps to distinguish them from cauda equina syndromes. In addition, higher spinal levels, namely the lower lumbar segments, may be involved. Autonomic symptoms may be similar to cauda equina lesions with overflow incontinence, fecal incontinence, and impotence.

Epidural abscess   Epidural abscesses, essentially another form of cord compression, deserve special mention. The symptoms of cord compression may be the same; however, long before neurologic symptoms set in, patients may demonstrate constitutional signs of infection (e.g., fever, elevated WBC count), as well as localizing signs of tenderness, pain, warmth, or erythema of the skin overlying the abscess. As a general rule, these are a consequence of previous instrumentation, such as spinal epidural anesthesia. They are treated with antibiotics and often require surgical drainage.

Case Conclusion This patient was taken to CT scan of the lower spine with IV contrast, which demonstrated an enhancing lesion within the cauda equina, approximately 5 cm. Further imaging with MRI demonstrated apparent involvement of the bilateral S2–S4 nerve roots within the mass. CT-guided lumbar puncture (to avoid injuring nerve roots tethered to the mass) demonstrated cells consistent with lymphoma. The patient was initiated on high-dose steroids, which caused marked improvement of his symptoms within several days, shortly after which antiretroviral therapy was initiated. The lymphoma will be treated with radiation and likely chemotherapy.

Thumbnail: Spinal Cord and Cauda Equina

Spinal Compression Syndromes

Signs	Cauda equina syndrome	Conus medullaris syndrome
UMN: Hyperreflexia Spastic paralysis	None (only LMN involvement)	Present (UMN involved)
LMN: Areflexia Flaccid paralysis	Should be present, unilateral or bilateral	May be present, unilateral or bilateral
Sensory loss	Yes, saddle anesthesia (or hemi)	Yes, saddle anesthesia (or hemi)
Pain	More likely	Less likely unless root involvement
Autonomic loss	Possible	Possible

Key Points

▶ The spinal cord contains motor, sensory, and autonomic fibers in close proximity, so both sides of the body may be affected by a single lesion, unlike the brain or peripheral nerves.

▶ Cauda equina syndrome and conus medullaris syndrome, though similar, should be distinguished by the presence or absence of spinal cord involvement, that is, UMN signs.

▶ Bowel or bladder function loss with saddle anesthesia always localizes a lesion to the spinal cord, and bilateral symptomatology is highly suggestive of it. Cord pathology should always be treated as an emergency.

Questions

1. A 45-year-old man is seen in the ED after trying to lift a heavy box and experiencing sudden severe back pain radiating down the back of both of his legs. On examination, he has loss of pinprick sensation surrounding the anus and down the back of both legs and shows a bilateral footdrop. Ankle jerks are absent. Strength is otherwise intact. What would a full-spine MRI be likely to show?
   A. 5-cm intrathecal mass compressing lumbar spinal cord between L2 and L3 nerve roots
   B. Compression fracture of S2 vertebra without impingement of spinal cord
   C. Severe spinal stenosis with inflammation of sacral nerve roots
   D. Lumbar disk prolapse at L2–L3 vertebral level
   E. Sacral spondylolisthesis at S2–S3 level

2. You are told that a 70-year-old patient has areflexia of the left ankle. Which lesions may explain this finding?
   A. Acute T12 complete cord transection
   B. Cauda equina syndrome
   C. Conus medullaris syndrome
   D. Benign age-related changes
   E. All of the above

3. A 31-year-old woman with known MS develops difficulty with voluntary voiding despite persistent dribbling of urine, as well as occasional fecal incontinence. She is noted to have bilateral hyperreflexic ankle jerks. On examination, a subtle degree of saddle anesthesia can be appreciated, as well as mild bilateral weakness of the foot muscles. What is the most likely cause?
   A. Cauda equina syndrome
   B. Bilateral peripheral neuropathy
   C. Lumbar disk prolapse
   D. Sacral spinal cord demyelinating lesion
   E. Amyotrophic lateral sclerosis

4. A 59-year-old male patient presents with bilateral weakness of the feet and difficulty walking. Examination is notable for mild weakness of intrinsic foot muscles bilaterally and absent ankle jerks bilaterally. He has no sensory deficit and denies bowel or bladder dysfunction; rectal tone is intact. What is a possible diagnosis?
   A. Amyotrophic lateral sclerosis (ALS)
   B. Conus medullaris syndrome
   C. Cauda equina syndrome
   D. Peripheral neuropathy
   E. Subacute combined systems degeneration (vitamin B_{12} deficiency)

> **HPI:** A 36-year-old woman has a healthy infant after a prolonged but otherwise normal spontaneous vaginal delivery. While recovering the following day, she discovers difficulty moving her toes and flexing her knees bilaterally and describes numbness along the back of her legs. She is able to walk with difficulty. She is gravida 2 para 2, without other significant history.
>
> **PE:** T 36.5°C   HR 85   BP 110/65
> She has bilateral weakness of the hamstring muscles and muscles of the foot. She has moderate anesthesia to pinprick on the posterior leg and thigh. Patellar reflexes are intact, but ankle jerks are absent (they were noted to be present before delivery). Quadriceps strength and rectal tone is intact.

Thought Questions

- What is the likely cause of her deficit?
- How did delivery cause this problem, and what other anatomic structures are likely to have played a role?
- What is the prognosis?

Basic Science Review and Discussion

The lumbosacral plexus is the network consisting of the L2–S3 spinal nerve roots, which **supplies sensorimotor function to the pelvis and lower extremities.** This plexus ultimately gives rise to the three major peripheral nerves of the lower extremity: the **sciatic, femoral,** and **obturator nerves,** which are described in more detail in Case 21. The lumbosacral plexus is in many ways analogous to the brachial plexus, although it is larger in scope and yet somewhat more simplified in design. Many of the nerves simply branch off nerve roots and are named for the muscles they innervate, making further description of little utility.

The location of the lumbosacral plexus allows many opportunities for compression against bony structures, with the pelvis offering several spots for characteristic nerve compression syndromes.

The lumbosacral plexus is often conceived of in two parts, the lumbar plexus and the sacral plexus. Each plexus is roughly divided into **anterior** and **posterior divisions.**

The Lumbar Plexus The lumbar plexus includes the L2–L5 nerve roots (other schemata may include L1). The L2–L4 roots are most involved, and each are divided into an anterior and posterior division.

The **obturator nerve** is formed by the anterior L2–L4 divisions, which serve the adductor (medial) compartment of the thigh.

The **femoral nerve** is formed by the posterior L2–L4 divisions, which serves the quadriceps (anterior) compartment of the thigh.

The **lateral femoral cutaneous nerve** is formed by the posterior L2 and L3 divisions, which serve cutaneous sensation of the lateral thigh. Arising from the lumbar region, it must descend inferiorly over the pelvic brim, run around the inside of the pelvis, and emerge from the anterior pelvis under the inguinal ligament. This affords numerous opportunities for compression, making compression neuropathy of the lateral femoral cutaneous nerve a relatively common problem.

The **lumbosacral trunk** is formed by a branch of L4 and the entirety of the L5 nerve root (L5's only contribution). It will form part of the sciatic nerve.

The Sacral Plexus The sacral plexus includes nerve roots from S1–S3, as well as the lumbosacral trunk, ultimately giving rise to the **sciatic nerve** (L4–S3 nerve roots). Each root, including the lumbosacral trunk, is divided into **anterior and posterior divisions.**

The **anterior** divisions form the **tibial** component of the sciatic nerve (L4–S3).

The **posterior** divisions of L4–S2 (S3 does not contribute) form the **common peroneal** component of the sciatic nerve. As the nerve roots combine within the pelvis to form the sciatic nerve, they give off numerous other branches which supply the gluteal, piriformis, gemellus, and quadratus femoris muscles, which are named for the muscles they supply.

The sciatic nerve passes through the greater sciatic foramen of the pelvis, then immediately next to the ischium (which may also lead to compressive injury), and into the lower extremity.

The S2 and S3 nerve roots also send branches to the pudendal (or coccygeal) plexus, which serves the lower pelvis and pudendum.

The S1–S4 nerve roots also give off parasympathetic branches, which form the pelvic splanchnic nerves and pelvic plexus, which governs pelvic parasympathetic function (bowel and bladder).

Lumbosacral Plexopathies and Associated Neuropathies

Upper lumbosacral plexus lesion   An upper lumbosacral plexus lesion generally involves the anterior and proximal aspects of the lower extremity, as the L4 and L5 nerve roots supply this general distribution. It may result in weakness of hip flexion and adduction and loss of sensation of the anterior lower extremity, as well as loss of patellar reflexes. It is difficult to distinguish from a femoral nerve palsy; the hip adductor weakness is generally seen only in a plexus lesion. Causative factors include abdominal masses or tumor leading to compression/infiltration, labor during birth, and abdominal surgery. Treatment involves decompression, often surgical, of any compressing mass or delivery of a pregnancy. Prognosis is generally suggested by improvement within 48 hours after decompression; patients with no improvement after 48 hours often do poorly and are likely to have permanent deficits, or will require months to years to recover.

Lower lumbosacral plexus lesion   Lower lumbosacral plexus lesions affect the distal and posterior lower extremity, which are innervated by the sacral nerves (S1–S3). Loss of ankle jerks and hamstring weakness, as well as foot weakness, will be seen. Anesthesia of the posterior and distal lateral lower extremity are also seen. This cannot be readily distinguished from sciatic nerve injury. Involvement of the sciatic nerve often results in sciatic pain at the site of entrapment of injury, whereas plexus lesions are more likely to be painless. Causative factors are similar to those for upper lumbosacral plexus lesions.

Lateral femoral cutaneous nerve entrapment (meralgia)
The lateral femoral cutaneous nerve's long arc around the bony pelvis and eventual emergence under the lateral aspect of the inguinal ligament render it vulnerable to compression. Patients may describe essentially congenital loss of thigh sensation since birth, or often it will come on with weight gain as the increased intra-abdominal fatty tissue exerts more pressure on this nerve. Lateral femoral cutaneous nerve dysfunction due to compression is fairly common and often improves when patients lose weight. The lateral femoral cutaneous nerve has no motor function, so meralgia is generally more of an annoyance than a functional disability.

Lumbosacral neuritis   Analogous to the brachial plexus and brachial neuritis, the nerve fibers of the lumbosacral plexus may become inflamed due a variety of factors, including infection (usually viral) or other illness. The result is diffuse, nonspecific pain and/or weakness of the lower extremities (unilateral or bilateral) that does not fit any particular nerve distribution. Treatment is again supportive, and the patients usually recover, although they are at increased risk of recurrence. Diabetes may also cause peripheral nerve or lumbosacral plexus dysfunction as a variant of ischemic neuropathy, which is less likely to recover.

Case Conclusion   Based on the pattern of posterior leg anesthesia and weakness in the setting of recent vaginal delivery, a lower lumbosacral plexus lesion was considered a likely diagnosis. The patient was able to perform physical therapy exercises and steadily made improvements in her walking, in addition to noting slow recovery of sensation in her posterior legs. Cesarean section can be offered for future pregnancies to avoid this complication, although it should be noted that lumbosacral plexus injury may occur in the setting of C-section surgery as well.

Thumbnail: Lumbosacral Plexus

Syndromes of Lumbosacral Plexus and Associated Nerves

Syndrome	Structure	Symptoms	Nerve roots
Upper plexus lesion	Upper plexus nerve roots	Weakened hip flexion, knee extension, anterior lower extremity anesthesia	L2–L5
Lower plexus lesion	Lower plexus nerve roots	Weaned knee flexion, hamstrings, foot muscles, posterior lower extremity anesthesia	S1–S3
Lateral femoral cutaneous nerve entrapment	Lateral femoral cutaneous nerve	Lateral hip anesthesia, no weakness	L2–L3
Lumbosacral neuritis	Lumbosacral plexus	Diffuse, nonspecific unilateral or bilateral lower extremity weakness and/or paresthesias	L2–S3

Key Points

▸ The lumbosacral plexus supplies essentially all of the motor and sensory function of the hips and lower extremities.

▸ The location of the lumbosacral plexus makes it vulnerable to compression against the bony pelvis, which may cause upper or lower plexopathy, as well as lateral femoral cutaneous nerve injury.

Questions

1. A 56-year-old woman is hospitalized for a spontaneous retroperitoneal hemorrhage while taking warfarin sodium (Coumadin). She is noted to develop weakness of right thigh flexion and knee extension, and anesthesia of the anterior right thigh, as well as the anterior leg. Right thigh adduction is also affected. What is the most likely cause?

   A. Right femoral nerve palsy secondary to compression
   B. Lumbosacral neuritis secondary to warfarin use
   C. Right lateral femoral cutaneous nerve compression
   D. Right upper lumbosacral plexopathy secondary to compression
   E. Cauda equina syndrome

2. An obese 35-year-old man visits the neurology clinic for annoying lack of sensation of the thigh. He has noticed intermittent "pins and needles" on the side of his thigh, on either side, for many years, but it has worsened over the past few years. His examination is notable for diminished sensation to light touch over both lateral thighs without loss of motor function. What is his diagnosis and prognosis?

   A. Upper lumbosacral plexopathy, unlikely to recover
   B. Lateral femoral cutaneous neuropathy, likely to resolve spontaneously
   C. Femoral nerve compression, unlikely to recover
   D. Lateral femoral cutaneous neuropathy, may improve with weight loss
   E. Lumbosacral neuritis, likely to resolve spontaneously

3. A 70-year-old woman with a pelvic mass for which she has declined further intervention begins to develop weakness of right knee flexion and ankle flexion. She notes some numbness along the back of her leg and around the foot. The problem started about 2 weeks ago and appears to be slowly progressing. What is a possible cause?

   A. Right upper lumbosacral plexopathy
   B. Right lower lumbosacral plexopathy
   C. Right lateral femoral cutaneous neuropathy
   D. Right femoral nerve compression
   E. Right obturator nerve compression

4. A surgeon removes a pelvic tumor found underneath the left inguinal ligament in an elderly man. After the operation, the patient complains of numbness in the left lateral upper thigh. He has no recognizable weakness on neurologic examination. What is a possible explanation?

   A. Femoral nerve transection secondary to surgery
   B. Upper lumbosacral plexopathy secondary to surgery
   C. Lateral femoral cutaneous nerve transection secondary to surgery
   D. Persistent side effect of general anesthesia
   E. Obturator nerve transection secondary to surgery

HPI: A 55-year-old male runner is seen at the doctor's office for worsening right leg pain brought on with running. He describes the pain as "shooting" down the back of his leg, running sometimes all the way down to his toes and the bottom of his foot. There is no history of trauma. He noted small fleeting episodes of this pain while running over the past couple of weeks, which have gradually worsened. He currently is not experiencing the pain, although it does intermittently occur when he walks as well. Previous medical history is unremarkable.

PE: T 37.1°C   HR 52   BP 130/75
He appears to have full strength of the hamstring muscles. He does have minimally decreased sensation on the lateral aspect of the right leg. When the right leg is passively raised to an angle of 30 degrees while he is lying on the table (straight leg raise test), he reexperiences the shooting pain.

Thought Questions

- Which nerve is most likely to be affected?

- What about the history and physical is suggestive that this nerve is involved?

- What anatomic structures is most likely to cause the problem?

- What is the prognosis?

Basic Science Review and Discussion

Much as was the case in the upper extremity, the nerves of the lower extremity are derived from a plexus of spinal nerves. The **lumbosacral plexus** is composed of spinal nerve segments L2–S3 and is discussed in greater detail in its own section. It gives rise to the three major peripheral nerves of the lower extremity: the femoral nerve, the obturator nerve, and the sciatic nerve, which are discussed in this case. The sciatic nerve, by far the largest of the three, divides into the tibial and common peroneal nerves.

The Femoral Nerve

Function   The femoral nerve is an upper lumbosacral plexus nerve, generated by the L2–L4 nerve roots. It runs along the iliopsoas muscle, exits the pelvis via the **femoral canal** (with the femoral artery and femoral vein) and then runs along the femur as it innervates the **quadriceps muscles.** The quadriceps muscles include the four major muscles of the anterior thigh: the vastus medialis, vastus intermedius, vastus lateralis, and the rectus femoris. The quadriceps extends the knee. The femoral nerve also flexes the hip via the sartorius and iliopsoas muscles. It provides sensation for the anterior thigh, proximal medial thigh, and medial leg (via the **saphenous nerve,** a pure sensory branch).

Dysfunction   The femoral nerve is most often affected by changes in the iliopsoas, pelvis, or femur, such as an ilio-

psoas abscess or hematoma, hip dislocation or surgery, or femoral fractures. This often presents with quadriceps weakness and possibly atrophy, as well as weakness of thigh flexion. Sensation of the anteromedial thigh and medial leg may be affected. The knee jerk or **patellar reflex** will be lost in the presence of significant quadriceps weakness.

The Obturator Nerve

Function   The obturator nerve is also an upper lumbosacral plexus nerve originating from the L2–L4 nerve roots. It runs through the **obturator canal** or **obturator foramen** of the pelvis and along the medial thigh to innervate the major **adductor muscles,** namely the adductor magnus, adductor longus, and gracilis muscles. It also serves to externally rotate the thigh via the obturator externus muscle (and the superior gemellus muscle). It provides sensation of the distal medial thigh (the proximal inner thigh being innervated by the femoral nerve).

Dysfunction   The obturator nerve is most vulnerable to compression against the bony pelvis within the obturator foramen, which occurs most commonly in women during labor. It may also be affected by pelvic fractures and many of the same factors that can damage the femoral nerve. Obturator nerve palsy predictably results in adductor weakness and weakness of external rotation of the thigh. Patients may note an inability to cross the affected leg onto the other and/or anesthesia of the distal inner thigh. The **adductor reflex** (jerk of adductor muscles when their tendons are struck proximal to the medial epicondyle of the femur) may be lost.

The Sciatic Nerve

Function   The sciatic nerve is the largest and the most significant nerve of the lower extremity. It is involved in the most common neuropathies of the lower limb: foot-drop and sciatica. It is derived from the lower lumbosacral plexus, L4–S3, and emerges from the posterior pelvis via the greater sciatic foramen. It is joined in this foramen by the posterior femoral cutaneous nerve, a pure sensory branch of the sciatic nerve, which serves the buttocks and posterior thigh. As the sciatic nerve runs within the pelvis, it abuts the **ischial tuberosity,** which may compress the nerve and result in **sciatica.** The sciatic nerve then runs down the posterior compartment of the thigh and innervates the **hamstring muscles,** which include the semimembranosus, semitendinosus, biceps femoris, and adductor magnus (also innervated in part by the obturator nerve). The hamstring muscles extend the hip joint and flex the knee joint. Within the popliteal fossa, the sciatic nerve divides into two major branches: the tibial nerve and common peroneal nerve.

Dysfunction: sciatica and other causes The sciatic nerve is most vulnerable to compression at the sciatic notch of the pelvis, immediately adjacent to the ischial tuberosity. Its close proximity to the ischium may result in friction and irritation with repetitive hip joint flexion/extension, which may be seen in athletes (especially runners) but may present in any patient spontaneously. This irritation of the sciatic nerve is known as **sciatica.** It usually presents with "shooting pain" along the posterior leg as far as the sole and even the plantar toes, following the cutaneous innervation of the sciatic nerve. Weakness resulting from sciatica is uncommon. It is usually treated by conservative management, including rest and anti-inflammatory medications.

Localized trauma in the area of the ischium may also result in sciatic nerve damage. For this reason, it is essential to administer intramuscular gluteal injections in the upper outer quadrant of the gluteal muscles. Injections placed in the medial inferior gluteal quadrant place the sciatic nerve at risk and have been known to produce permanent sciatic nerve injury.

However, it is worth noting that L5 or S1 radiculopathy (often from a herniated disk) may also present with pain similar to that seen in sciatica. It may be very difficult to clinically distinguish L5 or S1 radiculopathy from sciatic nerve entrapment. Radiculopathy, however, is more likely to result in demonstrable weakness. Both radiculopathy and sciatica may produce a **positive straight leg raise test,** which is pain in the sciatic nerve distribution when passively raising the patient's leg into the air. This maneuver places tension on the affected nerve roots and sciatic nerve, exacerbating the pain.

The Tibial Nerve

Function The tibial nerve is served by all of the nerve roots within the sciatic nerve, L2–S3. The tibial nerve (also referred to as the **posterior tibial nerve**) runs posterior to the tibia as it innervates the plantar flexor muscles of the leg. It then runs posterior and inferior to the medial malleolus, splitting into the **medial and lateral plantar nerves** on the sole of the

foot. It provides for **plantar flexion** via the muscles of the posterior leg (gastrocnemius, soleus, plantaris, and tibialis posterior muscles) and toe flexion (flexor digitorum longus and flexor hallucis longus). The medial and lateral plantar nerves innervate the intrinsic foot muscles.

Sensation of the sole of the foot is also provided by the medial plantar nerve (medial sole) and lateral plantar nerve (lateral sole of the foot). The tibial nerve otherwise has no cutaneous sensation.

Dysfunction The tibial nerve is most vulnerable to popliteal fossa trauma and tibial fractures, resulting in inability to plantar flex and intrinsic foot muscle weakness. Sensation on the sole of the foot may be lost. The ankle jerk (reflexive plantar flexion upon jerking the Achilles tendon) may be diminished or absent. **Tarsal tunnel syndrome** refers to entrapment of the tibial nerve against the medial malleolus of the tibia. It is compressed as it runs in the tarsal tunnel deep to the flexor retinaculum of the ankle, very much analogous to carpal tunnel syndrome of the median nerve. Tarsal tunnel syndrome results in a burning sensation of the sole of the foot and may also cause weakness of the intrinsic foot muscles. Surgery may be required to relieve the nerve compression.

The Common Peroneal Nerve

Function The common peroneal nerve is the other major branch of the sciatic nerve, diverging laterally from the tibial nerve to run over the head of the fibula. This overlap allows for a common nerve compression palsy to arise in various circumstances, namely **peroneal nerve palsy or foot-drop.** The peroneal nerve remains in the lateral compartment of the leg where it innervates the peroneal muscles, which control eversion, as well as the tibialis anterior, the major muscle involved in **dorsiflexion of the foot.**

Sensation of the anterolateral leg and foot is likewise controlled by the common peroneal nerve.

Dysfunction **Foot-drop** is the common name given to peroneal nerve palsy, as the inability to dorsiflex makes the foot "drop" or hang limp with each step, which makes the patient likely to trip. Patients with a foot-drop develop a circumducting gait to avoid tripping on the dragging foot. It may be caused by trauma to the fibular head or compression injury from lying on one side (during anesthesia or during critical illness). It may also arise spontaneously with predisposing factors such as poor nutrition, alcohol abuse, rapid weight loss, and so on. Patients usually recover some function over a period of weeks, although complete palsies are at greatest risk for permanent foot-drop. There is no treatment. Patients may wear a boot or brace that holds the foot perpendicular to the ankle to minimize dragging while walking.

Case Conclusion   The runner is advised that he has likely developed a case of sciatica. He admits that he had increased his mileage last week, which may have precipitated the episode. He is advised to abstain from running for several days and then gently resume as his symptoms permit. After taking a week off, he notes improvement in his symptoms. He is counseled that the sciatica may recur and that he should decrease his running if the symptoms recur or worsen.

Thumbnail: Nerves of Lower Extremity

Peripheral nerve	Motor function	Sensation	Dysfunction syndromes
Obturator nerve	Thigh adduction	Distal inner thigh	Inability to cross legs
Femoral nerve	Quadriceps	Anteromedial thigh; medial leg	Inability to extend knee
Sciatic nerve	Hamstrings, all leg muscles	Posterior thigh and lateral leg, foot	Sciatica
Common peroneal nerve	Dorsiflexion, eversion of foot	Lateral leg	Foot-drop (peroneal nerve palsy)
Tibial nerve	Plantar flexion, intrinsic foot muscles	Posterior leg, sole	Tarsal tunnel syndrome

Key Points

▸ The lower extremity is innervated by three major peripheral nerves: the obturator, the femoral, and the sciatic nerves. The sciatic nerve divides into the tibial and common peroneal nerves.

▸ The most common neuropathies of the lower extremity include foot-drop, sciatica, and tarsal tunnel syndrome. These may present spontaneously and are usually managed conservatively.

▸ Sciatica is difficult to differentiate from L5 or S1 radiculopathy, although cases with significant weakness are usually due to radiculopathy.

Questions

1. After what appears to be an uneventful spontaneous vaginal delivery with epidural anesthesia of a healthy female infant, a previously healthy 35-year-old woman is surprised to discover that she has difficulty crossing her right leg onto her left, and she cannot dorsiflex her right foot. Her epidural anesthesia has by now worn off. What nerve(s) is (are) most likely to be involved?

   A. Right sciatica
   B. Right femoral nerve injury
   C. Right common peroneal nerve injury
   D. Right sciatica and femoral nerve injury
   E. Right obturator and common peroneal nerve injury

2. A 70-year-old male patient presents with pain running along the back of his left lower extremity to the ankle. The left ankle jerk is diminished. Straight leg raise reproduces the pain on the left leg. He has weakness of plantar flexion. He notes that the pain started after lifting heavy boxes around the house. What is the most likely cause?

   A. Left sciatica
   B. Left S1 radiculopathy
   C. Left common peroneal nerve palsy
   D. Left tarsal tunnel syndrome
   E. Left femoral nerve palsy

3. After being struck on the head of the right fibula by a riot policeman's club, a now somber demonstrator discovers that he cannot run because his right foot is dragging. He is able to limp away and eventually pursue medical attention, where no fracture is seen on x-ray film. Over the next few hours, he regains the ability to walk normally. What is the most likely explanation?

   A. Transient tarsal tunnel syndrome due to tibial nerve injury
   B. Acute sciatica secondary to trauma
   C. Hairline fibular head fracture not seen on x-ray film
   D. Femoral nerve palsy secondary to trauma
   E. Common peroneal nerve palsy secondary to trauma

4. A 46-year-old woman on anticoagulation develops spontaneous abdominal pain. Abdominal CT scan shows a large retroperitoneal hematoma adjacent to the left iliopsoas muscle. She begins to complain of left thigh numbness. On examination, she has new profound weakness of the hip flexors and quadriceps muscles on the left. What has most likely happened?

   A. Left femoral nerve compression secondary to hematoma
   B. Left sciatic nerve compression secondary to hematoma
   C. Left obturator nerve compression secondary to hematoma
   D. Left L2 radiculopathy secondary to hematoma
   E. Left S2 radiculopathy secondary to hematoma

Case 14

1. D
2. C
3. B
4. A

Case 15

1. C
2. E
3. E
4. D

Case 16

1. B
2. E
3. B
4. E

Case 17

1. E
2. B
3. C
4. D

Case 18

1. B
2. C
3. C
4. A

Case 19

1. D
2. E
3. D
4. A

Case 20

1. D
2. D
3. B
4. C

Case 21

1. E
2. B
3. E
4. A

Part III

Special Senses, Cranial Nerves, and Brainstem

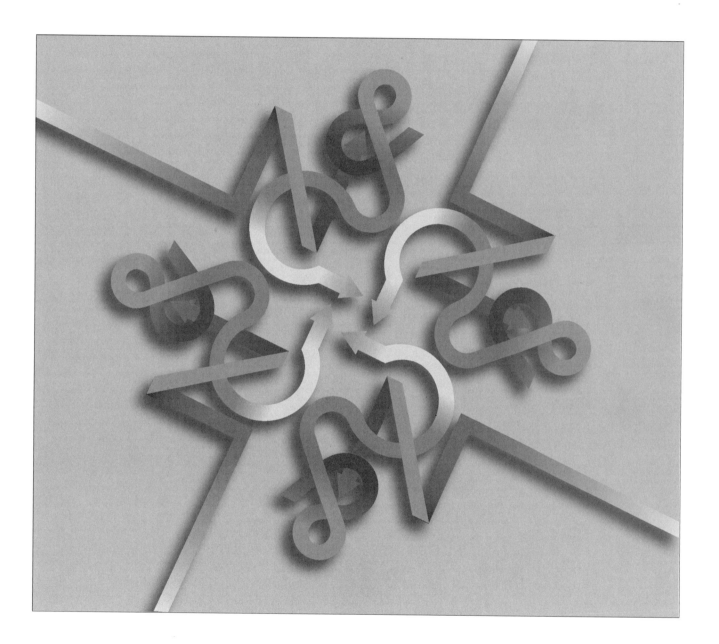

HPI: JK is a 74-year-old woman who is brought to your office by her family. They complain that she no longer seems to be acting like herself. Over the past several months, she has lost interest in her usual activities. She seems more withdrawn. Her appetite has deteriorated to the point where it is difficult to get her to eat enough. She had commented to her family in the remote past that food no longer seemed to have much smell or flavor. This was attributed to aging. She has been otherwise healthy.

PE: You note that she seems very withdrawn. Some frontal release signs are present. You decide to test her sense of smell and find that she is bilaterally anosmic. Her cranial nerves (CNs) are otherwise intact. Power, sensation, and coordination are all intact. Her reflexes are somewhat brisk, but symmetric. There are no long-tract signs.

Thought Questions

- Which brain region is implicated by the behavioral changes?

- What other functions are mediated by this area?

- What is the implication of the apparent loss of taste/olfaction?

- At what point along the taste and olfaction pathways are behavioral brain regions in proximity?

Basic Science Review and Discussion

Loss of smell (**anosmia**) and altered olfaction can present either unilaterally or bilaterally. The causes can be broadly divided into obstructive nasal or paranasal causes and central causes. Central causes may be related to neuronal dysfunction in the olfactory bulb, tract, pathways, or higher centers. **Infections of the respiratory tract** and paranasal sinuses are the most common causes of impaired olfaction. Various toxic substances, including **cigarette smoke,** and many medications also can impair olfactory function. Altered olfaction also can be seen in the context of head trauma, degenerative diseases, demyelinating disease, and in the setting of a variety of general medical and psychiatric disorders. Reduced sensitivity to odorants and impaired discrimination between odorants also can be seen as part of the aging process. However, loss of smell should always prompt an evaluation for potentially reversible or dangerous causes.

A number of tumors have been associated with olfactory loss (anosmia). Perhaps the most important to think about and recognize is **meningioma in the olfactory groove.** As we have seen in the present case, anosmia may be the only early clinical manifestation of these tumors. The deficit is often bilateral. If not detected early, these tumors can ultimately lead to frontal lobe damage, seizures, and visual impairment. This case focuses on a review of the compo-

nents of the olfactory system, collectively known as the **rhinencephalon.**

Organization of Olfaction

Olfactory receptors The **nasal mucosa** has two main systems for detecting diffusible chemical stimuli. **Free nerve endings** from the **trigeminal nerve** mediate the unpleasant experience associated with excessively high concentrations of odorants or excessively strong stimuli like ammonia. The remaining **olfactory receptors** are contained in the membranes of cilia extending into the olfactory mucous from the primary olfactory neurons of the **olfactory epithelium.** Airborne aromatic molecules become dissolved in the mucus overlying the olfactory epithelium. They diffuse through this mucus to interact with the **olfactory receptors** contained within the cilia of primary olfactory neurons. These are **bipolar neurons,** the central processes of which make up the true **olfactory nerve.**

The physiologic basis of olfaction remains relatively poorly understood, as compared to other sensory modalities. It is believed that several classes of olfactory receptor proteins exist. These proteins may preferentially bind specific aromatic molecules. These interactions are also concentration dependent, such that higher concentrations of a given odorant will elicit proportionally higher frequency responses from a given primary olfactory neuron. Different receptor cells are thought to express these proteins in varying proportions across the surface of the olfactory epithelium. The expression of receptor proteins can also vary over time. This is because the **primary olfactory neurons have a relatively short life span,** being replaced about once a month. These features give the olfactory epithelium the ability to respond selectively to a broad range of aromatic stimuli. This mechanism is analogous to the visual system, where a relatively small number of different retinal cones can mediate the detection of a nearly infinite number of colors. Information about odorants that bind to the receptors of primary olfactory neurons is transduced into electrical impulses, which are propagated centrally.

Olfactory neurons   The olfactory tract courses centrally from the **olfactory bulb,** along the inferior surface of the frontal lobe. This external structure looked like a nerve to early anatomists. We now know that these structures, like the optic nerves, are tracts rather than nerves (note that the first two CNs are not really nerves). The **olfactory nerves** are the short central processes of the primary olfactory neurons in the olfactory epithelium. These relatively short fibers exit the olfactory epithelium, pass through openings in the **cribriform plate,** and terminate on secondary olfactory neurons in the olfactory bulbs. Loss of smell can result from head **trauma** leading to injury of these nerve fibers as they pass through the cribriform plate.

The axons of the primary olfactory neurons terminate in the **glomeruli** of the olfactory bulb, where they contact the dendrites of **mitral cells, tufted cells,** and **periglomerular cells**. The latter function as local interneurons. The centrally projecting axons of mitral cells and tufted cells make up much of the **olfactory tract.** The remaining fibers in the olfactory tract originate on the contralateral side and provide feedback to the olfactory bulb. These **fibers synapse on granule cells** in the olfactory bulb. The axons of the granule cells then synapse onto their ipsilateral mitral cells and tufted cells. The granule cells also receive reciprocal input from these cells. Thus, the granule cells coordinate bilateral olfactory information.

Afferent axons from mitral cells and tufted cell axons project centrally through the olfactory tract. They have three main targets. The first target is **the anterior olfactory nucleus,** which is located at the boundary between the olfactory bulb and olfactory tract. Axons originating in this nucleus then continue centrally. The second target is located at the caudal end of the olfactory tract. This area includes the **olfactory trigone** and the **lateral olfactory nucleus.** Axons originating in these areas also continue centrally. The olfactory tract divides into two fiber bundles at the olfactory trigone (named for three fiber bundles, one

coming in and two going out). The **lateral olfactory stria** projects to the **primary olfactory cortex** via the **olfactory tubercle.** This is the third target of the fibers that originate in the olfactory bulb. The **medial olfactory stria** contains axons of neurons in the olfactory trigone. They cross the midline through the **anterior commissure** and project to granule cells in the contralateral olfactory bulb.

Primary olfactory cortex   The primary olfactory cortex is located in the **piriform cortex,** along the surface of the **medial temporal lobe.** This is illustrated in Figure 6-1. On gross brain specimens, this area corresponds to the **uncus.** The **amygdala** is located beneath this cortical region. Adjacent cortical regions include the **periamygdaloid cortex** and the **entorhinal cortex** (Brodmann's area 28). Associative olfactory processing takes place in these areas. Olfactory information from these areas projects to a wide variety of other brain regions including the limbic, thalamic, and brainstem targets. It is important to note that olfaction is the only sensory modality to reach its primary cortex without first passing through the thalamus, although this information does reach the thalamus eventually.

Clinical Correlation   This case has focused on anosmia resulting from olfactory groove meningioma. However, another important clinical entity to recognize is an olfactory hallucination occurring as an aura preceding seizures. These are generally unpleasant experiences. The smell of burning rubber is one commonly reported olfactory aura. **Uncinate seizures** are a manifestation of temporal lobe epilepsy in which olfactory auras are often reported. These seizures extend to involve the entorhinal, periamygdaloid, and piriform cortex of the uncus. This observation emphasizes that the clinical manifestation of seizure disorders tends to be related to the function of the cortical regions being affected by the electrical disturbance. Although seizures can manifest from all cortical areas, **temporal lobe epilepsy** is a particularly important syndrome with some unique features. Some of the most commonly encountered clinical manifestations of seizures are summarized later in this case (Thumbnail: Olfaction and Olfactory Nerve).

Case Conclusion   You order an MRI of the brain with contrast, which reveals a mass along the basal forebrain. This is consistent with the diagnosis of an olfactory groove meningioma. Meningiomas are relatively common intracranial neoplasms. They are usually slow-growing tumors that are most commonly encountered in the elderly. Their clinical manifestations depend on their local effect on cerebral function. In this case, involvement of the olfactory groove first compromised olfaction. Higher order frontal and prefrontal functions were affected later. She was referred for neurosurgical evaluation. Her lesion was removed. Unfortunately, her cognitive function remained impaired and she was no longer able to function independently. Had her anosmia prompted an earlier medical evaluation, JK's cognitive impairment might have been avoided.

Thumbnail : Olfaction and Olfactory Nerve

Clinical and Anatomic Seizure Correlations

Lobe	Region	Clinical features
Temporal lobe	Medial	Uncinate seizures Fear Unpleasant odor Déjà-vu Nausea or rising stomach Autonomic changes Unresponsive staring Orofacial automatisms Extremity automatisms
	Lateral	Auditory changes Aphasias Vertigo
Frontal lobe	Dorsolateral	Contralateral tonic postures Contralateral clonic activity Gaze, head, or eye deviation Fencing posture Speech arrest Expressive aphasia
	Orbitofrontal	Motor automatisms Incontinence
Parietal		Contralateral sensory changes Contralateral hemineglect Head or gaze deviation Receptive aphasia
Occipital		Flashes of light Changes in color vision Visual field deficits

Key Points

▶ Respiratory tract and sinus infections are the most common causes of anosmia.

▶ Anosmia may be the only early symptom of olfactory groove meningiomas.

▶ Free nerve endings of the trigeminal nerve mediate noxious olfactory experiences.

▶ The lateral olfactory stria projects to the primary olfactory cortex.

▶ The medial olfactory stria projects to the contralateral olfactory bulb.

▶ The primary olfactory cortex is in the piriform cortex of the medial temporal lobe.

▶ Olfaction is the only sensory modality to reach the cortex without passing through the thalamus.

Questions

1. A 36-year-old woman has had a syncopal event that is suspected to be a vasovagal reaction. An attempt is made to revive her by having her inhale ammonia vapors. Which CN mediates her reaction to this stimulus?
   A. Olfactory nerve
   B. Trigeminal nerve
   C. Facial nerve
   D. Glossopharyngeal nerve
   E. Vagus nerve

2. You evaluate a patient who has lost his sense of smell after a motor vehicle accident during which he sustained a significant head injury. Which structure is most likely responsible for his problem?
   A. Olfactory nerve
   B. Olfactory bulb
   C. Olfactory tract
   D. Olfactory stria
   E. Olfactory cortex

3. What is the anticipated life span of the average primary olfactory neuron?
   A. About 1 day
   B. About 1 week
   C. About 1 month
   D. About 6 months
   E. About 1 year

4. You evaluate a patient with epilepsy. She has very frequent episodes of déjà-vu. Her seizures are preceded by a strange smell and a rising sensation in the stomach. This is followed by a few minutes of unresponsive staring. This sometimes evolves into generalized convulsions. Which of the following is the most likely focus of her seizures?
   A. Parietal lobe
   B. Frontal lobe
   C. Occipital lobe
   D. Temporal lobe
   E. Multimodal associative cortex

> **HPI:** AF, a 23-year-old right-handed woman, presents to the ED with sudden onset of vision disturbance. She reports that the previous day she noticed some pain in the right eye, especially when looking around. This morning she awoke and realized she was unable to see on the right. She has never experienced anything like this before. She is otherwise in good health, does not take any daily medications, and reports no significant illnesses in first-degree relatives.
>
> **PE:** Her examination is remarkable for complete vision loss in her right eye with an absent pupillary response. She is noted to have a Marcus Gunn pupil on the right. She denies eye pain at this time. Her extraocular movements are full. Her visual field is intact in the left eye. CNs, fundi, power, sensation, coordination, and reflexes are otherwise intact.

Thought Questions

- How is what we see represented in the brain?
- Where is this patient's lesion?
- What other structures could be involved?
- What is the most likely diagnosis?
- What is the most potentially dangerous diagnosis?

Basic Science Review and Discussion

Acute **optic neuritis** can occur in isolation or can be a harbinger of future demyelinating disease. It is the most likely diagnosis in light of the examination and available data. Patients commonly present with monocular vision loss sometimes preceded by pain with movement of the eye. An afferent pupillary defect (**Marcus Gunn pupil**) can be found in the affected eye. The light input cannot be transmitted across the lesion, so the pupil of the affected eye does not constrict in response to light. However, it does constrict when light is presented to the intact eye because pupillary constriction is consensual (via bilateral third CN innervation). When the examiner swings a flashlight back and forth between the eyes, the pupil of the affected eye appears to dilate "paradoxically" in response to light. This is not active dilation but passive relaxation because the light is moving away from the intact eye.

Visual Fields The "visual field" is an image of everything the patient sees with the eyes at rest in the central position and is the sum of the visual fields of both eyes. Each eye has its own visual field and the two fields are mostly overlapped (spatial separation of the eyes and obstruction by the nose are the reasons for this incomplete overlap). Each visual field is projected onto its corresponding **retina** by light passing through the **cornea** and **lens**. In this process, the image is reversed and turned upside down. It is important to remember that the upper right portion of a visual field projects (upside down and backward) to the lower left portion of the corresponding retina. So, an object in the upper right quadrant of the "visual field" is "seen" by the lower left quadrant of each retina (the medial or nasal portion of the right retina and the lateral or temporal portion of the left retina). This relationship is maintained throughout the retina and the optic nerve.

Neuroanatomy of Visual System

Retina Visual processing begins in the retina, predominantly in the central portion, called the **macula.** The most sensitive part of the macula, the **fovea,** has the highest concentration of **cone photoreceptors.** They are responsible for **high-acuity central vision** and **color. Rod photoreceptors** are more prominent in the peripheral retina and mediate **low-acuity vision.** Energy from light is transduced to electrochemical energy by the photoreceptors, which are contained within the outer nuclear layer on the retina. Photoreceptors synapse onto **bipolar neurons** contained within the inner nuclear layer of the retina. These cells, in turn, synapse onto **ganglion cells** in the ganglion cell layer. Axons of the ganglion cells join to form the **optic nerve.** Numerous photoreceptors may converge on a single ganglion cell. The **receptive field** of a ganglion cell refers to the collective information from all the photoreceptors converging on that cell. However, there is minimal convergence within the fovea. This allows for higher acuity vision in this region.

Optic chiasm The medial half of each optic nerve (coming from the medial half of each retina and carrying information from the lateral half of each visual field) crosses the midline at the **optic chiasm** to become part of the contralateral **optic tract.** The lateral half of each optic nerve continues on as part of the ipsilateral optic tract. This means that information from each half of the visual field (the sum of what both eyes see on one side) is carried by the contralateral optic tract (upside down and backward). This relationship is maintained throughout the remainder of the visual system, all the way to the level of the primary visual cortex.

Lesions that compress the optic chiasm cause loss of peripheral vision in the lateral half of the visual field of each eye (a bitemporal visual field deficit). Pituitary tumors can cause this visual deficit. This can also be seen in pregnancy, when the pituitary gland can become significantly enlarged.

Thalamus The optic tract ends in the **LGN** of the thalamus, where further processing of visual information occurs. The LGN has six layers. Axons from the ipsilateral retina project to layers 2, 3, and 5. Axons from the contralateral retina project to layers 1, 4, and 6. Layers 1 and 2 **(magnocellular layers)** respond to low contrast and are involved in the detection of motion. The remaining layers **(parvocellular layers)** respond to high contrast and color.

Optic radiations From the LGN, the visual system projects to the **primary visual (calcarine) cortex** via the **optic radiations.** Information from the lower portion of the visual field is carried within the upper portion of the corresponding optic tract and along the **geniculocalcarine fibers** of the optic radiations. These fibers project straight back from the

LGN to the superior portion of the visual cortex (the area above the calcarine sulcus). Information from the upper portion of the visual field is carried within the lower portion of the corresponding optic tract. Within the optic radiations, the fibers carrying this information follow a less direct route, looping somewhat anteriorly and superiorly through the temporal lobe **(Meyer's loop)**, before ending in the inferior portion of the visual cortex (the area below the calcarine sulcus). The organization of the visual cortex is discussed in Case 5. Figure 23-1 summarizes the visual pathways leading to the occipital cortex.

Visual Field Deficits A loss of vision in one half of the "visual field" **(homonymous hemianopia)** can be localized to a contralateral lesion involving the optic tract, LGN, or visual cortex. Clinicians refer to these deficits as "field cuts." As a general rule, cortical homonymous hemianopias tend to be more congruous (the shape of the visual defect is the same in both eyes) than lesions involving the optic tracts. Lesions in the optic radiations would not be expected to cause complete hemianopias because these fibers are spread too far apart anatomically. It is important to note that temporal lobe lesions can involve Meyer's loop and thus, lead to a loss of vision in the contralateral upper and outer quadrant of the visual field **(homonymous quadrantanopia)**. Such "pie in the sky" lesions tend to spare central vision. These deficits are reviewed in Figure 23-1 and in Thumbnail: Vision and Optic Nerve, later in this case.

Vision Loss Sudden vision loss is a particularly disturbing symptom for patients and can be localized to lesions anywhere from the eye (globe) to the visual cortex. Ocular causes include corneal disease, refractive error, cataracts, and glaucoma. These often manifest as blurring, but vision loss can also be seen. Double vision is most commonly associated with disturbance of extraocular movement. Lesions affecting the retina or visual pathways generally are associated with visual field defects, called **scotomas.** Diseases affecting the retina, especially the macula, often present with a **positive scotoma** (a dark spot in the field of vision). Diseases affecting the optic nerve often present with a unilateral **negative scotoma** (a "blind spot"). Lesions affecting the optic chiasm, optic tract, or visual cortex affect vision in both eyes.

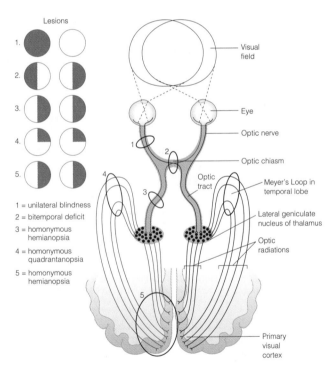

Figure 23-1 Visual system.

Case Conclusion   Optic neuritis is generally self-limited, with peak disability within days to weeks. Most patients regain normal vision within the first 6 months. Subclinical demyelination may manifest as a decrease in visual acuity under certain stressors, such as fever (Uhthoff's phenomenon). As a general rule, about half of patients who present with a single demyelinating event, like optic neuritis, will ultimately be diagnosed with MS. The risk is higher in the setting of supportive imaging or CSF laboratory data, and lower in the absence of such findings. The differential diagnosis in this case should include acute angle-closure glaucoma and amaurosis fugax (sudden, transient monocular loss of vision "like a curtain coming down," suggesting vascular compromise of the optic nerve and retina). Trauma, vitreous hemorrhage, retinal detachment, orbital infection, tumor, or pseudotumor and intracranial mass lesions would also have to be considered.

AF was admitted to the hospital and lumbar puncture was performed. MRI scan was ordered and revealed increased signal and contrast enhancement in the right optic nerve. CSF studies were normal. A 3-day course of IV methylprednisolone was initiated. After discharge, her vision gradually returned to normal over 8 weeks.

Thumbnail: Vision and Optic Nerve

Visual System Lesions

Location	Lesion	Clinical features
Anterior to chiasm	Refractory error	Blurring
	Cataract	Blurring, dimming
	Glaucoma	Blurring, peripheral vision loss
	Orbital pseudotumor	Blurring, pain, proptosis
	Macular degeneration	Positive scotoma centrally
	Amaurosis fugax	Scotoma "like a curtain coming down"
	Optic neuritis	Negative scotoma centrally
Optic chiasm	Pituitary adenoma	Bitemporal peripheral vision loss
Posterior to chiasm	Optic tract/LGN lesions	Incongruous homonymous hemianopia
	Optic radiation lesions	Homonymous quadrantanopia
	Primary visual cortex lesions	Congruous homonymous hemianopia
	Associative visual cortex lesions	Higher order visual defect (visual agnosia, alexia)

Key Points

▶ A Marcus Gunn pupil "dilates paradoxically" in response to light (afferent pupillary defect).

▶ Lesions that compress the optic chiasm cause bitemporal visual field deficits.

▶ Meyer's loop describes the optic radiations arising from the ventral portion of the optic tracts, which loop anteriorly in the temporal lobe.

▶ Lesions of Meyer's loop cause homonymous quadrantanopsias.

▶ Lesions involving the optic tract, LGN, or visual cortex cause homonymous hemianopias.

Questions

1. A 36-year-old man presents with difficulty reading for 1 day. Examination reveals a left centrocecal scotoma. Peripheral vision is relatively spared, as is vision in the right eye. He also is noted to have brisk reflexes and a positive Babinski's sign on the left. Where is the lesion?

   A. Midbrain on the left, involving oculomotor nerve and corticospinal tract
   B. Left optic nerve and right cervical spinal cord
   C. Left optic nerve and left cervical spinal cord
   D. Left optic nerve and left pons
   E. Optic chiasm and right internal capsule

2. An 18-year-old girl with intractable epilepsy and documented right MTS by MRI undergoes an anterior temporal lobectomy. Postoperatively, she is seizure free but reports difficulty seeing the television. Where is the television located?

   A. Eye level and to the left
   B. Near the ceiling and to the right
   C. Centrally, beyond the foot of the bed
   D. Near the ceiling and to the left
   E. Eye level and to the right

3. A 23-year-old woman who is 15 weeks into her first pregnancy is referred to your office because of vision problems. She reports that, at times, she has been seeing things out of the corner of her eye. On further discussion, you discover that she also has been more prone to bump into things lately. Her examination is nonfocal. What is the most likely explanation?

   A. An electrical disturbance of the visual cortex related to migraine
   B. Substance abuse, check the urine drug screen
   C. An electrical disturbance of the visual cortex related to seizure
   D. Compression of the optic chiasm
   E. Demyelination in the optic tracts

4. A 63-year-old man with a history of diabetes, hypertension, and intermittent atrial fibrillation has sudden onset of vision loss in his left eye. He says it was as though someone pulled down a curtain over his eye. His symptoms resolved after about 20 minutes. Which structure was most likely to have been affected?

   A. Optic nerve
   B. Retina
   C. Optic chiasm
   D. Optic tract
   E. Visual cortex

HPI: You are asked to evaluate ME, a 46-year-old right-handed woman, in the ED. She complains of blurred vision, which developed suddenly while she was typing a letter at work. She has never experienced anything like this before. You determine that in addition to blurring, she complains of seeing double when she tries to look to the right. She is otherwise alert, oriented, and medically stable. She has a history of type 2 diabetes that she controls with an oral agent. She smokes half a pack of cigarettes per day and has done so for the past 25 years.

PE: Her BP is 176/89 mm Hg. Her general examination is unremarkable. Her neurologic examination reveals her left eye to be deviated downward and laterally. She has ptosis on the left. Her pupils are unequal, measuring 3 mm on the right and 6 mm on the left. Her left pupil does not respond to light. She is able to count fingers with each eye independently. Her examination is otherwise nonlateralizing and nonlocalizing with full power, equal reflexes, and no long-tract signs.

Thought Questions

- Where is the lesion?

- How is extraocular movement controlled?

- How does each extraocular muscle contribute?

- What is the innervation of each muscle?

- Where in the brainstem does each nerve originate?

Basic Science Review and Discussion

The key to interpreting the case presented is that ME's third nerve palsy occurred in isolation and the pupil was spared. Disorders that result in disruption of extraocular movement can occur anywhere from the level of the brainstem to the orbit itself. However, as a general rule, a lesion is likely to be located peripherally when a CN appears to be affected in isolation. Although many brainstem processes can lead to eye findings, other signs and symptoms often accompany them because other structures are affected. Similarly, disorders affecting the cavernous sinus, retro-orbital space, or orbit also would be expected to have other associated signs and symptoms. **Infarction of the third nerve** classically presents as a **painful, pupil-sparing third nerve palsy.** This is most often seen in those patients at risk of small-vessel disease (diabetes, hypertension, tobacco use). **Third nerve palsy** resulting from compression by a **posterior communicating artery aneurysm** or other mass does not spare pupillary function. This is because extrinsic compression of the third nerve first affects the most superficial (parasympathetic) fibers, causing the pupil to dilate. This is also seen in the setting of third nerve compression by **uncal herniation.** A systematic approach to the anatomy mediating control of eye movements is helpful in the evaluation of patients presenting with eye findings.

Control of Eye Movement   The control of extraocular movement is mediated by CNs III, IV, and VI. The **superior oblique muscle** is innervated by the fourth or **trochlear nerve** (SO4). The **lateral rectus muscle** is innervated by the sixth or **abducens nerve** (LR6). All of the other extraocular muscles are innervated by the third or **oculomotor nerve.** The actions of each of the extraocular muscles in the control of eye movement are summarized in Figure 24-1. The third nerve also mediates innervation to the **levator palpebrae muscle,** as well as **parasympathetic autonomic innervation to the eye.** Sympathetic autonomic innervation to the eye, as with all targets in the head, is mediated by sympathetic nerves originating in the **superior cervical (stellate) ganglion** at the top of the sympathetic chain. These nerves travel along the carotid artery, its branches, and CN branches to reach their targets.

Fourth (trochlear) nerve   The cell bodies of the neurons whose axons make up CN IV are located in the trochlear nucleus. The trochlear nuclei are paired nuclei on either side of the midline located dorsally in the midbrain tegmentum at the border with the pons. The fourth nerve (one on each side) exits the brainstem dorsally, crosses the midline, and goes anteriorly, wrapping itself around the brainstem. The fourth nerve is often listed as the longest of the CNs for this reason. It passes through the cavernous sinus and enters the orbit through the superior orbital fissure. Its only target is the contralateral superior oblique muscle. This muscle is responsible for intorsion ("top" of iris rotates toward the nose). It also helps direct downward gaze when the eye is adducted. Patients with fourth nerve palsies have vertical diplopia.

Sixth (abducens) nerve   The cell bodies of the neurons whose axons make up CN VI are located in the abducens nucleus. The abducens nuclei are paired nuclei on either side of the midline located dorsally in the pontine tegmentum (in the "floor" of the fourth ventricle). Fascicles from these nuclei course ventrally and caudally, exiting the brainstem near the midline at the junction of the pons and medulla. The sixth nerve (one on each side) then courses

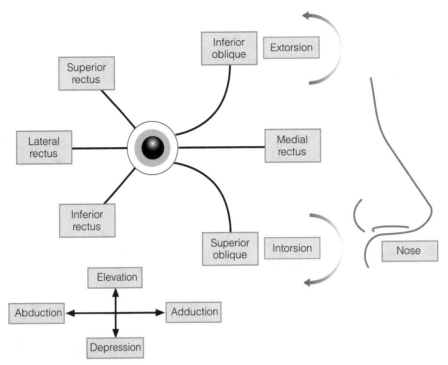

Figure 24-1 Overview of extraocular movement illustrated in the right eye. Note: The superior oblique and inferior oblique muscles intort and extort the eye (respectively). They also mediate depression and elevation of the adducted eye. The superior rectus and inferior rectus muscles elevate and depress the abducted eye. All four muscles work together when the eye is in mid position.

rostrally through the interpeduncular fossa, into the cavernous sinus, and enters the orbit through superior orbital fissure. The axons that make up the sixth nerve are often said to have the longest course (includes both fascicle and nerve) of any of the CNs. Thus the sixth nerve is sometimes listed as the longest of the CNs (note the confusion between this and the fourth nerve). Its only target is the ipsilateral lateral rectus muscle. This muscle is responsible for directing lateral gaze. Lateral gaze palsy is covered in Case 30.

Third (oculomotor) nerve The cell bodies of the axons that make up the third nerve are located in a cluster of nuclei located near the midline in the **midbrain tegmentum.** The fascicles of the third nerve course anteriorly, sometimes passing through the red nucleus and/or the substantia nigra. They penetrate the **cerebral peduncle,** perpendicular to its pyramidal fibers. The third nerve emerges from the cerebral peduncle, passing through the interpeduncular fossa. It passes between the **superior cerebellar and posterior cerebral arteries** adjacent to the **posterior communicating artery.** It then goes through the cavernous sinus and enters the orbit through the superior orbital fissure. The third nerve innervates all other extraocular muscles as well as the levator palpebrae muscle. It also provides parasympathetic innervation to the eye. Throughout its course, the parasympathetic fibers are on the exterior surface of the nerve. The association between each oculomotor subnucleus and the

muscle it innervates is summarized on the next page (Thumbnail: Extraoccular Movement). Note that the medial and central subnuclei innervate contralateral targets. These fibers cross within the midbrain, close to their origin.

Autonomic innervation to the eye The ANS is discussed in more detail in Case 10. However, autonomic innervation to the eye warrants extra attention. The eye receives **parasympathetic** autonomic innervation from the **Edinger-Westphal nucleus** and **sympathetic** autonomic innervation from the **superior cervical ganglion.** Preganglionic parasympathetic axons originating in the Edinger-Westphal nucleus travel along the **surface of CN III** and terminate in the **ciliary ganglion.** Postganglionic parasympathetic axons originating in the ciliary ganglion travel along **short ciliary nerves** to reach the eye. The primary targets of parasympathetic innervation to the eyes are the **ciliary muscles,** which are responsible for changing the shape of the lenses during **accommodation,** and the **sphincter pupillae muscles,** which are responsible for **miosis** (pupillary constriction). The **pupillary light reflex** is a reflex arc mediated, in part, by this system. Light entering the eye causes a retinal response that is conveyed by the optic nerve to the midbrain. These fibers pass through the LGN of the thalamus but do not synapse there. The information is conveyed to the Edinger-Westphal nucleus. Reactive pupillary constriction is then mediated by the parasympathetic portion of CN III. The same type of reflex arc conveys information mediating the **accommodation reflex.** This is the reflex that allows the eye to focus on near objects.

Postganglionic sympathetic axons originate in the paraspinous **sympathetic chain.** These nerves extend along the surface of large arteries to reach targets within the head. Sympathetic innervation also reaches the eyes via the **ciliary nerves.** The primary targets of sympathetic innervation to the eyes are the **dilator iridis muscles,** which contract to cause **mydriasis** (pupillary dilation). There is also a small amount of sympathetic innervation to the **ciliary muscles,** which counteracts the parasympathetic effect and opposes accommodation.

Case Conclusion   ME was admitted to the hospital to exclude posterior communicating artery aneurysm and brainstem infarction as causes for her symptoms. An MRI of the brain revealed only scattered small-vessel disease. Cerebral angiography was performed and no evidence of aneurysm was found. Routine laboratory studies were remarkable only for moderately elevated nonfasting serum glucose level. The fact that this patient retained pupillary responses suggests an intrinsic nerve problem sparing the most superficial nerve layers. A diagnosis of diabetic third nerve palsy was made.

Thumbnail: Extraocular Movement

Subnuclei of the Oculomotor Nucleus and Their Targets		
Subnucleus	**Projection**	**Muscle**
Dorsal	Ipsilateral	Inferior oblique
Intermediate	Ipsilateral	Inferior rectus
Ventral	Ipsilateral	Medial rectus
Medial	Contralateral	Superior rectus
Central	Bilateral	Levator palpebrae
Edinger-Westphal	Bilateral	Sphincter pupillae, ciliary muscles

Key Points

- Only the "superior muscles" are innervated contralaterally.
- Each superior oblique muscle is innervated by the contralateral trochlear nucleus.
- Each superior rectus muscle is innervated by the medial subnucleus of the contralateral oculomotor nuclear group.

- The remaining muscles mediating eye movement are innervated ipsilaterally.
- Parasympathetic and levator palpebrae innervation is bilateral.
- The trochlear and abducens nerves each innervate only one muscle.

Questions

1. A 36-year-old man presents with sudden onset of the worst headache of his life. Examination reveals a dilated pupil on the left as compared to the right. Diplopia can be elicited with extreme right lateral gaze and he reports some difficulty reading. Where is the lesion?

   A. Compressive lesion, right sixth nerve
   B. Intrinsic lesion, left third nerve
   C. Compressive lesion, left third nerve
   D. Compressive lesion, right third nerve
   E. Intrinsic lesion, left sixth nerve

2. A 56-year-old diabetic man presents to the ED with fever and altered mental status. His sinuses have been troubling him for several months. He began complaining of headache several days ago, particularly left facial pain. He is noted to be proptotic, with periorbital edema, ptosis, and ophthalmoparesis on the left. He has impaired sensation on the upper half of the face on the left. What is the most likely anatomic involvement?

   A. Brainstem, an infarction or mass lesion
   B. Orbit, orbital pseudotumor
   C. Cavernous sinus, a thrombosis related to mucormycosis
   D. Meninges, subacute meningitis
   E. Pituitary adenoma

3. You evaluate a patient with unusual eye findings including restricted upward gaze. When he tries to look up, his eyes seem repeatedly to converge and retract deeper into his sockets (convergence-retraction nystagmus). His pupils do not constrict in response to light but do constrict when he focuses on near objects, like the tip of his nose. Which of the following structures is most likely being compressed?

   A. Ventral midbrain
   B. Dorsal midbrain
   C. Oculomotor nerve
   D. Optic nerve
   E. Pituitary gland

4. You evaluate a patient who complains of difficulty walking down stairs. You determine that he has vertical diplopia, which he relieves by tilting his head to the right. Which muscle is affected?

   A. Right superior rectus muscle
   B. Right inferior oblique muscle
   C. Left inferior oblique muscle
   D. Right superior oblique muscle
   E. Left superior oblique muscle

HPI: JM is a 67-year-old right-handed man who presents to the ED complaining of double vision and left-sided weakness. His symptoms started about 9 hours before presentation. He initially thought his symptoms would subside, but they did not. His wife insisted he go to the hospital when she returned home and found him unable to stand without support. He has never had any similar symptoms in the past. He reports that he is a smoker. He states that he takes medication for cholesterol level and high BP. He has been told to take daily aspirin but does not do so because he doesn't want to take too many pills.

PE: His presenting BP is 176/90 mm Hg. Vital signs are otherwise unremarkable. On examination, his right eye is deviated downward and laterally. There is ptosis on the right. Pupils are unequal, the right pupil being larger and non-responsive to light in either eye. He has marked left-sided weakness, rated 2/5 in both the upper and the lower extremity, as well as drooping of the left lower face. Coordination on the left is impaired but proportional to the power deficit and reflexes are relatively symmetrical. He has an extensor plantar (Babinski's sign) on the left.

Thought Questions

- How many lesions does this patient have?
- Where do the two involved systems "cross paths"?
- What is the vascular supply for this area?
- Can you identify some other nearby structures?

Basic Science Review and Discussion

The most important clinical point in this case is that JM has had an acute onset of "crossed" findings. He has disturbance of oculomotor function on one side with contralateral extremity weakness. As a general rule, crossed findings implicate brainstem involvement until proven otherwise. This is because many pathways decussate at different levels within the relatively small brainstem. Thus, a single brainstem lesion can manifest with different findings on either side of the body. A cerebral etiology would require bilateral lesions, which are usually associated with some degree of altered mentation. The exception to the rule is encountered when bilateral cerebral dysfunction presents as an acute lesion superimposed on an old contralateral lesion. This is called **pseudobulbar palsy** because it gives the false impression of brainstem (bulb) disease.

There are many eponymous brainstem syndromes. Each is characterized by a specific combination of CN and long-tract deficits. It is not important to memorize each of these syndromes. The most common tested are **Wallenberg's syndrome** and **Weber's syndrome.** It is important, however, to understand brainstem anatomy well enough to localize a lesion on the basis of clinical findings. In this case, JM has **Weber's syndrome** (ipsilateral third nerve palsy with contralateral hemiparesis). Some of the subsequent cases in this section focus on other brainstem syndromes. They are also summarized in Case 30 (see Thumbnail: Pons). Rather than memorize each syndrome, try to use the information that is provided as a tool for reviewing brainstem anatomy.

Developmental Anatomy The organization of the brainstem is best reviewed within the context of CNS development. Remember that the nervous system starts as a **neural plate.** On this flat surface, motor systems develop medially from a structure called the **basal plate.** The medial portion of the basal plate gives rise to **somatic motor** structures (innervating skeletal muscle). The lateral portion of the basal plate gives rise to **visceral motor** structures (innervating smooth muscle, cardiac muscle, and glands). Sensory systems develop from the lateral portion of the neural plate, called the **alar plate.** Within the alar plate, **visceral sensory** systems (conveying information from the viscera and taste pathways) are relatively medial. **Somatic sensory** systems (conveying information from skin, skeletal muscles, connective tissues, and the inner ear) are located laterally. This organization is summarized in Figure 25-1. Although these organizing principles refer mainly to brainstem nuclei, the long tracts (motor and sensory pathways) that pass through the brainstem are similarly organized.

The boundary between motor and sensory structures (between the basal plate and the alar plate) is defined by the **sulcus limitans.** As the edges of the neural plate fold up to form the **neural tube,** motor systems remain medial and

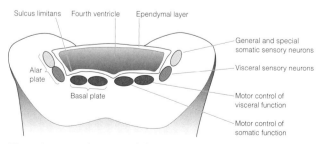

Figure 25-1 Development of the neural tube.

ventral within the tube while sensory systems are located more laterally and dorsally. This organization is maintained through adulthood. It is clinically significant because paramedian and dorsolateral regions of the brainstem tend to differ in their vascular supply. Thus, a paramedian process, as seen in the present case, is associated with predominantly motor deficits. A dorsolateral process, on the other hand, may be associated with predominantly sensory, autonomic, and vestibular deficits while sparing motor systems. **Wallenberg's syndrome,** discussed in a subsequent case, is an example of this.

Brainstem and Midbrain Anatomy The brainstem includes the **midbrain, pons, and medulla** and contains the nuclei for most of the CNs (excluding the first two). The role of these nuclei is analogous to the role of the spinal cord for sensory and motor systems. Unlike the spinal cord, some CNs have uniquely motor or uniquely sensory function. The functions of all the CNs are summarized later in this case (see Thumbnail: Midbrain). The CNs, pons, and medulla are discussed in greater detail separately. This case focuses on the midbrain. The rostral boundary of the **midbrain (mesencephalon)** is defined by the **diencephalon** (thalamus, subthalamus, hypothalamus, and third ventricle). The caudal boundary of the midbrain is defined by the **metencephalon** (pons, cerebellum, and fourth ventricle). The midbrain is subdivided into the **tegmentum,** which includes the areas ventral to the **cerebral (sylvian) aqueduct,** and the **tectum** (dorsal to the aqueduct).

Ventral midbrain The **tegmentum** contains several important structures. The **oculomotor nuclear group** is located medially in the "center" of the rostral midbrain. The fibers that make up the **oculomotor nerve** exit this nucleus ventrally, sometimes passing through portions of the **red nucleus, substantia nigra, and cerebral peduncles.** Note that all of these paramedian structures have predominantly

motor function. Figure 25-2 illustrates these structures in cross section. At this level, the **occulomotor nerve** controls predominantly ipsilateral function, while the **corticospinal tract** is above the pyramidal decussation and controls contralateral motor function. The paramedian vascular supply for this area originates from branches of the basilar artery. A lesion in this area, as in the presented case, produces ipsilateral disruption of occulomotor function (third nerve palsy) and contralateral hemiparesis (corticospinal tract involvement), resulting in **Weber's syndrome.** Different eponyms are applied if this syndrome is combined with tremor (from involvement of the red nucleus or substantia nigra) or ataxia (from involvement of the decussation of the superior cerebellar peduncles). The main sensory pathways passing through the midbrain (**medial lemniscus and spinothalamic tracts**) are dorsolateral to the motor structures discussed earlier. They are less likely to be involved by midbrain lesions.

There are several other important midbrain structures. The **trochlear nucleus** is immediately caudal to the occulomotor nucleus, near the midbrain-pons border. Fibers making up the **trochlear nerve** exit dorsally, cross the midline, and wrap around the midbrain on their way to the orbits. The occulomotor and trochlear nerves are the only CNs that originate from the midbrain. They are both involved in the control of eye movement. Monoaminergic nuclei within the midbrain, pons, and reticular formation are important in the control of movement (**substantia nigra, red nucleus**), motivation (**ventral-tegmental area**), mood (**raphe nuclei**), and arousal (**locus ceruleus**). These systems are discussed separately.

Dorsal midbrain The most important structures of the rostral midbrain **tectum** are the **superior colliculi.** Each superior colliculus receives direct, mostly contralateral input

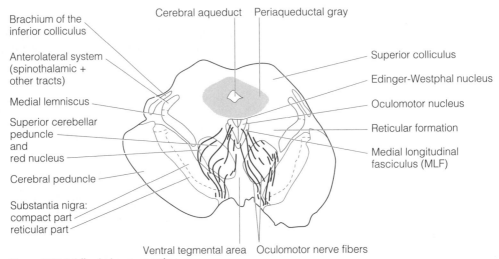

Figure 25-2 Midbrain in cross section.

from the retina via branches of the optic tracts. Many other cortical and subcortical areas also project to the superior colliculi. Output from the superior colliculus goes to the pulvinar of the thalamus and, from there, to higher order visual association cortex. Many brainstem nuclei also receive input from the superior colliculi. Their primary function is the **coordination of eye and head movements** that bring objects of interest into central vision. This area is also responsible for **"blind sight"** (the ability to perceive objects in a dark room without "seeing" them). Immediately ventral to the superior colliculi, the **periaqueductal gray matter** surrounds the cerebral aqueduct. Nuclei in this

region are involved in central analgesia mechanisms. The center for **vertical gaze** is also located in this area. Dorsal midbrain lesions (usually pineal gland tumors) can present with impairment of upward gaze (Parinaud's syndrome).

The caudal midbrain tectum is made up of the **inferior colliculi,** which represent a major brainstem auditory relay center. Auditory information enters the brainstem via the pontine cochlear nuclei projects to the superior olivary nuclei and from there to the inferior colliculi via the **lateral lemniscus.** The auditory system is discussed in more detail separately.

Case Conclusion   The patient was given aspirin, IV fluids, and supportive care. Thrombolysis was not an option given the delayed presentation. MRI of the brain confirmed an infarction involving the right ventromedial midbrain. Abundant diffuse small-vessel disease was evident on imaging. Antiplatelet therapy was continued and the patient was transferred to acute rehabilitation once stabilized.

Thumbnail: Midbrain

Cranial Nerves

Nerve	General sensory	Visceral sensory	Special sensory	Somatic motor	Branchial motor	Visceral motor	Major functions
Olfactory			x				Smell
Optic			x				Vision
Oculomotor				x		x	Motor and parasympathetic to eye
Trochlear				x			Superior oblique muscle
Trigeminal	x				x		Facial sensation, muscles of mastication
Abducens				x			Lateral rectus muscle
Facial	x		x		x	x	Motor to face, glands of head, taste anterior two thirds of tongue
Vestibulocochlear			x				Hearing balance
Glossopharyngeal	x	x	x		x	x	Stylopharyngeus muscle, parotid gland, carotid body, sensation posterior one third of tongue
Vagus	x	x			x	x	Motor, parasympathetic, and sensory for pharynx, larynx, and viscera
Spinal accessory					x		Sternocleidomastoid and trapezius
Hypoglossal				x			Intrinsic tongue muscles

Key Points

- Crossed findings implicate the brainstem first.
- Bilateral hemispheric disease can mimic a brainstem process.
- Motor systems are located ventromedially in the brainstem.
- Sensory systems are located dorsolaterally in the brainstem.

- Only two CNs originate from the midbrain, both are purely motor nerves.
- The superior colliculi are involved in the visual system.
- The inferior colliculi are involved in the auditory system.

Questions

1. A 45-year-old man presents with gradual onset of problems with vision. On examination, his pupils are not reactive to light but constrict when gaze is focused on near objects. His pupils are otherwise slightly dilated. Extraocular movements are intact except for the fact that he cannot look up. Where is the lesion?

    A. Midbrain tegmentum
    B. Midbrain tectum
    C. Bilateral oculomotor nerves
    D. Horizontal gaze center (para-pontine reticular formation [PPRF])
    E. Interpeduncular fossa

2. A 73-year-old woman complains of tremor in her right hand, which has developed gradually over several months. She also notes that her writing has changed in quality. On further assessment, it is determined that she has had several falls. On examination, she is easily pulled off balance and has a shuffling gait. She has a tremor in her right upper extremity that is more prominent at rest. Her tone is increased on the right. What is the most likely structure involved?

    A. Right cerebral peduncle
    B. Left cerebral peduncle
    C. Midbrain tectum
    D. Decussation of the superior cerebellar peduncles
    E. Substantia nigra

3. You evaluate a 15-year-old boy who complains of vision problems. You determine that he has limited upward gaze. Which part of his brainstem is most likely to be affected?

    A. Midbrain tegmentum
    B. Dorsal pons
    C. Dorsal medulla
    D. Midbrain tectum
    E. Ventral pons

4. You evaluate a 73-year-old man with left-sided weakness and right-sided sensory loss. He tells you that he had a thalamic hemorrhage several years ago but has new symptoms today. Where is his new lesion?

    A. Spinal cord
    B. Dorsolateral medulla
    C. Ventral midbrain
    D. Right cerebrum
    E. Right cerebellum

HPI: FP, a 52-year-old man, comes to your office for evaluation of headache. He reports that several times per day he experiences sharp pain on the right side of the face and jaw. The pain lasts only a few seconds but is so severe that it cannot be ignored. The problem first developed several weeks ago, and his spells are getting more frequent. He has gone to his dentist who found nothing wrong and referred him to you. Lately, he has noticed that his symptoms can be triggered by stimulation of a spot on his right jaw. He has since stopped shaving. He denies any other problems or illnesses. He has not had any rashes. His examination is unremarkable.

Thought Questions

- Does this patient have a peripheral or central process?
- What is the most likely structure to be involved?
- What functions are mediated by this structure?

Basic Science Review and Discussion

FP presents with brief, episodic, lancinating pain involving the right side of the face. The upper face and eye are spared. There are no visible skin lesions. In this age-group, the most likely diagnosis is **trigeminal neuralgia,** a clinical entity whose etiology is not clearly defined. The absence of other associated signs or symptoms makes the possibility of a central lesion less likely, especially in the setting of a spared first division of the trigeminal nerve. A mass lesion compressing the trigeminal nerve should be excluded. Migraine can present with unilateral head pain and belongs in the differential. Cluster headache can also present with unilateral head pain but is usually localized to the first branch of the trigeminal nerve rather than sparing it. As always, an understanding of the anatomy involved is important for the clinical evaluation.

Anatomy of Trigeminal Nerve   CN V is the only CN to exit from the body of the **pons.** It does so from the midlateral surface, originating as two roots: a larger sensory root and a smaller motor root. The roots come together to form the nerve, which enters the **trigeminal ganglion.** The trigeminal ganglion has a purely sensory function, analogous to the dorsal root ganglia along the spinal cord. As its name implies, the trigeminal nerve has three main divisions that emerge from the trigeminal ganglion before exiting the skull. Some studies have implicated anatomic compression of the trigeminal ganglion or its main divisions as a possible cause for trigeminal neuralgia. Surgical decompression has been used in some cases but has not gained wide use. Chemical or radioablation is reserved for intractable cases not responsive to conservative medical management because of the resulting permanent sensory disturbance. These procedures are generally limited to the most affected of the three major divisions of the trigeminal nerve.

Divisions of trigeminal nerve   The first division is the **ophthalmic nerve (V1),** which conveys purely sensory information. It passes through the **cavernous sinus** and exits the skull through the **superior orbital fissure.** It has several branches including lacrimal, frontal, ciliary, and meningeal branches. The ophthalmic nerve conveys sensory information from the upper face, eye, cornea, and nose. The meningeal branch conveys sensory information from the tentorium cerebelli. Although the ophthalmic division of the trigeminal nerve mediates purely sensory information, small sympathetic nerves that originate in the superior cervical ganglion and ascend along the internal carotid artery follow the ciliary branches to reach the eye. The patient in this case did not have any pain or abnormality associated with the ophthalmic division of the trigeminal nerve. However, there are a few clinical syndromes associated with this nerve. Herpes-zoster ophthalmicus is one example. Although herpes zoster can affect any nerve and most commonly affects thoracic spinal nerves, herpes-zoster ophthalmicus is an important entity to recognize because vesicular involvement of the cornea can lead to loss of vision.

The second division is the **maxillary nerve (V2),** also a pure sensory nerve. It generally passes through the cavernous sinus before exiting the skull through the **foramen rotundum.** It has several branches including zygomatic, infraorbital, pterygopalatine, and meningeal branches. The maxillary nerve conveys sensory information from the middle face, nose, upper lip, and pharynx. The meningeal branch of the maxillary nerve conveys sensory information from the meninges of the anterior and middle cranial fossae. The maxillary nerve is often involved in trigeminal neuralgia (also called **tic douloureux** because the severe sudden pain can cause patients to wince).

The third division is **the mandibular nerve (V3).** The mandibular nerve has both a sensory and a motor component. It exits the skull through the **foramen ovale.** It has several branches including buccal, lingual, auriculotemporal, inferior alveolar, and meningeal branches. The mandibular nerve conveys sensory information from the lower face, lower lip, buccal mucosa, and anterior two thirds of the tongue. Nerve fibers that convey taste information from the anterior two thirds of the tongue also are contained within the lingual nerve for a short distance.

Rather than continuing to the trigeminal nucleus, these fibers leave the mandibular nerve as the **chorda tympani,** passing through the petrotympanic fissure and joining CN VII. The meningeal branch of the mandibular nerve also conveys sensory information from the meninges of the anterior and middle cranial fossae. The mandibular nerve also has several branches that innervate the **muscles of mastication.** These represent the only motor function mediated by the trigeminal nerve.

Brainstem trigeminal nuclei   The trigeminal nerve enters the brainstem on the midlateral surface of the pons. Within the pons, there are two **trigeminal nuclei:** a motor nucleus and a sensory nucleus. Both are located within the **pontine tegmentum** and are medial to the middle cerebellar peduncle, lateral to the medial longitudinal fasciculus (MLF), ventral to the superior cerebellar peduncle, and dorsal to the medial lemniscus. In keeping with the brainstem organizational principles previously discussed, the motor trigeminal nucleus is medial to the sensory nucleus.

The **motor trigeminal nucleus** is restricted to the pons. Its role is analogous to the anterior horn of the spinal cord. UMNs whose cell bodies are located within the primary motor cortex project to this nucleus where they synapse onto the LMNs. Each motor nucleus receives bilateral cortical input. Output from the motor nucleus projects out the ipsilateral trigeminal nerve, along the mandibular division, to reach the **muscles of mastication.** Because these nuclei **receive bilateral cortical input,** UMN lesions of the muscles of mastication are rarely seen.

The **sensory trigeminal nucleus has three components.** The rostral portion of the trigeminal sensory nucleus extends into the midbrain. This mesencephalic portion of the trigeminal nucleus is responsible for proprioceptive input from the muscles of mastication. The neurons of the **mesencephalic trigeminal nucleus** are unique in that they are the only primary sensory neurons known to exist within the CNS, rather than within sensory ganglia. Their peripheral processes come directly from the muscles of mastication without synapsing in the trigeminal ganglion. Their central processes project primarily onto the neurons of the motor trigeminal nucleus, forming a monosynaptic arc that mediates reflexes such as the jaw jerk. The **principle sensory trigeminal nucleus is located within the pons** and is primarily responsible for tactile sensation from the face, analogous to the dorsal columns of the spinal cord. The **nucleus of the spinal tract of the trigeminal nerve extends caudally through the medulla and into the upper segments of the spinal cord.** It is primarily responsible for pain and temperature sensation from the face, analogous to the anterolateral sensory system of the spinal cord. Both the principle trigeminal nucleus and the nucleus of the spinal tract of the trigeminal nerve contain second-order sensory neurons. They receive input from primary sensory neurons in the trigeminal ganglion. The central projections from neurons within the trigeminal nuclei decussate within the pons to join the contralateral ascending spinothalamic pathways as the **trigeminal lemniscus.** Upon reaching the thalamus, nerve fibers from the trigeminal system synapse onto third-order sensory neurons in the **ventral posterior medial nucleus,** which then project to the primary sensory cortex.

Clinical Correlation   As mentioned previously, the constellation of symptoms in this patient is most consistent with trigeminal neuralgia. This clinical entity may be triggered by focal stimulation and is often responsive to carbamazepine. In younger patients, particularly in younger women, demyelinating disease should be considered as a cause for trigeminal neuralgia. Migraine can present with hemicranial pain, but attacks are more prolonged, pain is described as throbbing, and there are often other associated features (photophobia, phonophobia, nausea). Herpes zoster also can present with facial pain. In the acute phase, pain can precede vesicular eruption, but our patient is well into the subacute phase of his syndrome. In a patient with a history of herpes zoster, postherpetic neuralgia can present as severe facial pain that is generally more persistent. Trauma is another important potential cause for trigeminal nerve dysfunction. New-onset facial pain in an older individual should always raise the suspicion for tumor and an imaging study of the head should be performed.

Case Conclusion   Routine laboratory studies were unremarkable. An MRI of the head with contrast was obtained and was also unremarkable. The patient was started on carbamazepine at the initial visit based on a presumptive diagnosis of trigeminal neuralgia. The dose was gradually increased with good response. Several months later the medication was weaned and the patient remained free of symptoms.

Thumbnail: Trigeminal Nerve

Major Branches of the Trigeminal Nerve

Divisions	Main branches
Ophthalmic (V1)	Lacrimal Frontal Nasociliary Meningeal
Maxillary (V2)	Zygomatic Infraorbital Pterygopalatine Meningeal
Mandibular (V3)	Buccal Auriculotemporal Lingual Inferior alveolar Meningeal Motor branches (to muscles of mastication)

Key Points

▸ Trigeminal nerve has predominantly sensory function.

▸ The motor component of the trigeminal nerve innervates the muscles of mastication.

▸ Proprioceptive information goes to the mesencephalic trigeminal nucleus.

▸ Tactile sensation information goes to the principle trigeminal nucleus in the pons.

▸ Pain and temperature information goes to the spinal trigeminal nucleus in the medulla and upper spinal cord.

Questions

1. A 40-year-old woman presents with brief severe headaches over the right eye. They occur several times per day and are associated with runny nose, sweating, and reddening of the eye. What structure is involved?
   A. Maxillary sinus
   B. Ophthalmic nerve
   C. Trigeminal ganglion
   D. Ophthalmic artery
   E. Ciliary ganglion

2. A 72-year-old hypertensive man has been having brief spells that he describes as tingling on the right side of his face. They have generally lasted only minutes at a time. This morning he awoke to find a similar sensation involving his left arm and leg. The symptoms have persisted throughout the day and he is getting worried. Where is his lesion?
   A. Dorsal pontine tegmentum on the left
   B. Ventral pontine tegmentum on the left
   C. Dorsal pontine tegmentum on the right
   D. Ventral pontine tegmentum on the right
   E. Trigeminal ganglion on the right

3. A 34-year-old man presents with left facial droop and diminished sensation on the left side of the face. Both the upper and the lower face are affected. His ability to taste is also diminished on the left side of the tongue. Which structure is affected?
   A. Trigeminal nerve on the right
   B. Trigeminal nerve on the left
   C. Pons on the left
   D. Facial nerve on the left
   E. Cerebral cortex on the left

4. Another 34-year-old man presents with a left facial droop involving both the upper and lower face. Taste is diminished on the left side of the tongue. Which muscles are spared?
   A. Orbicularis oculi and frontalis
   B. Levator palpebrae and frontalis
   C. Masseter and levator palpebrae
   D. Orbicularis oculi and masseter
   E. Frontalis and masseter

HPI: A 35-year-old otherwise healthy woman presents to your office complaining of an inability to close her left eye. She had been in good health (other than a case of the flu several weeks ago) when she noticed upon waking the previous day that her left eye would not close all the way and was somewhat irritated. Her family notes that the left side of her face doesn't seem to move as much as the right, and the left corner of her mouth appears to droop. She also complains that she is not able to taste food on the left side of her tongue.

PE: Her examination is notable for a fairly noticeable left facial droop with a decreased left nasolabial fold, and slightly increased size of the palpebral fissure on the left versus the right. When asked to close her eyes, her left eye looks upward, but the lids are not able to completely close. She is unable to appreciate sweet taste on the left side of her tongue. Otherwise, her examination is completely benign.

Thought Questions

- What area of the nervous system has been affected?

- How is motor innervation of the face controlled?

- How is taste appreciated?

- What is her prognosis?

Basic Science Review and Discussion

Control of Facial Muscles and CN VII Motor function of the face is almost completely governed by CN VII (the facial nerve), with the exception of the levator palpebrae superioris, which is controlled by CN III. It is the lack of opposition to levator palpebrae that resulted in this patient's inability to close her eye (normally closure is performed by the orbicularis oculi). In addition, CN VII also (at some points in its course) contains fibers for taste, sensation of the ear, and some of the autonomic fibers controlling salivation.

Facial motor function originates in the **motor cortex,** located in the precentral gyrus of the frontal lobe. Motor fibers projecting to the pons (also known as *corticobulbar fibers*) coalesce with all other motor fibers, forming the corona radiata and then the internal capsule, then passing through the cerebral peduncles. After entering the brainstem, the corticobulbar fibers (which control all motor function governed by CNs) diverge to the various CN nuclei, crossing the midline in most cases. The **corticospinal** fibers progress onward to the spinal cord.

The pons contains the **facial nucleus,** in which the UMNs (in this case, the corticobulbar fibers to the facial nucleus) synapse to the LMNs, whose cell bodies essentially make up the facial nucleus. The facial nucleus is separated into two basic halves, one of which projects to the lower face and one of which projects to the upper face. Because these parts are innervated differently, they are discussed separately.

The projections from the facial nucleus exit the brainstem to form the majority of the **facial nerve, or CN VII.**

The facial nucleus The facial nucleus is concerned only with motor function, namely that of the head and neck. The **lower half** of the facial nucleus receives axons solely from the contralateral motor cortex. These "singly innervated" LMNs project fibers (axons) that exit the brainstem to form part of the facial nerve. They innervate the lower half of the face and neck, generally at and below the level of the nose.

Because the lower half of the face is innervated only by the contralateral cortex, it is susceptible to both UMN and LMN lesions, which include stroke and Bell's palsy (discussed subsequently).

The **upper half** of the facial nucleus receives bilateral projections from the motor cortex: both the ipsilateral and contralateral cortex synapses with these LMN cell bodies. These "dual-innervated" LMNs then run to the muscles of the upper half of the face. As a result, processes that affect the UMN only (stroke) generally do not cause upper facial weakness, because the opposite cortex also projects to the upper half of the facial nucleus, and thus may compensate. As a result, only LMN processes (Bell's palsy) affect strength in the upper portion of the face.

CN VII Fibers from both the upper and the lower half of the facial nucleus coalesce to form the facial tract, which loops around the abducent nucleus in the dorsal pons. This loop forms a dorsal bulge on the floor of the fourth ventricle known as the **facial colliculus.** These motor fibers then exit the ventral pons at the pontomedullary junction. These motor fibers have joined with other autonomic, taste, and sensory fibers before exiting the brainstem. CN VII comprises this complex collection of nerve fibers outside of the brain. Upon leaving the brainstem, CN VII enters the **internal auditory meatus** and the **facial canal** within the skull.

The facial canal leaves little room for expansion in its tighter segments, resulting in the possibility of facial nerve compression if CN VII should become swollen or inflamed (to be discussed later).

Motor Fibers   The first motor branch diverges within the facial canal to the **stapedius** muscle of the inner ear. The stapedius dampens tympanic membrane vibration, which is helpful when excessively loud noises are encountered. Remaining motor fibers exit the skull via the **stylomastoid foramen.** Branches are sent to the **posterior digastric belly** and **stylohyoid** muscles. They then weave through the parotid gland and divide into the five major motor branches of the facial nerve: **cervical, mandibular, buccal, zygomatic,** and **temporal.** These innervate the platysmas and muscles of facial expression.

Sensory Fibers   The sensation of the outer ear is governed by sensory fibers whose cell bodies are located in the **geniculate ganglion** (so named because it lies in the curve, or **genu,** of the facial canal) after joining the other facial nerve fibers in the facial canal. These sensory fibers enter the brainstem as part of CN VII, and then diverge to the **spinal trigeminal nucleus.** (General sensory fibers associated with CNs generally project to the spinal trigeminal nucleus.)

Taste Fibers   Taste of the anterior two thirds of the tongue, in addition to taste of the hard and soft palates, is governed by fibers that also form part of CN VII. These gustatory fibers initially run or "hitchhike" with the lingual branch of the trigeminal nerve before diverging to form the **chorda tympani.** The **chorda tympani** is an important branch of CN VII, which enters the skull at the **petrotympanic fissure** and then runs through the middle ear, adjacent to the tympanic membrane (thus giving it its name) before joining the rest of CN VII in the facial canal. It synapses in the geniculate ganglion and then continues with CN VII into the brainstem, where the gustatory fibers run to the **nucleus solitarius,** which governs taste. The nucleus solitarius also projects onto the superior salivary nucleus, which governs salivation and lacrimation (discussed later in this case).

Autonomic Fibers (Secretory Function)   The autonomic fibers of CN VII essentially control all major salivary and mucous glands of the head, with the important exception of the parotid gland. This is accomplished by projections from the **superior salivary nucleus,** which join the facial tract as it exits the brainstem. These autonomic fibers form two branches that diverge from CN VII in the facial canal.

The first branch is the **greater superficial petrosal nerve.** It enters the pterygoid canal and then synapses in the pterygopalatine (or sphenopalatine) ganglion. Postganglionic nerve fibers leave the ganglion and follow a complicated course ("hitchhiking" on different branches of CN V) en route to the lacrimal glands of the orbit and mucous glands of the nose and pharynx.

The second branch runs with the chorda tympani to synapse in the submandibular ganglion, which sends postganglionic fibers to the submandibular and sublingual salivary glands.

Clinical Presentations of Facial Weakness   Because of the anatomy described earlier in regards to the upper and lower halves of the facial nucleus, UMN lesions present differently from LMN lesions.

UMN lesions   Processes affecting the facial aspect of the motor strip are only evident in their exclusive projections to the lower half of the contralateral facial nucleus. As a result, they generally present with contralateral weakness of the lower half of the face, with relative preservation of periorbital and forehead muscles. Patients present with a droop of the mouth and diminished nasolabial fold on the affected side. Stroke (cerebrovascular accident [CVA]) is the most common cause of UMN dysfunction, but brain tumors, MS, and head trauma are other possibilities, to name a few.

LMN lesions   Lesions affecting the facial nerve itself, the final common pathway to the innervation of facial musculature, **affect motor function of the entire side of the face,** including the periorbital muscles and the forehead. They may also affect taste on the ipsilateral tongue due to compromise of the chorda tympani fibers, and theoretically salivation and sensation of the ear may be affected, although these are less obvious. The presence or absence of upper facial weakness often allow LMN versus UMN lesions to be distinguished clinically.

Bell's Palsy   *Bell's palsy* refers to an acute hemifacial palsy of unknown cause. It occurs in about 30 patients per 100,000 per year (rare) and is more likely in diabetics and pregnant patients (third trimester or 1 week postpartum). Patients will present with a partial or complete paralysis of both the upper and the lower half of one side of the face. This presentation can be caused only by LMN dysfunction, because UMN lesions spare the upper half of the face. There are other causes of hemifacial palsy, including trauma, severe otitis media, Lyme disease, tumor, sarcoidosis, and HIV. However, most patients with acute hemifacial palsy will not have any clear etiology, and aggressive diagnostic testing is generally unnecessary unless the problem persists more than 2 weeks.

Although Bell's palsy refers to unknown causes by definition, some evidence suggests that most cases are caused by a neuritis secondary to HSV-1 infection. HSV-1, when present, resides within CN ganglia and may periodically reactivate, often resulting in vesicular eruptions (cold sores) and possibly facial nerve inflammation. This inflammatory response causes swelling. The facial canal is constrictive and compression of CN VII may follow, resulting in dysfunction and hemifacial paralysis. It may also cause loss of taste and salivation on the affected side, although many patients will not notice this.

Most patients with Bell's palsy (about 70%) will completely recover. A good rule of thumb is that patients with an incomplete palsy will recover (about 95%), whereas significantly fewer of those with a complete palsy (60%) recover. In severe cases, regeneration of the facial nerve may be inappropriate, leading to tearing of the eye when salivation should occur. This is known as **"crocodile tears."** Treatment is usually supportive, although medium-dose oral steroids and antiherpetic agents (acyclovir or valacyclovir) are sometimes used.

> **Case Conclusion**   Because both the upper and the lower portion of her face was clearly involved, it is clear that the LMN (the peripheral nerve) is the culprit. The patient was diagnosed with a Bell's palsy in light of the lack of other cranial neuropathies or physical findings. She was given a 2-week regimen of oral prednisolone and valacyclovir and allowed to go home. She was also told to tape her eye closed at night and to use eyedrops to keep it moist, because she is unable to close it. Within 3 weeks, she reported return of eye closure and some use of her face, and she regained complete use of her face after 2 months.

Thumbnail: Taste and Facial Nerve

Facial Nerve and Selected Cranial Nerve Functions

Cranial nerve	Motor function	Sensory function	Autonomic function	Other
VII	Facial muscles; stapedius	External ear	Salivary, lacrimal; nasal glands	Taste anterior two thirds of the tongue
V	Mastication	Face, eyes, mouth	None	
IX	Stylopharyngeus	External ear; middle ear; pharynx	Parotid gland; carotid sinus	
X	Pharynx, larynx	External ear; pharynx, larynx	Parasympathetic; of internal viscera	

Key Points

▶ The facial nucleus receives bilateral projections to its upper half, such that central or UMN lesions affect only the lower contralateral facial quadrant. Facial hemiplegia involving the upper and lower face results from lesions of the LMN, often within the facial canal.

▶ CN VII is a complex nerve that controls almost all voluntary facial musculature, sensation of the ear, secretory function of the eye, nasopharynx, and salivary glands (except the parotid), and taste of the anterior two thirds of the tongue.

▶ Bell's palsy refers to idiopathic acute facial hemiplegia. It is thought to often be caused by facial neuritis, leading to compression in the facial canal, generally due to HSV-1 reactivation. Patients usually fully recover.

Questions

1. You meet a patient in the hospital who has an isolated schwannoma of the left facial nerve, which has completely compromised all function of all the nerve fibers just as they exit the brainstem. What symptoms do you expect this patient to have?

   A. Left hemifacial palsy (upper and lower), decreased taste on anterior left tongue, hyperacusis left ear, decreased sensation external left ear, decreased secretion of left salivary and nasal glands

   B. Left lower facial palsy, decreased taste on anterior left tongue, hyperacusis left ear, decreased sensation external left ear, decreased secretion of left salivary and nasal glands

   C. Right hemifacial palsy (upper and lower), decreased taste on anterior right tongue, hyperacusis right ear, decreased sensation external left ear, decreased secretion of left salivary and nasal glands

   D. Asymptomatic

   E. Left hemifacial palsy (upper and lower) only

2. A 75-year-old man with a history of left lower facial droop due to stroke and recurrent left-sided otitis media is noted to have diminished taste on the anterior left tongue. Sensation is otherwise intact. What is the most likely explanation?

   A. Congenital absence of taste buds on the left tongue

   B. Infarction of cerebral taste pathways from stroke

   C. Benign changes related to aging

   D. Involvement of chorda tympani from otitis media

   E. New onset Bell's palsy

3. A 70-year-old male patient has a persistent left hemifacial droop secondary to a parotid gland tumor that was excised 5 years ago. What other deficiencies would he be expected to have?

   A. Lack of taste left anterior tongue

   B. Lack of salivation left salivary glands

   C. Lack of sensation left face

   D. No other deficits

   E. Left hyperacusis

4. A 46-year-old woman developed an apparent Bell's palsy several months ago with residual right hemifacial droop. Over time, the droop slowly improves, but she begins to note that her right eye tears when she eats or salivates. What is a possible explanation?

   A. Inappropriate regeneration of salivary autonomic fibers to lacrimal glands

   B. Recurrence of Bell's palsy

   C. Conjunctivitis

   D. Hyperlacrimation syndrome

   E. Normal prodrome of recovery

HPI: HM, a 56-year-old right-handed man, comes to your office complaining of hearing loss and ringing in the right ear. He reports that his symptoms were initially subtle. In retrospect, he admits to diminished hearing over the past year. More recently, he becomes dizzy at times, although this is mild. He also reports that food just doesn't taste the same anymore. His health has been good in all other respects.

PE: His examination reveals asymmetry on the Weber test, with sound heard better on the left. Air conduction is louder than bone conduction bilaterally on the Rinne test. He has a subtle right lower facial droop and diminished taste sensation on the right side of the tongue. The remainder of the examination is unremarkable.

Thought Questions

- Where is this patient's lesion?
- What are the structural implications of the examination findings?
- What other structures could be involved?
- Can you describe the auditory pathways involved?

Basic Science Review and Discussion

Hearing loss can be divided into central and peripheral causes. **Central hearing loss** is usually relatively mild unless the cochlear nuclei are involved. **Peripheral hearing loss** can be either **conductive** (sound not getting to the inner ear) or **sensorineural** (sound gets in but cannot be conveyed centrally). In the **Weber test,** a tuning fork is held at the midline on the skull. The sound is perceived asymmetrically if there is a deficit. Sound is louder in the affected ear with a conductive deficit but louder in the intact ear with a sensorineural deficit. In the **Rinne test,** conduction of sound waves in bone and air are compared. Bone conduction is louder only in the setting of a conductive deficit. This patient's complaint and examination findings suggest a sensorineural hearing loss on the right. The LMN facial weakness and loss of taste on the right implicate the right facial nerve. Given the absence of other associated symptoms, the lesion is more likely to be extra-axial and involving CN VII and VIII on the right.

A slow-growing mass lesion in the cerebellopontine angle could produce this clinical syndrome. The mass lesion most often associated with this location is an **acoustic neuroma.** These tumors usually begin on the vestibular portion of the eighth nerve but grow slowly enough that hearing loss is seen more often than vertigo as an initial manifestation. Acoustic neuromas can occur either sporadically or in association with **neurofibromatosis.** This is the most common of the neurocutaneous syndromes (associated with both neurologic deficits and characteristic skin lesions). Two types of neurofibromatosis are recognized. Both are inherited in a dominant pattern. Type 1 (von Recklinghausen's disease) is primarily peripheral in its manifestation. Type 2 is more commonly associated with CNS manifestations. Bilateral acoustic neuromas are classically associated with neurofibromatosis type 2.

Sound Reception The auricle of the ear concentrates sound toward the external acoustic meatus. These sound waves cause vibration of the **tympanic membrane,** which converts the sound wave energy into mechanical energy. Movement of the tympanic membrane sets the ossicles in motion. Within the tympanic cavity, two muscles exert control over the sensitivity of this system. The **tensor tympani muscle,** innervated by the trigeminal nerve, can reduce tympanic membrane flexibility. The **stapedius muscle,** innervated by the facial nerve, can reduce ossicle motion. The first of the **ossicles,** the **malleus,** is attached to the tympanic membrane. The **stapes** is attached to the membrane covering the oval window. The **incus** connects the malleus to the stapes. Movement of the stapes causes movement of the membrane covering the **oval window** of the cochlea.

Cochlea The **cochlea** is a coiled tube with three fluid-filled compartments (scalae) divided by two membranes (Figure 28-1). **Reissner's membrane** separates the **scala vestibuli** from the **scala media.** The **basilar membrane** separates the **scala media** from the **scala tympani.** The scala media is completely isolated from the other two compartments and contains potassium-rich **endolymph.** The scala vestibuli and scala tympani are connected through an opening at the apex of the cochlea, called the **helicotrema.** The **oval window** is at the proximal end of the scala vestibuli. The **round window** is at the proximal end of the scala tympani. The flexible membrane covering the round window accommodates the piston-like movement of the stapes against the membrane of the oval window (as one moves in, the other moves out). The resulting fluid waves set the basilar membrane in motion. The **organ of Corti,** which transduces this motion into electrochemical energy, is located within the basilar membrane. The shape of the basilar membrane is

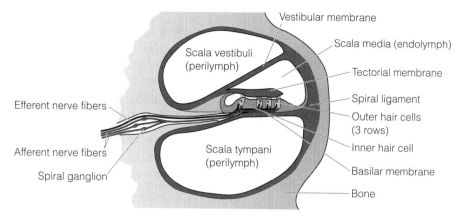

Figure 28-1 Cochlea in cross section.

such that it is stiffer near the base of the cochlea and more flexible at the apex. This allows for sound frequency differentiation. Higher frequencies are best detected at the cochlear base, and lower frequencies are best detected at the apex. This **tonotopic organization** starts in the cochlea and is maintained all the way up to the **primary auditory cortex.**

Organ of Corti The organ of Corti converts mechanical energy into electrochemical energy. It contains one row of inner **hair cells** and three rows of outer **hair cells.** The **cilia** of the hair cells are attached to an overlying **tectorial membrane** and are surrounded by potassium-rich endolymph. Movement of the basilar membrane and hair cells relative to the tectorial membrane cause bending of the cilia, which causes **potassium ion channels** within them to either open or close. Altered potassium conductance changes the membrane potential of the hair cells. The hair cells are direction sensitive. Movement in one direction causes relative hair cell depolarization, and movement in the opposite direction causes relative hyperpolarization. The hair cells are in synaptic contact with the peripheral processes of bipolar (primary) sensory neurons in the **spiral ganglion.** The hair cell membrane potential modulates neurotransmitter release from hair cells onto these dendrites.

Sensory neurons The **primary auditory sensory neurons** are glutamatergic bipolar neurons in the **spiral ganglion** of the cochlea, which receive input from **cochlear hair cells.** The central projections from these neurons make up the cochlear portion of the eighth nerve. They enter the skull at the internal auditory meatus and enter the brainstem near the cerebellopontine angle, at the pontomedullary junction. They terminate on secondary sensory neurons in the **dorsal and ventral cochlear nuclei.** The cochlear nuclei are

located in the dorsolateral pons, near the inferior cerebellar peduncle, and lateral to the vestibular nuclei.

Afferent auditory pathways The cochlear nuclei have bilateral central projections. Ipsilateral projections enter the **lateral lemniscus** on the same side. Three acoustic striae (the **dorsal, intermediate, and ventral striae**) project to the contralateral side of the brainstem. The dorsal and intermediate pathways decussate more dorsally in the pons and enter the lateral lemniscus directly. The ventral pathway (also called the **trapezoid body**) decussates more ventrally in the pons, terminating in the **superior olivary nuclear group** and reticular formation. Tertiary auditory neurons from these areas then project into the **lateral lemniscus.** The lateral lemniscus terminates in the **inferior colliculus.** Neurons in the inferior colliculus project to the **medial geniculate nucleus of the thalamus.** Neurons from this nucleus then project to the **primary auditory cortex** (discussed in Case 6).

Organization of Sound Processing Beginning at the level of the cochlear nuclei, **auditory pathways have bilateral representation.** This means that unilateral deafness can only be caused by a peripheral lesion (cochlea, eighth nerve) or a lesion involving the cochlear nuclei (which would likely involve other structures too). Any higher lesion in the auditory pathways may cause mild diminished hearing bilaterally but would not cause unilateral deafness. Auditory pathways are further complicated by feedback loops at every level of processing. Integration of auditory input from the two ears allows **localization of sounds in space.** Neurons in the auditory cortex are organized in columns, as is the case in other cortical sensory areas. Columns may respond preferentially to a given frequency or to sound from one side or the other. Further processing of auditory input occurs in higher associative cortices.

Case Conclusion An MRI scan was ordered and revealed an enhancing mass near the cerebellopontine angle on the right. The patient was referred for neurosurgical evaluation and resection of the mass. The eighth nerve on the right could not be spared. Postoperatively, the patient was left with permanent unilateral deafness on the right. He was initially vertiginous, but this ultimately resolved with vestibular therapy. His facial nerve deficits also resolved.

Thumbnail: Auditory System and Vestibulocochlear Nerve

Peripheral Hearing Loss

	Conductive	Sensorineural
Structures involved	Outer or middle ear	Cochlear or retrocochlear
Frequencies affected	Same for all frequencies	High frequencies affected
Speech discrimination	Intact	Impaired
Tinnitus	May be present	Usually present
Causes	Usually acquired (structural, trauma, toxic, tumors)	Congenital or acquired (noise, aging, inflammation, infection, trauma, toxic, tumor)

Key Points

▶ Unilateral deafness suggests a peripheral, neural, or nuclear lesion.

▶ Conductive hearing loss is cause by lesions in the external or middle ear.

▶ Sensorineural hearing loss is cause by lesions in the inner ear or nerve.

▶ The auditory system is tonotopically organized.

▶ In the Weber test, a tuning fork is held at the midline on the skull. Sound is louder in the affected ear with a conductive deficit and louder in the intact ear with a sensorineural deficit.

▶ In the Rinne test, conduction of sound waves in bone and air are compared. Bone conduction is louder than air conduction in the setting of a conductive deficit.

Questions

1. A 30-year-old woman presents with sudden onset of hearing loss and tinnitus on the right. She asks if this could be a manifestation of her MS. Where might her lesion be located?
   A. Trapezoid body
   B. Left superior olivary nuclei
   C. Right cochlear nuclei
   D. Right lateral pons
   E. Left lateral lemniscus

2. A 63-year-old man comes to the ED complaining of gradual loss of hearing on the left. This is confirmed objectively. The Weber test reveals asymmetric findings with sound louder on the left. The Rinne test reveals bone conduction to be louder than air conduction on the left. What is the most likely explanation?
   A. Excessive cerumen buildup, his ears need to be cleaned
   B. Probable exposure to an aminoglycoside
   C. Tumor in the cerebellopontine angle on the left
   D. Too many rock concerts
   E. Increased endolymph pressure and distended semi-circular canals

3. A 53-year-old man complains of attacks of vertigo associated with fullness in the ears and impaired hearing. This is worse on the right than the left. These attacks can last hours and have been occurring on and off for several years. More recently, he has noticed trouble hearing between attacks too. What is the most likely explanation?
   A. Excessive cerumen buildup, his ears need to be cleaned
   B. Probable exposure to an aminoglycoside
   C. Tumor in the cerebellopontine angle on the left
   D. Too many rock concerts
   E. Increased endolymph pressure and distended semi-circular canals

4. A 28-year-old man comes to the ED with sudden onset of a left facial droop. He complains that sounds are louder on the left than the right. You determine that he has impaired taste sensation on the right side of the tongue. What is the explanation for his hearing problem?
   A. Impaired tensor tympani muscle function on the left
   B. Impaired stapedius muscle function on the right
   C. Impaired tensor tympani muscle function on the right
   D. Impaired stapedius muscle function on the left
   E. Tumor in the cerebellopontine angle on the left

HPI: JW, a 53-year-old right-handed woman, presents to your office complaining of attacks of severe vertigo. The attacks occur unexpectedly and are not precipitated by any particular movement. The first few minutes are the worst. During that time, the room spins, she cannot stand, and she often vomits. The symptoms gradually subside over a few hours, but she can remain "off balance" for days afterward. When you ask, she admits that she sometimes has ringing and a sensation of fullness in the right ear during the attacks. She has been having some trouble with her hearing over the past few years, particularly on the right, but has not given it much thought because this seems to run in her family. She has not had an attack for several weeks.

PE: She has a normal neurologic examination, with no evidence of nystagmus, and her symptoms cannot be provoked in the office.

Thought Questions

■ Where is this patient's lesion?

■ What are the structural implications of her symptoms?

■ What other structures could be involved?

■ How is the vestibular system organized?

Basic Science Review and Discussion

JW has paroxysmal attacks of severe **vertigo** associated with hearing loss but no other neurologic symptoms. One would be inclined to suspect a peripheral vestibular process. The duration of the spells, hearing loss, associated symptoms, and family history are all suggestive of **Ménière's disease.** Attacks of benign positional vertigo **(BPV)** often are shorter in duration and usually are associated with a particular provocative head position. **Vestibular neuritis** and other peripheral inflammatory conditions are often associated with spells of longer duration, may be provoked by movement, but generally are not associated with a specific head position. **Central vertigo** is less likely to be episodic and is far more likely to be associated with other neurologic deficits. Lesions within the brainstem usually involve multiple structures and result in multiple deficits. Central vestibular pathways also project widely within the nervous system. However, a larger number of centrally mediated and systemic conditions can be associated with disturbance of balance.

Detection of Movement   The **vestibular apparatus** is a collective term for the fluid-filled labyrinthine structures involved in the detection of movement. It includes **three semicircular canals,** which are arranged perpendicular to each other, as well as to the **utricle** and **saccule.** The semicircular canals are involved in the detection of **angular acceleration,** and the utricle and saccule are involved in the detection of **linear acceleration.**

Each semicircular canal responds maximally to movement in a specific plane. The lateral canal responds to head turning. The anterior canal responds to head nodding. The posterior canal responds to lateral head tilting. Vestibular detection of motion is direction specific and each canal is functionally related to its contralateral counterpart. Movement that causes increased activity in one canal will generally cause decreased activity in the corresponding contralateral canal. Lesions on one side of the vestibular system result in a subjective sensation of motion, called **vertigo.**

The physiologic basis for the detection of motion is very similar to the system previously described for the cochlea. In fact, the endolymph of the cochlear duct (scala media) is continuous with the endolymph of the vestibular structures. Motion is detected by **ciliated hair cells** bathed in endolymph. Movement of the head in space causes movement of endolymph within these structures (this is analogous to a turning glass of ice water in which the ice cubes turn at a different rate than the glass). This motion causes bending of hair cell cilia and subsequent altered conductance through their membrane ion channels. The hair cells of the semicircular canals are located in the ampulla of each canal, in the **crista ampullaris.** Hair cells of the utricle and saccule are similarly arranged in structures called **maculae.** Hair cells in the macula of the utricle respond to linear acceleration along the long axis of the body. Hair cells in the macula of the saccule respond to linear acceleration along the dorsoventral axis of the body.

Sensory Neurons   The primary vestibular sensory neurons are glutamatergic bipolar neurons in the **superior and inferior vestibular ganglia.** Their peripheral processes receive input from the vestibular hair cells. The central projections from these neurons make up the vestibular portion of the eighth nerve. They enter the skull at the internal auditory meatus and enter the brainstem near the cerebellopontine angle, at the pontomedullary junction. Most of these fibers terminate on secondary sensory neurons in the **vestibular**

nuclei. However, some of these fibers extend directly into the cerebellum through the inferior cerebellar peduncles.

Vestibular Nuclei There are four vestibular nuclei on each side of the brainstem **(superior, medial, lateral, and inferior vestibular nuclei).** They are located dorsolaterally in the caudal pons, in the floor of the fourth ventricle, and adjacent to the inferior cerebellar peduncle. Secondary sensory neurons within these nuclei project widely throughout the nervous system. They are reciprocally connected to each of their major targets, including the contralateral vestibular nuclei, the cerebellum, the spinal cord, and the nuclei controlling eye movement. There is also a minor projection to the thalamus. Conscious perception of vestibular information is thought to be mediated by the posterior insular cortex.

Vestibular Projections

Vestibulocerebellar system Fibers from the vestibular nuclei enter the cerebellum through the inferior cerebellar peduncles. Cerebellar efferents reach the vestibular nuclei via both the superior and the inferior cerebellar peduncle. This **vestibulocerebellar system** mediates equilibrium of the body and is involved in the control of eye movement. The cerebellum is discussed in greater detail in Case 13.

Vestibulospinal system The **vestibulospinal tracts** originate in the vestibular nuclei and project to all levels of the spinal cord. They help mediate the body's reflexive reactions to movement in space by activating primarily extensor (antigravity) muscles. This is the system that mediates the reaction to the feeling that one's chair is about to fall backward. There is also a separate vestibular projection to the cervical spinal cord through the **MLF,** which is involved in coordinating head movement with eye movement (e.g., making it possible to watch a tennis match).

Vestibulo-ocular system The vestibular nuclei receive input from the visual system and project to the nuclei controlling eye movement through the **MLF.** This system helps to coor-dinate eye movement with head movement to maintain the image of an object of interest focused on the fovea in the retina. As previously described, damage to the vestibular system on one side causes disequilibrium of vestibular input, which is interpreted as motion by the nervous system (vertigo). This results in compensatory slow eye movement opposite to the direction of perceived motion followed by rapid (saccadic) correction. This repetitive process is called **nystagmus.** Nystagmus is named for the direction of the fast phase by convention.

Testing the **vestibulo-ocular reflex (VOR)** is important in the evaluation of the comatose patient. This can be done by oculocephalic testing (if there is no head or neck trauma) or by caloric testing. Passive head turning in an unconscious patient should elicit reflexive movement of the eyes toward the contralateral side such that the direction of gaze remains fixed. This represents a positive **doll's eyes response** (referring to dolls with moving eyes). This terminology is confusing to those more familiar with dolls whose eyes are motionless and has been largely abandoned in favor of the term *VOR.* If intact, this reflex suggests that the brainstem is intact from the level of the vestibular nuclei at the pontomedullary junction up to the third and fourth nerve nuclei in the midbrain. When the VOR is absent, the eyes do not move as the head is turned and the direction of gaze changes. The VOR is normally suppressed in the awake patient, so the absence of the VOR either indicates an awake patient with an intact brainstem or a comatose patient with a brainstem lesion.

The VOR can also be evaluated by **caloric testing.** Cold water infusion into the ear creates a convection current within the semicircular canals on one side and the illusion of motion. The eyes will deviate toward the cold ear and a compensatory nystagmus will develop. The direction of the nystagmus (named for the fast phase) will be away from the cold ear. The opposite will occur with infusion of warm water. The mnemonic *COWS* (cold opposite, warm same) refers to the nystagmus, not to the direction of initial eye deviation.

Case Conclusion JW was diagnosed with a vestibulopathy, possible related to Ménière's disease. Audiology testing was performed and confirmed a mild degree of sensorineural hearing loss, which was more prominent on the right and consistent with the presumptive diagnosis of Ménière's disease. A low-salt diet was recommended because this has been reported to slow the progression of Ménière's disease in some cases. The patient will be followed clinically for signs of deterioration, which would require referral for surgical evaluation.

Thumbnail: Vestibular System

Vertigo		
	Peripheral	**Central**
Duration	Relatively short	Relatively long
Nausea	Severe	Moderate
Imbalance	Moderate	Severe
Hearing loss	Common	Rare
Induced nystagmus	Unidirectional Suppressed by fixation Latency up to 40 seconds	Variable direction Not suppressed by fixation No latency
Reproducible	Inconsistently	Consistently
Fatigable with therapy	More so	Less so
Recovery	Days to weeks	Months or longer
Other neurologic deficits	Rare	Common
Causes	Vestibular neuritis BPV Ménière's disease Post-traumatic Vestibular toxicity (especially aminoglycosides) Ramsey Hunt's syndrome Many others (more rare)	Migraine Stroke Tumors Familial

Key Points

▶ Semicircular canals are involved in the detection of angular acceleration.

▶ The utricle and saccule are involved in the detection of linear acceleration.

▶ BPV is shortest in duration (<1 minute) and associated with a particular provocative head position.

▶ Vertigo of Ménière's disease is short in duration (minutes) and is associated with ear fullness and hearing impairment.

▶ Vestibular neuritis is associated with spells of longer duration (minutes to hours) and may be provoked by movement but is not associated with a specific head position.

▶ Central vertigo lasts longer (days to months), is less likely to be episodic, and is far more likely to be associated with other neurologic deficits.

Questions

1. A 25-year-old female patient with a known history of MS presents with sudden onset of vertigo and tinnitus in the right ear. Where might her lesion be located?
   A. Right dorsolateral pons
   B. Cerebellum
   C. Right vestibular nuclei
   D. Right MLF
   E. Left MLF

2. A 56-year-old man complains of sudden onset of severe dizziness "like the room was spinning," which he first noted while checking his car tire pressure. His symptoms resolved quickly but recurred for several seconds when turning in bed this morning. He has no other symptoms and his hearing is normal. Where is the problem?
   A. Utricle
   B. Eighth nerve
   C. Vestibular nuclei
   D. Semicircular canal
   E. Saccule

3. You are asked to evaluate a patient who was found down and comatose. On CN testing, you note that several CN reflexes are absent. You decide to check cold calorics. You infuse cold water into the right ear and the eyes tonically deviate to the right, then a leftward nystagmus develops. Once this has resolved, you infuse cold water into the left ear. No response is seen. Which of the following is most likely affected.
   A. Pons on the left
   B. Pons on the right
   C. Midbrain on the left
   D. Midbrain on the right
   E. Inner ear on the right

4. A patient develops chronic vertigo after high doses of an aminoglycoside. Which of the following structures was affected?
   A. Utricle
   B. Saccule
   C. Semicircular canal
   D. Hair cells
   E. Eighth nerve axons

HPI: A 32-year-old female school teacher comes to your office for evaluation. She has been having episodic double vision for several days. She first noticed it while writing on her chalkboard and trying to look over her right shoulder at her class. It also occurs when she tries to back up her car. It has never occurred with central gaze. She has never experienced anything like this before and is otherwise healthy. You ask if she has had difficulty reading and she denies it.

PE: Her examination is remarkable for impaired left eye adduction on right lateral gaze with associated diplopia. All other extraocular movements are intact in both eyes. Interestingly, when you ask her to watch your finger as you move it closer to her face (vergence testing), both eyes adduct equally and diplopia is denied. Pupillary responses are intact bilaterally and her examination is otherwise unremarkable.

Thought Questions

- Does this patient have a peripheral or central lesion?

- What is the most likely structure to be involved?

- What functions are mediated by this structure?

Basic Science Review and Discussion

The patient presents with episodic diplopia in association with right lateral gaze. Although she is unable to adduct her left eye with right lateral gaze, the eye does adduct with vergence. This apparent paradox defines the deficit as an **internuclear ophthalmoplegia (INO)** and localizes the lesion to the left **MLF**. The MLF provides a functional connection between the pontine abducens nucleus on one side and the contralateral mesencephalic oculomotor nucleus, allowing for the coordination of conjugate eye movements.

Coordination of Horizontal Gaze Remember that extraocular movement is mediated by three CNs, two of which (third and fourth) are located in the midbrain and one of which (sixth) is located more caudally, in the pons. The **abducens nucleus** is located at the midpontine level and is relatively medial and dorsal within the pontine tegmentum. Its location beneath the floor of the fourth ventricle is anatomically analogous to the location of the third and fourth CN nuclei with respect to the cerebral aqueduct in the midbrain. Although these different CN nuclei have unique control over their respective muscles, their actions must be coordinated to maintain conjugate gaze. The pathway connecting these three CN nuclei, the **MLF,** allows for this coordination to take place. Brainstem regulatory fibers projecting down to the medulla and spinal cord are contained within a caudal extension of the MLF.

Whereas the **MLF** is needed for **coordination of lateral gaze,** it is not needed for vergence (bilateral medial rectus activation). Vergence is mediated within the midbrain and would not be affected by a pontine MLF lesion. This explains why this patient has impaired left eye adduction only on right

lateral gaze. The MLF runs along the dorsomedial aspect of the pontine and mesencephalic tegmentum and is so close to the midline that central lesions can sometimes cause a bilateral INO. Another important clinical syndrome to recognize is the **one-and-a-half syndrome.** This occurs when a single lesion affects both the abducens nucleus and the MLF on the same side. The result is a loss of ipsilateral abduction and an ipsilateral INO. Thus, the only horizontal gaze movement to remain intact is abduction in the contralateral eye. Think of the one-and-a-half syndrome as one in which three fourths of the horizontal gaze movements are lost and in which the lesion is on the same side as the most affected eye. Coordination of horizontal gaze is also facilitated by the **horizontal gaze center,** located adjacent to the abducens nucleus in the **PPRF.** The PPRF also can be involved in the one-and-a-half syndrome. Although it is important to recognize these clinical scenarios, the location of the lesions can also be determined by understanding the anatomy of the pons.

Pontine Anatomy

External features and cranial nerves The **basilar pons** makes up the central portion of the brainstem. It is bounded rostrally by the mesencephalon, caudally by the medulla, and dorsally by the fourth ventricle and cerebellum. It contains the continuation of both ascending and descending pathways. The major sensory and motor systems are discussed separately. Their location in the pons remains relatively similar to their location in other parts of the brainstem and spinal cord. One exception to this is the medial lemniscus. As it ascends through the pons, it shifts gradually from its medial location in the medulla to a more dorsolateral position, twisting like a ribbon. The pons also contains the nuclei of the fifth, sixth, seventh, and eighth CNs, portions of the reticular formation, and the ventral pontine nuclei. Figure 30-1 illustrates the location of some of the major structures one should be able to recognize.

The **fifth CN** is the only one to emerge from the surface of the basilar pons. Its sensory nucleus extends rostrally into the midbrain and caudally into the cervical spinal cord.

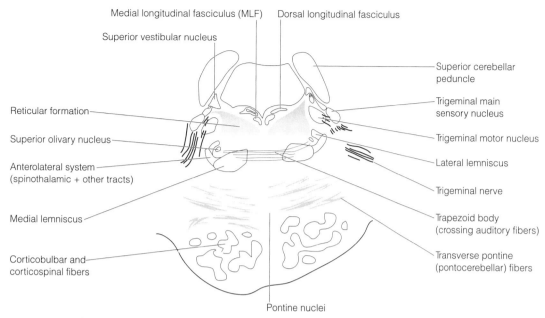

Figure 30-1 Mid-pons in cross section.

Nerve fibers exiting the **sixth nerve nucleus** travel caudally and ventrally to traverse the pontine tegmentum and exit the brainstem near the midline. Because they loop caudally before exiting the brainstem, these CN fibers are thought to have the longest intracranial course. The **seventh and eighth CNs** also exit from the border of the pons and the medulla. The sixth nerve (motor function) exits most medially, and the eighth nerve (sensory function) exits most laterally. The seventh nerve has both motor and sensory functions and exits between the other two. These CNs, their nuclei, and their associated systems have already been discussed in other cases. However, the present case uses conjugate eye movement as an example to emphasizes how different brainstem structures need to work in a coordinated manner.

Cerebellar connections The pons is a bulbous structure extending from the ventral surface of the midbrain. This bulge is caused by many small **pontine nuclei,** which are interspersed among the fascicles of the corticospinal and corticobulbar tracts. The primary function of the pons is as a relay station between the cerebrum and the cerebellum. Descending corticopontine fibers terminate onto the pontine nuclei. These nuclei then give off transverse fibers that decussate before ascending dorsally into the cerebellum through the **middle cerebellar peduncle,** the main cerebellar afferent pathway. Reciprocal cerebellar output exits primarily through the **superior cerebellar peduncle,** which decussates at the border between the pons and midbrain and represents the main cerebellar efferent pathway. **The inferior cerebellar peduncle (restiform body)** is also predominantly an afferent cerebellar pathway. It conveys information from the spinal cord and medulla. A small component of the inferior cerebellar peduncle **(juxtarestiform**

body) conveys cerebellar fastigial efferents, which project to brainstem nuclei. Cerebellar systems are discussed in more detail separately. However, the cerebellar peduncles and pontine nuclei are important to consider here because their injury in disorders of the pons manifests as ataxia.

Vascular supply of the pons Like other parts of the brainstem, the vascular supply to the pons can be divided broadly into **paramedian branches of the basilar artery, short circumferential branches,** and **long circumferential branches.** Different clinical syndromes are associated with disruption of these vessels. As a general rule, paramedian and short circumferential branches are implicated when weakness is present because motor systems tend to be concentrated ventromedially. Sensory disturbance with sparing of motor function, on the other hand, implicates longer circumferential branches. Involvement of facial sensation often implicates a more rostral level of dysfunction, whereas involvement of the sixth, seventh, or eighth nerve implicates a more caudal pontine process.

Internuclear ophthalmoplegia As previously mentioned, INO is caused by disruption of the MLF. The MLF provides a functional connection between the sixth CN nucleus on one side and the contralateral third CN nucleus. This communication allows for conjugate eye movement in the horizontal plane. The two most likely causes for small pontine lesions like this would be small-vessel ischemia and demyelinating disease. Mass lesions such as tumors or vascular malformations would be less likely. In our young female patient, demyelinating disease is most likely. A vascular etiology also would have to be considered, particularly if the patient had a history consistent with coagulopathy or connective tissue disease.

Case Conclusion   Routine laboratory studies were unremarkable. A hypercoagulability work-up also turned out to be unrevealing. An MRI of the head was obtained and revealed multiple brainstem and periventricular white matter lesions. The patient was admitted to the hospital for a course of IV methylprednisolone. A lumbar puncture was performed and CSF studies were consistent with a demyelinating process. The patient reported that she had had episodes of transient sensory and motor deficits over the past few years but was afraid to seek medical attention. The diagnosis of MS was made. An immunomodulatory agent was started in the out-patient setting.

Thumbnail: Pons

Midbrain and Pontine Syndromes

Midbrain syndromes	Structures	Deficits
Weber's	Third nerve; cerebral peduncle	Ipsilateral third nerve palsy; contralateral hemiparesis
Parinaud's	Superior colliculi; periaqueductal gray	Light-near pupillary dissociation; paralysis of upgaze
Pontine syndromes	**Structures**	**Deficits**
Medial (paramedian basilar artery branches)	Fascicles of pyramidal tract; cerebellar pathways; MLF; PPRF	Contralateral hemiparesis; ipsilateral ataxia; ipsilateral INO; horizontal gaze paresis
Lateral (AICA and long circumferential arteries)	Medial lemniscus; descending autonomic fibers; trigeminal nucleus; cerebellar pathways	Contralateral hemianesthesia; ipsilateral Horner's syndrome; ipsilateral facial hemianesthesia; ataxia
Caudal (short and long circumferential arteries)	Seventh nerve; sixth nerve; eighth nerve	Ipsilateral LMN facial palsy; ipsilateral lateral rectus palsy; ipsilateral deafness; vertigo
INO (small-vessel lacuna)	MLF	Ipsilateral adduction palsy on contralateral gaze
One-and-a-half syndrome (small-vessel lacuna)	Sixth nerve nucleus; MLF; PPRF	Ipsilateral lateral rectus palsy; ipsilateral INO; functionally, contralateral INO
Dysarthria, clumsy hand, and other small-vessel lacunae	Fascicles of pyramidal tract; pontocerebellar fibers	Partial corticospinal disorders occurring because pyramidal fascicles are separated by pontine nuclei, so only some affected
Locked-in syndrome	All motor systems; below pontine lesion	Retained awareness; retained eye movements; unable to speak or move

Key Points

▶ Crossed findings implicate the brainstem.

▶ Crossed findings involving the fifth, sixth, seventh, or eighth CN implicate the pons.

▶ Coordination of conjugate horizontal gaze is mediated by the MLF and PPRF.

▶ Vertigo and ataxia implicate the cerebellum, its peduncles, and/or the vestibular system.

▶ Pontine syndromes most commonly present with mixed long-tract, cerebellar, and CN findings.

Questions

1. A 73-year-old woman presents to the ED with sudden onset of left face and right extremity numbness. She is noted to be profoundly ataxic on examination. What other finding might one expect to find?

   A. Tongue deviation to the left
   B. Right eye deviated down and out
   C. Smaller pupil on the left
   D. Left eye deviated down and out
   E. Smaller pupil on the right

2. A 66-year-old man presents complaining of vision problems manifesting as double vision when he looks to the left. This has been going on for several hours. On examination, he fails to adduct the right eye on left lateral gaze. On right lateral gaze, his eyes do not cross the midline. His reading ability is relatively spared. What structures are involved?

   A. Left sixth nerve nucleus and right PPRF
   B. Right sixth nerve nucleus and left MLF
   C. Left sixth nerve nucleus and left MLF
   D. Right sixth nerve nucleus and right MLF
   E. Right sixth nerve nucleus and left PPRF

3. Branches from which of the following vessels would be affected in a patient with a pontine lacunar infarction?

   A. Basilar artery
   B. PICA
   C. AICA
   D. Vertebral artery
   E. SCA

4. Which of the following CNs would be least affected by a large lateral pontine demyelinating plaque?

   A. Facial nerve
   B. Abducens nerve
   C. Trigeminal nerve
   D. Trochlear nerve
   E. Vestibulocochlear nerve

HPI: You are asked to see HS, a 56-year-old truck driver, who awoke in his truck this morning with profound dizziness, several hours ago. He felt as though he was falling to the right. He reports that the room is still spinning. He is nauseated and has been vomiting. He has a history of mild hypertension, no diabetes, and he smokes two packs of cigarettes per day. He reports only chronic back and neck pain, which he attributes to his long hours on the road. This is usually responsive to ibuprofen. When his pain gets really bad, he sees a chiropractor.

PE: His BP is 176/94 mm Hg and remaining vital signs are stable. His speech is hoarse and slurred. He has nystagmus, which is most prominent on rightward gaze. He has ptosis on the right. His pupils are unequal (2 mm on the right and 5 mm on the left). He reports right-sided facial pain. He has full strength throughout but is clumsy in the right upper extremity. Pain and temperature sensation is impaired in the extremities on the left. He is able to stand with assistance but is easily pulled off balance and feels as though he will fall to the right.

Thought Questions

- What are the affected structures?
- Where are these structures located?
- Could a single lesion affect all of these structures?
- Where would that lesion be located?
- Does this area have a common vascular supply?

Basic Science Review and Discussion

Brainstem syndromes often involve both long tracts and CN nuclei. However, the CN and long-tract findings are often **crossed** so the CN deficit is ipsilateral to the lesion and the long-tract deficit is contralateral to the lesion. Also, because of the structures involved, brainstem syndromes are more likely than supratentorial lesions to present with disturbance of extraocular movement, LMN CN findings, ataxia, vertigo, or coma. Applying these rules to the presented case, the patient's symptoms localize to the right lateral medulla.

External Medullary Anatomy and Motor Pathways The medulla is the most caudal portion of the brainstem and represents a transition between spinal cord and brainstem anatomy. It has several distinctive external features. The **pyramids** are longitudinally arranged fascicles visible on the ventral surface, on either side of the midline. They contain the axons of cortical UMNs that make up the **corticospinal tract.** These fibers cross the midline at the **pyramidal decussation,** immediately rostral to the cervicomedullary junction. The **inferior olives** are oval protrusions located dorsolateral to the pyramids. They contain the inferior olivary nuclei, which project to the cerebellum via the **inferior cerebellar peduncles.**

Vascular supply to the medulla comes primarily from the two **vertebral arteries** and their branches. Medially, **paramedian branches** supply paramedian structures, like the pyramids. Each vertebral artery also has a relatively prominent medial branch that together with its contralateral counterpart, makes up the **anterior spinal artery.** The most prominent lateral branch of each vertebral artery is the **PICA.** It supplies the dorsolateral aspect of the medulla and part of the cerebellum. Other **circumferential branches** also supply the lateral medulla to some extent.

Sensory pathways The sensory pathways of the dorsal columns-medial lemniscus system are located dorsally in the medulla. Each **dorsal column** terminates in its associated nucleus. The **nucleus gracilis** is more medial, in the dorsal medulla (at the "top" of what was the neural tube during development). It receives the central projections of cervical and upper thoracic dorsal root ganglion neurons. The **nucleus cuneatus** is more lateral but still in the dorsal medulla. It receives the central projections of lower thoracic, lumbar, and sacral dorsal root ganglion neurons. Both of these nuclei convey sensory information regarding **vibration, proprioception, and light touch.** These nuclei give rise **to arcuate fibers** that cross the midline ventral to the central gray matter to form the ascending contralateral **medial lemniscus** in a location dorsal to the pyramidal tract. This major sensory decussation is located rostral to the pyramidal decussation. The **spinothalamic pathways,** which convey sensory information regarding pain, temperature, and crude touch, decussate within the spinal cord and ascend laterally through the brainstem. In the medulla, these fibers are located dorsolateral to the pyramidal tract, inferior olivary nuclei, and MLF. The **medial lemniscus** remains near the midline throughout the medulla but gradually rotates laterally and dorsally, joining the spinothalamic tracts in their dorsolateral location at the level of the pons.

Other medullary long tracts Three other long tracts in the medulla warrant discussion. The **MLF,** which plays an important role in mediating conjugate horizontal gaze, also extends into the medulla and spinal cord. It conveys infor-

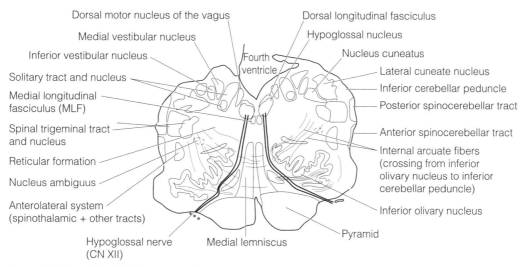

Figure 31-1 Rostral medulla in cross section.

mation from brainstem nuclei caudally. The MLF is located dorsolateral to the pyramidal tract. The **anterior and posterior spinocerebellar tracts** convey information from the spinal cord to the cerebellar vermis via the superior and inferior cerebellar peduncles, respectively. Both are located superficially on the lateral surface of the medulla, dorsolateral to the pyramidal tracts, and inferior olivary nuclei. Finally, the **spinal nucleus and tract of the trigeminal nerve** are located dorsal to the spinocerebellar pathways and ventral to the nucleus cuneatus. These relationships are illustrated in Figure 31-1.

Lower Cranial Nerves

Glossopharyngeal and vagus nerves: motor   The sixth, seventh, and eighth CNs emerge from the border between the pons and the medulla. They are discussed in Case 30. The **ninth (glossopharyngeal), tenth (vagus), and eleventh (spinal accessory) CNs** all exit as rootlets from the medulla just lateral to the inferior olive and medial to the inferior cerebellar peduncle. They are organized in numerical order from the most rostral (ninth) to the most caudal (eleventh). All three of these nerves exit the skull through the **jugular foramen.** The lower CNs share many common features, including many of the same CN nuclei. The vagus nerve provides all motor control to the muscles of the pharynx, larynx, and to the palatoglossus muscle of the tongue. The only pharyngeal muscle to receive innervation from the glossopharyngeal nerve is the stylopharyngeus muscle. The motor output for both of these nerves originates in the **nucleus ambiguous,** which is located between the spinal trigeminal nucleus and the inferior olivary nuclei. The nucleus ambiguous is in proximity to the hypoglossal nucleus, which controls motor function of most of the tongue muscles. Disruption of these nerves can lead to **hoarseness, dysarthria,** and **dysphagia.**

Glossopharyngeal and vagus nerves: autonomic   The ninth and tenth CNs also have **parasympathetic** components. The glossopharyngeal nerve provides preganglionic parasympathetic innervation from the **salivatory nucleus** to the otic ganglion, which then innervates the parotid gland. The vagus nerve provides preganglionic parasympathetic innervation from the **dorsal motor nucleus of the vagus nerve** to the smooth muscle and glands of the pharynx, larynx, thorax, and abdominal viscera proximal to the splenic flexure.

Glossopharyngeal and vagus nerves: sensory   The ninth and tenth CNs also have important sensory functions. Visceral sensation from the **carotid body** and **carotid sinus** is conveyed by the glossopharyngeal nerve to the **nucleus solitarius** via the inferior petrosal ganglion. Visceral sensation from larynx, trachea, esophagus, stretch receptors in the **aortic arch,** chemoreceptors in the **aortic bodies,** and the thoracic and abdominal viscera is conveyed by the vagus nerve to the nucleus solitarius via the inferior vagal ganglion. The nucleus solitarius, nucleus ambiguous, vagal dorsal motor nucleus, and surrounding reticular formation are thought to be important in the medullary control of respiratory and cardiovascular function.

Tactile, pain, and temperature information from the posterior one third of the tongue, the external ear, and the internal surface of the tympanic membrane is conveyed by the glossopharyngeal nerve to **the spinal nucleus of the trigeminal nerve** via the superior petrosal ganglion. Tactile, pain, and temperature information from skin behind the ear, external acoustic meatus, part of the external surface of the tympanic membrane, and the pharynx is conveyed by the vagus nerve to the spinal nucleus of the trigeminal nerve via the inferior and superior vagal ganglia. Finally, **taste** from the posterior one third of the tongue is conveyed by the glossopharyngeal nerve to the **nucleus solitarius** via the inferior petrosal ganglion. Note that with a few exceptions, the glossopharyngeal nerve has mostly sensory function.

Spinal accessory nerve   The eleventh CN is a pure motor nerve. It has a cranial portion and a spinal portion. The cranial portion originates in the nucleus ambiguous and joins the vagus nerve to provide innervation to the larynx. The spinal portion originates in the anterior horn of the upper cervical spine, enters the skull through the foramen magnum, and then joins the cervical portion to form the eleventh CN. The spinal portion of the eleventh CN innervates the ipsilateral sternocleidomastoid and upper trapezius muscles.

Hypoglossal nerve   The boundary between the pyramid and the olive forms a groove, or *sulcus.* The **twelfth CN (hypoglossal nerve)** is the only CN to emerge from this sulcus. Its only function is motor control of the tongue muscles. The hypoglossal nucleus is also a paramedian structure but is located more dorsally within the medullary tegmentum, in the gray matter beneath the floor of the fourth ventricle. Its fibers extend ventrally, traversing most of the medulla, to exit between the pyramidal tract and the inferior olivary nuclei. One of the hallmarks of LMN hypoglossal nerve dysfunction is **tongue deviation** to the side of the lesion with protrusion, caused by unopposed action of the contralateral **genioglossus muscle.** Thus, medullary lesions involving the hypoglossal nerve may present with ipsilateral tongue weakness and contralateral extremity hemiparesis (involvement of the pyramidal tract

above its decussation). In UMN lesions (e.g., internal capsule), the tongue weakness and extremity hemiparesis occur on the same side. This difference can be helpful in localizing the cause of hemiparesis.

Clinical Correlation   Altered pain and temperature sensation on the right side of the face and left extremities suggests a brainstem syndrome because of **crossed findings.** The right trigeminal nucleus or tract is involved below its decussation. Ascending spinothalamic fibers also are involved, but they decussate in the spinal cord. Vertigo and nystagmus implicate the vestibular nuclei and/or cerebellum. The cerebellum or cerebellar peduncles are also implicated by the tendency to fall to the right. Dysarthria, dysphagia, and hoarseness implicate the lower CNs and nuclei within the medulla. The eye findings can be misleading. The patient has a **Horner's syndrome.** This does not localize to the third nerve. Instead, it suggests disruption of the sympathetic system. Remember that sympathetic control begins in the hypothalamus and that these fibers pass through the brainstem on their way to the spinal cord. There is no prominent weakness, suggesting that the pyramidal system is spared. Thus, one would conclude that this is a **lateral medullary syndrome.** Also called the **Wallenberg syndrome,** this clinical presentation is one of the more commonly encountered brainstem syndromes. It is classically associated with a **PICA** occlusion but, in the clinical setting, a **vertebral artery** occlusion is far more common. Midline medullary structures, like the corticospinal tracts, are often spared because they receive blood from paramedian branches of the contralateral vertebral artery.

Case Conclusion   In the current case, the patient presented several hours after the onset of a lateral medullary syndrome. Elements of the history were suggestive of a vertebral artery dissection. Specifically, the recent chiropractic neck manipulation raises this possibility (an unusual but not rare complication). Neck trauma of any kind should always raise the suspicion of vertebral artery dissection. However, this patient had other potential etiologies as well. His smoking history and hypertension puts him at increased risk for small-vessel disease. His sedentary lifestyle and likely long hours of sitting in the same position should raise the possibility of deep vein thrombosis and paradoxical embolism. An MRI scan of the brain confirmed his lateral medullary infarction. A magnetic resonance angiography (MRA) of the neck confirmed vertebral artery dissection. The patient received supportive care, IV hydration, and anticoagulation.

Thumbnail: Medulla and Lower Cranial Nerves

Medullary Syndromes

Medullary syndromes	Structures	Deficits
Wallenberg's	Trigeminal nucleus or tract; ascending spinothalamic tract; vestibular nuclei and/or cerebellum; cerebellum or peduncles and lower CNs; descending sympathetics	Ipsilateral facial sensory deficit; contralateral hemianesthesia; vertigo and nystagmus; lateropulsion; dysarthria, dysphagia, hoarseness; ipsilateral Horner's syndrome
Jackson's, Vernet's, and Avellis'	Pyramid; lower CNs in various combinations	Contralateral hemiparesis; dysarthria, dysphagia, hoarseness; ipsilateral sternocleidomastoid, trapezius, and tongue weakness
Ventral medullary	Pyramid; ± twelfth CN	Contralateral hemiparesis; ± ipsilateral tongue

Key Points

▸ Crossed findings implicate the brainstem first.

▸ Vertigo and nystagmus implicate the vestibular nuclei and/or cerebellum.

▸ Dysarthria, dysphagia, and hoarseness implicate the lower CNs.

▸ A Horner's syndrome can be caused by lesions of the descending sympathetic fibers.

▸ Wallenberg's syndrome most often is associated with vertebral artery compromise.

▸ The nucleus ambiguous is the motor nucleus for CN IX, X, and XI.

▸ The hypoglossal nucleus is the motor nucleus for CN XII.

▸ Preganglionic parasympathetics of the ninth nerve originate in the salivatory nucleus.

▸ Preganglionic parasympathetics of the tenth nerve originate in the dorsal motor nucleus.

▸ Visceral sensory input carried by the ninth and tenth CNs goes to the nucleus solitarius.

▸ Tactile sensory input carried by the ninth and tenth CNs goes to the spinal trigeminal (CN V) nucleus.

Questions

1. You have determined that a 63-year-old woman has had a stroke. You note that she is weak in the extremities on the right. Her tongue deviates to the left. Her deficits include a lesion involving which of the following?

   A. Right UMN to the genioglossus muscle
   B. Right LMN to the genioglossus muscle
   C. Left UMN to the genioglossus muscle
   D. Left LMN to the genioglossus muscle
   E. Left MCA territory

2. You have determined that your patient has lost taste sensation over the posterior one third of the tongue on the left. Which structure receives this input?

   A. Nucleus ambiguous
   B. Nucleus solitarius
   C. Salivatory nucleus
   D. Dorsal motor nucleus
   E. Spinal trigeminal nucleus

3. A patient becomes quadriparetic following cerebral angiography. His facial strength is preserved. A branch of which of the following vessels has been compromised?

   A. Anterior cerebral artery
   B. Basilar artery
   C. Vertebral artery
   D. MCA
   E. PCA

4. You evaluated a suspected stroke patient. During the examination, you note left hemiparesis in both extremities. The tongue deviates to the left. Where is this patient's lesion?

   A. Medulla on the right
   B. Midline medullary process
   C. Internal capsule
   D. Spinal cord
   E. Medulla on the left

Case 22

1. B
2. A
3. C
4. D

Case 23

1. C
2. D
3. D
4. A

Case 24

1. C
2. C
3. B
4. E

Case 25

1. B
2. E
3. D
4. D

Case 26

1. B
2. C
3. D
4. C

Case 27

1. A
2. D
3. D
4. A

Case 28

1. D
2. A
3. E
4. D

Case 29

1. A
2. D
3. A
4. D

Case 30

1. C
2. D
3. A
4. D

Case 31

1. D
2. B
3. C
4. C

Part IV

Ventricles, Vasculature, and Meninges

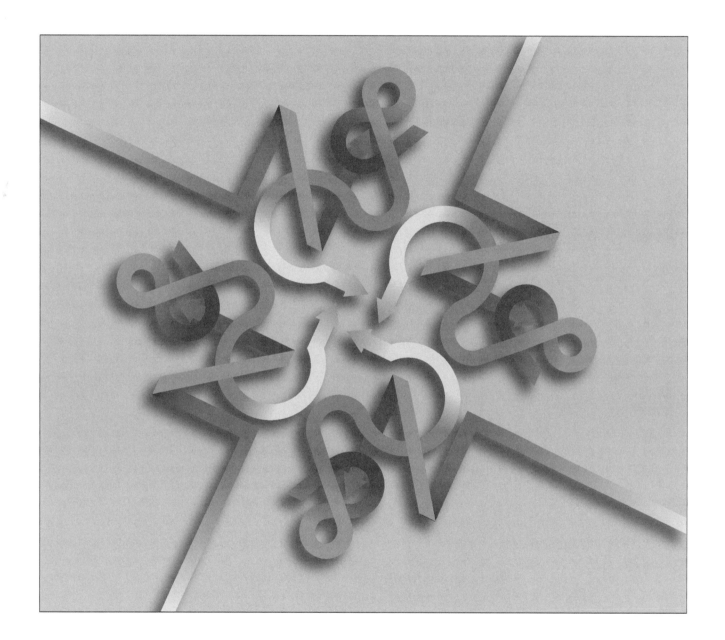

HPI: As a pediatrician, you are called to the nursery to evaluate a newborn baby boy. His mother presented to the ED the previous night in active labor; she had received no prenatal care and was unsure of her due date. The patient was delivered by cesarean section after an arrest of descent during labor. On delivery, he weighed 2800 grams but had a head circumference of 39 cm (>90th percentile).

PE: The patient's skull is markedly misshapen, the anterior fontanelle is bulging, the sutures are abnormally separated, tone is increased overall, and the baby seems less alert than normal. Imaging reveals very dilated lateral ventricles with compression of the gray matter; the cerebral aqueduct appears stenotic.

Thought Questions

- What is CSF?
- Where is CSF generated in the CNS?
- What is the path of CSF flow through the CNS?
- What pathologies can arise in the ventricular system?

Basic Science Review and Discussion

This baby has a noncommunicating hydrocephalus. Hydrocephalus is dilation of the ventricles, often seen with increased intracranial pressure (ICP) or increased CSF pressure. To correctly diagnose and treat hydrocephalus, one must understand the normal generation and flow of CSF, as well as ways in which normal flow is commonly altered.

Cerebrospinal Fluid The brain and spinal cord are cushioned by a fluid layer of **CSF.** CSF serves not only to mechanically cushion the CNS, but also to provide a well-regulated environment of electrolytes and also to wash away toxins to maximize function. Normally, CSF is clear. One way to determine the status of the CNS is to sample the CSF through a **lumbar puncture.** The presence of blood or bacteria in the CSF signifies pathology, such as hemorrhage or infection.

Ventricular System CSF is synthesized within hollow areas in the brain called **ventricles.** The walls of each ventricle are lined with a specialized tissue, **choroid plexus,** containing in-foldings of vessels covered by specialized cells. These **ependymal cells** have modified cilia, which aid in the secretion of CSF, as well as tight junctions, which form the blood-CSF barrier.

CSF circulation begins in the two **lateral ventricles.** The left and right ventricles communicate via the **interventricular foramina of Monro** with one central **third ventricle.** The third ventricle is at the midline, lying between the medial walls of the diencephalon. Fluid flows from the third ventricle through the **aqueduct of Sylvius** to the fourth ventricle. CSF leaves the brain from the fourth ventricle through two lateral

foramina of Luschka and the medial **foramen of Magendie.** (Remember: *l*ateral *L*uschka and *m*edial *M*agendie)

Once outside the brain and spinal cord, the CSF is contained between the pia mater and the arachnoid layer in the **subarachnoid space.** Pockets of CSF in this space exist normally; they are called **cisterns.** (It is a normal cistern that one samples when doing a spinal tap on a patient.) CSF leaves the CNS at the sagittal sinus, where arachnoid villi in the sinus wall absorb the fluid.

Clinical Correlation **Hydrocephalus** is dilation of the ventricles. Most often, it is the result of some dysfunction of normal CSF circulation. In newborns, hydrocephalus is present in approximately 1 per 1000 births, often the result of an anatomic abnormality or a perinatal infection, such as toxoplasmosis. Hydrocephalus can occur in patients of all ages for various other reasons.

There are two general forms of hydrocephalus: noncommunicating and communicating. **Noncommunicating hydrocephalus** occurs when there is an obstruction within the ventricular pathway. This causes CSF pressure within the ventricles to build up, eventually dilating the ventricles and compressing the gray matter. Noncommunicating hydrocephalus can result from causes such as mass lesions compressing any of the foramina or congenital aqueductal stenosis. In contrast, **communicating hydrocephalus** occurs when there is elevated CSF pressure not resulting from an obstruction in the ventricular pathway. This occurs when blockage in the subarachnoid space prevents normal flow and reabsorption of CSF outside the brain, such as with postmeningeal adhesions. In normal pressure hydrocephalus the ventricles dilate to accommodate increased CSF volume, making the CSF pressure as measured on a lumbar puncture appear normal. In this disease, more commonly seen in elderly patients, CSF is no longer absorbed normally by the arachnoid villi, often secondary to hemorrhage of the meninges. These patients are characterized by a triad of progressive dementia, ataxic gait, and incontinence (as in the mnemonic of the three *w*'s: "wacky, wobbly, and wet"). Generally, noncommunicating hydrocephalus should make one think of pathology within the brain, whereas communicating hydrocephalus indicates pathology around the brain.

Other less common forms of hydrocephalus have their own designations. Although they are rarer clinically, their definitions can be useful on the USMLE. **Hydrocephalus ex vacuo** refers to the apparently enlarged ventricles seen in patients with HD or degeneration of the caudate nucleus. Because tissue is lost as the basal ganglia atrophy, the space in this region fills with CSF, increasing the overall volume of the ventricles. **Pseudotumor cerebri,** also known as **benign intracranial hypertension,** is a syndrome seen most commonly in young, obese women. The syndrome's name refers to its presentation, which is easily mistaken for a brain tumor. In this disorder, the arachnoid villi develop increased resistance to CSF outflow, resulting in increased ICP and manifesting as papilledema, headache, and deteriorating

vision. On first inspection, this can be confused with the presentation of a mass lesion within the cranium.

Treatment for hydrocephalus is targeted at the primary cause of disease and at relieving ICP to maintain mental function and prevent permanent damage to gray matter. Mildly progressing cases may be treated with diuretics, which can lower ICP and alleviate symptoms. More severe cases require surgical intervention, most often ventriculoperitoneal shunting, in which a shunt is placed to drain CSF from the ventricles into the peritoneal cavity. This shunt is left in place to maintain normal ventricular pressure, although it may require replacement and adjustment in cases of obstruction or infection.

Case Conclusion The patient is evaluated by the neurosurgery team, who agree with your assessment of noncommunicating hydrocephalus. Because of the relatively severe and early presentation, surgical treatment is recommended. The patient receives a ventriculoperitoneal shunt and within days of surgery has normal cranial size with normal fontanelles and no deformity. The baby becomes much more alert and interactive with his environment after surgery, responding well to stimuli. He begins long-term care with a neurologist to follow his development and ensure continued function of the shunt.

Thumbnail: Ventricular System

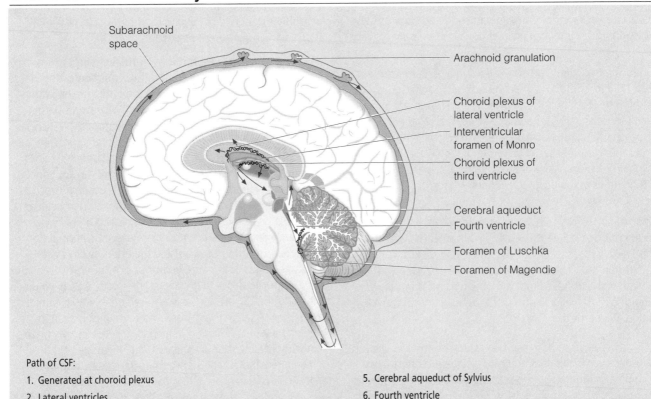

Path of CSF:

1. Generated at choroid plexus
2. Lateral ventricles
3. Interventricular foramina (of Monro)
4. Third ventricle

5. Cerebral aqueduct of Sylvius
6. Fourth ventricle
7. Foramen of Luschka (lateral) or Magendie (medial)
8. Subarachnoid space

Key Points

▸ CSF helps cushion the brain and spinal cord, maintain a balanced CNS environment, and wash away toxins.

▸ CSF is generated by ependymal cells of the choroid plexus.

▸ CSF flows from lateral to third to fourth ventricles, then to the subarachnoid space.

▸ Hydrocephalus is dilation of the ventricles, often with increased CSF pressure.

▸ Noncommunicating hydrocephalus occurs when an obstruction blocks the ventricular pathway; communicating hydrocephalus occurs when there is no block within the ventricles.

Questions

1. Which of the following pathologies could result in a noncommunicating hydrocephalus?
   A. HD
   B. Posterior fossa tumor
   C. Meningeal adhesions
   D. A and C
   E. All of the above

2. A 77-year-old man is brought to the ED by a visiting family member who found him confused and slightly disoriented. Assessment includes a lumbar puncture, which showed an opening pressure of 190 mm H_2O (normal range: 180 to 200 mm H_2O). Which of the following pathologies is likely given this information?
   A. Pseudotumor cerebri
   B. Bulky cerebral tumor
   C. Meningeal fibrosis secondary to subarachnoid hemorrhage
   D. A and C
   E. All of the above

3. A patient has a bulky posterior fossa tumor at the level of the midbrain, immediately inferior to the tentorium at midline. If it were to cause CSF obstruction, the patient would most likely have which of the following?
   A. Dilation of the lateral ventricles
   B. Dilation of the foramen of Magendie
   C. Dilation of the fourth ventricle
   D. Dilation of the third ventricle
   E. All of the above

4. Which of the following is the primary structure creating the blood-CSF barrier?
   A. Choroid plexus
   B. Modified cilia
   C. Tight junctions
   D. Arachnoid granulations
   E. Arachnoid villi

HPI: A 75-year-old woman who has not been able to speak or use her right side for the past hour is seen in the ED. She was at home with her family around 8 p.m. when she developed a droop on the lower right side of her face, then dropped a pen from her writing (right) hand. She slumped over to her right side and appeared unable to speak, although she retained consciousness. Her eyes were deviated to the left.
History is notable for hypertension and hypercholesterolemia.

PE: T 98.3°F   HR 92   BP 165/85   RR 15   SaO$_2$ 95% at room air
She is a bewildered elderly woman with a right lower facial droop and plegic right arm. She does not phonate or follow commands. She winces but does not move the right arm in response to painful stimuli, but abruptly and purposefully moves her right leg. Movement on the left side and the rest of her other CNs is unaffected.

Thought Questions

- Where is the lesion?

- What is the diagnosis?

- Why is her leg relatively spared?

Basic Science Review and Discussion

The Anterior Cerebral Circulation The anterior or **carotid** circulation is composed of the internal carotid arteries (ICAs), the circle of Willis, and the middle cerebral arteries (MCAs) and anterior cerebral arteries (ACAs).

The **ICAs** are relatively straightforward and do not have the multiple branches for which the external carotid arteries are well known. The important branch derived from the ICA is the **ophthalmic artery,** which supplies the optic nerve and retina. Internal carotid disease may thus cause inadequate blood flow to the retina, which may result in **amaurosis fugax** (transient monocular blindness). After giving off the ophthalmic branch, the ICA rises superiorly to join the circle of Willis, and metamorphoses into the MCA.

The **circle of Willis** is a circular ring of adjoining arteries ultimately supplied by the ICAs and the basilar artery (Figure 33-1). This circular connection allows compensation for vascular insufficiency on one side by allowing the other side's blood flow to cross over the midline. This is accomplished via the anterior and posterior communicating arteries (ACom and PCom). The **MCA**, originating from the circle of Willis, then forms multiple branches supplying the temporal lobe, the parietal lobe, and the superior and lateral aspects of the frontal lobe (Figure 33-2). Both the cortex and subcortical white matter are supplied by the MCA. The MCA also gives off perforating arteries, which supply the corona radiata, internal capsule, and much of the basal ganglia. The **ACA** runs anteriorly from the circle of Willis to supply the medial aspect of the frontal lobe, curving superiorly and posteriorly as it does so. It often runs posteriorly enough to supply the medial parietal lobe as well.

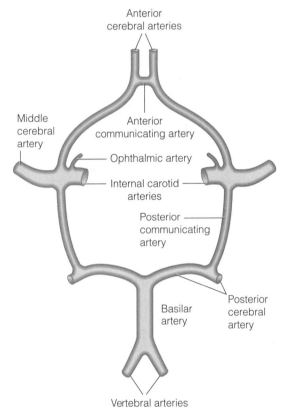

Figure 33-1 Circle of Willis (simplified).

The PCAs also originate from the circle of Willis and are discussed in Case 34.

Organization of the Cortex by Vascular Territory It is worthwhile to recognize which areas of the brain are supplied by which vessels, to recognize different types of strokes.

The **MCA** supplies the motor strip (precentral gyrus) pertaining to the face, trunk, and upper extremity, but not the leg. It also supplies the postcentral gyrus, which controls sensation in the same areas. The MCA supplies **the frontal eye fields,** which control conjugate horizontal eye

Of note, the **PCA** supplies the occipital lobes, which govern the contralateral hemifield of vision, as well as association visual cortex.

Clinical Discussion   This patient has had a **left MCA stroke** until proven otherwise. Her constellation of symptoms fit the areas of the cerebrum supplied by the left MCA: the motor cortex involving the face and arm (located laterally and superiorly, respectively) and Broca's and Wernicke's areas, resulting in a **global aphasia.**

The **language centers** of the cortex are located on the **left side** of the brain in more than 99% of right-handed patients (note that she was using her right hand to write). The sparing of her leg also suggests an MCA stroke. The motor cortex projecting to the leg is located on the medial aspect of the motor strip, which is supplied by the ACA and thus spared by MCA infarcts.

Differential Diagnosis   Other considerations should involve the motor system as well. A stroke of the left internal capsule or corona radiata will cause right-sided face and arm weakness but will often involve the leg because all the motor fibers of the internal capsule coalesce into a small area sharing the same vascular supply. Language involvement would also be less likely. A seizure that involved primarily the left frontal cortex, which was not witnessed, could result in plegia as a result of the postictal hypofunction of the cortex. This phenomenon has been described as **Todd's paralysis, and it usually resolves within 24 hours.** Hemorrhage of the left frontal lobe, as well as a subdural or epidural hematoma compressing primarily the left frontal lobe, might appear in similar fashion. A mass or tumor might compress or impinge on the frontal lobe, but this usually presents gradually rather than abruptly.

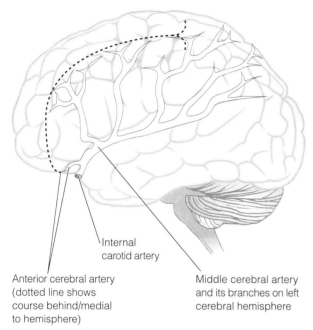

Internal
carotid artery

Anterior cerebral artery
(dotted line shows
course behind/medial
to hemisphere)

Middle cerebral artery
and its branches on left
cerebral hemisphere

Figure 33-2 Middle cerebral artery.

movement. Injuries to the frontal eye field result in a gaze preference **toward the side of the lesion; for example,** left MCA strokes cause patients to look toward the left. Perforating arteries from the MCA supply the basal ganglia and the anterior thalamus. The MCA also supplies the language centers: **Broca's area** in the posterolateral frontal lobe and **Wernicke's area** in the adjacent anterior temporal lobe.

The **ACA** supplies the medial aspect of the motor strip and the medial aspect of the sensory strip in the parietal lobe. These areas control motor function and sensation of the lower extremity, respectively.

Case Conclusion   Thankfully, head CT showed no hemorrhage, and the patient was given IV tissue plasminogen activator (TPA). IV TPA may be given up to three hours after the onset of symptoms in stroke patients without evidence of hemorrhage. She began to regain some use of her right arm and began to follow commands. Head MRI demonstrated infarct in the left frontal, temporal, and parietal cortices, with sparing of the medial frontal lobe and occipital lobe (ACA and PCA territories, respectively).

Thumbnail: Anterior Circulation

Vessel	Territory supplied	Ischemic syndrome
ICA/ophthalmic artery	Retina	Amaurosis fugax (transient monocular blindness)
MCA	Lateral motor strip	Contralateral face and arm weakness
	Lateral sensory strip	Contralateral face and arm anesthesia
	Internal capsule	Contralateral face, arm, leg weakness
	Frontal eye fields (frontal lobe)	Gaze preference toward affected side
	Broca's area (frontal lobe)	Expressive (motor) aphasia
	Wernicke's area (temporal lobe)	Receptive (sensory) aphasia
ACA	Medial motor and sensory strips	Contralateral leg weakness and anesthesia

Key Points

- ▶ The anterior circulation (internal carotid system) serves the retina, frontal lobe, parietal lobe, temporal lobe, internal capsule, and basal ganglia via the MCA and the ACA.
- ▶ Anterior circulation stroke syndromes may be discerned by involvement of the leg (ACA territory) and the development of aphasias (suggests cortical involvement).
- ▶ The circle of Willis allows blood supply from any of its supply vessels to run to any of its outflow vessels.

Questions

1. A 72-year-old man is brought in by his family for "not speaking right." Starting 2 days ago, his children noticed that he tends to put inappropriate words together or makes up words that do not exist (paraphasias). He also does not seem to understand everything that they tell him. Upon examination, you notice a subtle right lower facial droop and weakness of the right arm. He has no difficulty walking. What is a head CT most likely to show?
   A. Infarction of Wernicke's area (left anterior temporal lobe) and the left motor cortex
   B. Brainstem infarct involving left facial nucleus and hypoglossal nucleus
   C. Infarction of Broca's area (left lateral frontal lobe) and left motor cortex
   D. Left ACA infarct
   E. Right posterior frontal lobe infarct with some involvement of parietal and temporal lobes

2. A 36-year-old right-handed healthy woman develops abrupt difficulty in producing words, essentially becoming completely mute over the course of a few minutes. Motor function and comprehension are retained. She takes oral contraceptives and is an avid smoker. Her medical history is notable only for a patent foramen ovale. What is the most likely cause?
   A. Paradoxical fat embolism to left temporal lobe, causing embolic infarct
   B. Thromboembolism to left posterior frontal lobe, causing embolic infarct
   C. Right frontal lobe hemorrhage
   D. Acute right internal carotid occlusion
   E. Septic emboli to left parietal lobe, causing hemorrhagic infarct

3. An 85-year-old man complains of the complete inability to see out of the left eye for the past 15 minutes. He describes a "shade" or "blind" that appeared to abruptly cover his vision. Vision of the right eye is relatively unaffected. Physical examination shows a pale retina on the left side. What is the most likely explanation?
   A. Ocular migraine
   B. Acute left ophthalmic artery occlusion
   C. Acute right occipital lobe infarct
   D. Acute left occipital lobe infarct
   E. Elevated ICP

4. A 79-year-old woman is noticed in the nursing home to have difficulty using her right leg over the past several days. She does not complain of any pain. The leg's appearance has not changed. She has diffuse weakness affecting both flexors and extensors in both the thigh and the leg, as well as the foot. What is the most likely diagnosis?
   A. Left ACA occlusion
   B. Pelvic mass impinging on right sciatic and femoral nerves
   C. Left MCA occlusion
   D. ACom occlusion
   E. Left deep femoral venous thrombosis

> **HPI:** RS is a 63-year-old right-handed man with a history of tobacco use, diabetes, and atrial fibrillation. He has had two myocardial infarctions. He is brought to the ED because his wife can no longer control his behavior. Over the past 2 days, he has become progressively more argumentative. He insists that his wife must stop contradicting his mother. However, the wife reports that his mother passed away many years ago. He states that he does not want to be evaluated because "you can't trust those doctors," but she has talked him into this visit. Since this morning, he has been more confused. He has been falling and has been unable to get up on his own power. He reports that he has been seeing double all day.
>
> **PE:** His BP is 189/100 mm Hg. His examination is remarkable for a homonymous left visual field deficit when each eye is tested separately. He has ptosis on the right. His right pupil is deviated downward and laterally. He has bilateral impairment of upward gaze. His reflexes are symmetric and his toes are up-going bilaterally.

Thought Questions

■ What structures are responsible of each of the symptoms?

■ How are they anatomically related?

■ What is their vascular supply?

■ Could a single lesion cause all of these deficits?

Basic Science Review and Discussion

The posterior circulation of the brain and brainstem covers a large territory containing varied structures and pathways. However, a systematic approach to the vascular territories and functional systems can help to localize lesions and define clinical syndromes. This patient has a right homonymous hemianopsia, implicating the left visual cortex or optic tract. He has a right third nerve palsy but also has bilateral impairment of upward gaze. He has bilateral long-tract signs. He is also confused, agitated, and delusional. This combination of findings can initially appear confusing. However, a systematic review can identify a single lesion at the top of the basilar artery. This case focuses on the posterior circulation of the brain and brainstem, which is derived from the vertebral arteries, the basilar artery, and their branches. The posterior circulation is connected to the anterior circulation through the circle of Willis. The anterior circulation is discussed in Case 33.

Vertebral Arteries

Cervical portion Each **vertebral artery** originates from the proximal portion of the corresponding **subclavian artery.** They ascend and move posteriorly, entering the cervical vertebrae for which they are named in the midcervical region. From this point, they continue to ascend through the transverse foramina of each of the upper cervical vertebrae. The vertebral arteries are particularly susceptible to damage

resulting from neck injury because of their proximity to the cervical vertebrae. Abrupt turning movements of the neck, as may be seen even with mild trauma or chiropractic cervical manipulation, can sometimes lead to **vertebral artery dissection** (tearing of the intimal layer of the arterial wall, leading to obstruction and/or formation of emboli) and **posterior circulation infarctions.** Throughout the neck, the vertebral arteries give off **spinal branches** to the spinal cord, as well as branches to the soft tissues of the neck. At the atlanto-occipital junction, they turn medially across the superior surface of the atlas and then enter the skull and penetrate the dura mater through the foramen magnum. Each gives off a **posterior meningeal branch** in this area.

Cranial portion The vertebral arteries enter the posterior fossa through the foramen magnum and course along the ventrolateral aspects of the medulla oblongata. Although many branches come off of the vertebral arteries, they can be divided broadly into three categories. (1) Medial branches provide blood supply to the most ventral and medial aspects of the neuraxis. The largest of these are the two branches (one from each vertebral artery) that come together to form the **anterior spinal artery.** It courses caudally in the midline, along the ventral aspect of the spinal cord. Small **paramedian branches** of the vertebral arteries and anterior spinal artery represent the primary vascular supply to the pyramidal tracts and overlying paramedian portions of the medulla (medial lemniscus, MLF, hypoglossal nucleus). Lateral branches from the vertebral arteries can be further divided into short circumferential branches and long circumferential branches. (2) The (unnamed) **short circumferential branches** provide the vascular supply to the ventrolateral aspects of the medulla. (3) The **long circumferential branches** provide the vascular supply to the dorsal and dorsolateral aspects of the medulla, the dorsal spinal cord, and the ventrocaudal cerebellum. The two most important lateral branches of the vertebral arteries are the **posterior spinal artery** and the **posterior inferior cerebellar artery (PICA).** In addition to supplying the dorsal spinal cord and posterior inferior cerebellum, respectively, small branches from these important arteries supply the dorsal and dorsolateral medulla. One of the most important eponymous brainstem syndromes, the **lateral medullary syndrome of Wallenberg,** is classically attributed to occlusion of the PICA on one side. This syndrome is described separately in detail. In practice, a vertebral artery occlusion is more likely to be seen in the context of Wallenberg's syndrome.

Basilar Artery   The two vertebral arteries join at the pontomedullary junction, near the midline, to form the **basilar artery.** The basilar artery continues along the ventral aspect of pons, up to the level of the midbrain. Branches from the basilar artery supply the pons, the midbrain, the remainder of the cerebellum, and the posterior and inferior portions of the diencephalon (thalamus, hypothalamus) and cerebral hemispheres. As was the case with branches from the vertebral arteries, branches of the basilar artery can be divided broadly into (1) **paramedian,** (2) **short circumferential,** and (3) **long circumferential branches.** As a general rule, paramedian branches supply predominantly motor structures, which are more medial. Circumferential branches, on the other hand, supply predominantly sensory structures, which tend to be located dorsolaterally. These vascular territories help define the symptoms associated with brainstem stroke syndromes. Rather than trying to remember a long list of symptoms for each syndrome, ask yourself what the involved vascular territory might be. Then consider the CNs and long tracts that are likely to be involved.

Lower and middle branches   **Paramedian branches** of the basilar artery supply the corticospinal and corticobulbar fibers of the ventral pons, as well as the pontine nuclei interspersed among them. **Short circumferential branches** of the basilar artery supply more lateral aspects of the ventral pons, including pontocerebellar fibers, ascending sensory pathways, and descending sympathetic fibers that project from the hypothalamus to preganglionic autonomic neurons in the spinal cord. **Long circumferential branches** of the basilar artery supply dorsal and dorsolateral portions of the pons, including structures in and near the floor of the fourth ventricle. These structures include nuclei of the pontine CNs, portions of the cerebellar peduncles, and portions of the ascending sensory pathways. As in the medulla, one can predict the clinical manifestations associated with disruption of each of the pontine vascular territories based on the affected structures.

The basilar artery also gives off several important large paired branches. Beginning at the caudal end, the first branch is the **anterior inferior cerebellar artery (AICA).** The AICA supplies portions of the inferior aspect of the cerebellum and portions of the cerebellar peduncles and contributes to the supply of the dorsolateral pons. The **labyrinthine artery** originates immediately rostral to the AICA and supplies the structures of the inner ear. Small and unnamed

pontine branches dominate the midbasilar region. The basilar artery ends at the level of the midbrain.

Terminal branches   The basilar artery gives off another pair of large, important branches, the **superior cerebellar arteries (SCAs),** at the level of the midbrain. The SCA supplies the remainder of the cerebellum. The basilar artery then bifurcates into the right and left **posterior cerebral arteries (PCAs).** The PCA supplies the posterior and inferior aspects of the cerebral hemispheres, including ventral temporal lobe and most of the visual cortex in the occipital lobe. Each PCA also receives flow from the anterior circulation via its corresponding posterior communicating artery (PCom). It is important to note that the third CN passes between these two vessels as it exits the midbrain. Mass lesions in this area, such as an aneurysm involving either of these arteries (or more likely the PCom), can compress the third nerve and cause an isolated **third nerve palsy.** Penetrating branches from these large vessels supply most of the diencephalon including the hypothalamus, the subthalamus, and the thalamus. The most prominent branch of the PCA is the **posterior choroidal artery,** which supplies the posterior aspect of the thalamus, the pineal gland, and the choroids plexus of the third ventricle and inferior portions of the lateral ventricles.

As was the case for the medulla and the pons, the vascular supply of the midbrain itself can be divided broadly into (1) **paramedian,** (2) **short circumferential,** and (3) **long circumferential branches.** These penetrating branches are derived from all of the large vessels discussed earlier (basilar artery, SCA, PCA, PCom). The paramedian branches supply the most medial portions of the cerebral peduncles, the occulomotor nuclear group, and portions of the red nucleus and substantia nigra. Infarction in this territory results in another important brainstem syndrome. **Weber's syndrome** is characterized by unilateral third nerve palsy with associated contralateral hemiplegia. It is discussed in more detail in Case 25. Short circumferential branches supply more lateral aspects of these same structures. Long circumferential branches supply the midbrain tectum. Infarction in this territory can lead to Parinaud's syndrome and restricted upgaze, as seen with the patient in the present case.

Top-of-the-basilar syndrome   RS had findings that were localized to many areas, including the visual cortex, midbrain, and diencephalon. Although relatively nonspecific, the altered mentation was most likely related to thalamic involvement. Several of the thalamic subnuclei are interconnected with the limbic system and prefrontal cortex. They are involved in the modulation of emotional behavior and the coordination of that behavior with sensory experience. The term **peduncular hallucinosis** is used to describe the confusion often associated with the top-of-the-basilar syndrome. The clinical manifestations of this syndrome can vary dramatically, depending on the location and extent of the lesion and the presence of collateral vascular supply to critical areas.

Case Conclusion Shortly after presentation, the patient became comatose and required intubation. CT angiography confirmed occlusion of the distal basilar artery. Although the exact time of symptom onset could not be defined, the prognosis in the absence of intervention was felt to be poor. The endovascular team was activated and intra-arterial thrombolysis was performed. Blood flow was restored. Follow-up MRI scans confirmed a large region of infarction involving the midbrain, thalami, and left visual cortex. The patient remained comatose, requiring extensive supportive care. The prognosis remained grim and the family decided to withdraw supportive measures.

Thumbnail: Posterior Circulation

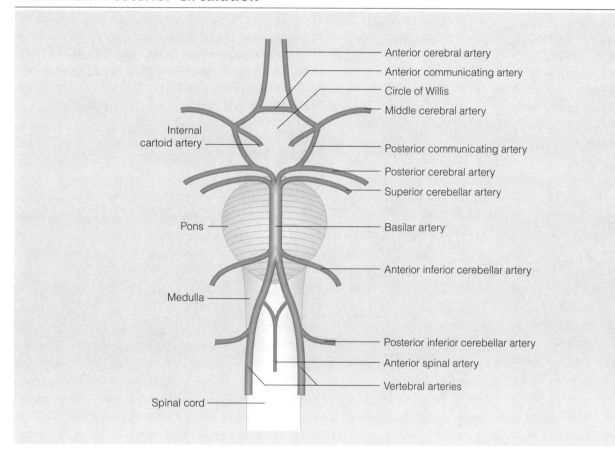

Key Points

▶ Within the posterior circulation, vascular territories can be broadly defined on the basis of paramedian, short circumferential, and long circumferential branches.

▶ Paramedian branches supply predominantly motor structures.

▶ Short circumferential branches supply predominantly ventrolateral tracts and intrinsic nuclei.

▶ Long circumferential branches supply dorsal and dorsolateral structures.

▶ Large, named branches contribute to these territories.

Questions

1. A 60-year-old man has a right vertebral artery occlusion. Which of the following symptoms is he most likely to have?

   A. Right-sided weakness
   B. Loss of pain and temperature on the left
   C. Left-sided Horner's syndrome
   D. Left-sided weakness
   E. Loss of pain and temperature on the right

2. A 73-year-old woman has complete loss of sensation on the left (hemianesthesia) involving the face, arm, trunk, and leg equally. She has full strength. Which artery is most likely involved?

   A. Left vertebral artery
   B. Right PCA
   C. Right vertebral artery
   D. Left PCA
   E. Basilar artery

3. A 67-year-old man has had sudden loss of vision in his right visual field. Which arterial distribution is most likely involved?

   A. Left vertebral artery
   B. Right PCA
   C. Right vertebral artery
   D. Left PCA
   E. Basilar artery

4. A 45-year-old man presents with right-sided weakness. His symptoms quickly resolve to the point at which his only objective neurologic deficit is a mild degree of finger-to-nose dysmetria on the right. His MRI scan reveals a rather large new infarction. Which vascular territory is most likely affected?

   A. Left vertebral artery
   B. Right PICA
   C. Right vertebral artery
   D. Left MCA
   E. Left PICA

HPI: BM is a 45-year-old right-handed man who collapsed while jogging in the desert today. He normally runs 15 miles every other day. Today was a particularly hot day. He has been stabilized in the ED. Rehydration has been initiated, but he remains unresponsive. When he was found, he complained of severe headache.

PE: He does not respond to voice, he withdraws to noxious stimulation but does so more briskly on the right, his CN reflexes are intact, and he has bilateral Babinski's signs.

Thought Questions

■ What structures are responsible of each of the symptoms?

■ How are they anatomically related?

■ What is their vascular supply?

■ Could a single lesion cause all of these deficits?

Basic Science Review and Discussion

The presence of lateralized findings on the neurologic examination implicates the CNS. The level of consciousness suggests that both cerebral hemispheres may be affected, although the left hemisphere seems more involved. In cases with such acute presentation, a vascular cause must be considered first. Given the apparent dehydration, one would suspect the possibility of a **dural venous sinus thrombosis.** Venous drainage of the brain and brainstem can be broadly divided into the dural venous sinuses and the veins that drain into them. This case focuses on the dural venous sinuses themselves. The cerebral veins that drain into the dural sinus system are discussed further in Case 36. The cavernous sinus is considered in more detail in Case 37.

Dural Sinus System   The vessels and sinuses that mediate venous drainage of the brain can be divided into those vessels draining superficial cortical regions and those draining deep regions. As a general rule, superficial regions of the cerebrum are drained by the superior sagittal sinus and the cavernous sinuses. The deeper regions of the cerebrum are drained by a system of lesser known veins and sinuses. The fundamental difference between the dural sinuses and the cerebral veins is that the veins drain the brain parenchyma and travel through the subarachnoid and subdural spaces, whereas the venous sinuses are all intradural. Dural sinuses are contained between the **periosteal and meningeal layers** of the **dura mater.** The dural venous sinuses are firm structures. They are lined with endothelium, and unlike systemic veins, they lack valves. They are located along the large fissures of the brain. Most of the dural sinuses drain posteriorly toward the **confluence of the sinuses** near the occipital pole

or inferiorly toward the **jugular veins.** The dural sinuses are a **low-pressure system** with slow-moving blood. They are susceptible to congestion and thrombosis during hypercoagulable states. Sinus thrombosis should always be considered in the setting of headache in such patients. **Dehydration, pregnancy, oral contraceptives,** and **tobacco** are all associated with hypercoagulability and are often favored in test questions.

Superficial drainage   The largest of the dural venous sinuses, the **superior sagittal sinus,** is located within the **falx cerebri** along the superior aspect of the interhemispheric fissure. It is the most likely sinus to be affected by thrombosis in the clinical setting. The superior sagittal sinus receives blood from the superficial cerebral veins. It also receives venous blood from the scalp through **emissary veins** that penetrate the skull. Along its course, the superior sagittal sinus also receives CSF from the subarachnoid space via **arachnoid granulations** that penetrate the meningeal layer of the dura mater. The function of the arachnoid granulations is discussed in further detail within the context of CSF flow and the ventricular system. The superior sagittal sinus is smaller anteriorly, in the area of the prefrontal cortex, and gets larger posteriorly. It terminates posteriorly at the **confluence of the sinuses,** in the **tentorium cerebelli** near the occipital pole.

Deep drainage   The **inferior sagittal sinus** is parallel to its superior counterpart but drains deeper cerebral tissue. It also is contained within the **falx cerebri** but is located more deeply within the interhemispheric fissure and is situated along the superior surface of the corpus callosum. The **great cerebral vein of Galen** drains even deeper tissue. The inferior sagittal sinus and the vein of Galen come together to form the **straight sinus** at the anterior boundary of the **tentorium cerebelli.** The straight sinus continues posteriorly, through the tentorium cerebelli, to the confluence of the sinuses. Thus, all venous drainage from superior aspects of the cerebrum arrives at the confluence of the sinuses via the superior sagittal sinus and the straight sinus.

The **transverse sinuses,** one on each side, drain blood laterally from the confluence of the sinuses toward the jugular veins. They are the second most likely sinuses to be affected by thrombosis. They are usually asymmetric, and in most people, the right one is larger. The transverse sinuses follow the contour of the skull, along the tentorium cerebelli, between the cerebral and cerebellar hemispheres. At the boundary between the occipital and petrosal bones, the transverse sinus is joined by the **superior petrosal sinus** to form the sigmoid sinus. The **sigmoid sinus** curves inferiorly, medially, then inferiorly again and is joined by the **inferior petrosal sinus** at the jugular foramen to form the **jugular vein.**

Clinical Correlation Dural venous sinus thrombosis is most commonly associated with hypercoagulability related to either intrinsic or acquired processes. Some of the more commonly encountered clinical situations include dehydration, pregnancy, oral contraceptive use, and tobacco use. Thrombosis can also occur in association with infections and direct infection spread. Frontal sinusitis can lead to superior sagittal sinus thrombosis. Sphenoid sinusitis can lead to **cavernous sinus thrombosis.** This important clinical condition is discussed further in Case 37. The most common presenting symptom is headache. Altered mentation and nausea are also seen often. Other symptoms vary, depending on the sinus involved and the extent to which the adjacent brain parenchyma is affected. Diagnosis is on a clinical basis and is supported by venography. The most important differential considerations are cerebral infarction or hemorrhage on an arterial basis. Dural sinus thrombosis can cause ischemia and infarction of adjacent tissue. Hemorrhage can also occur in these areas. Treatment is primarily with heparin anticoagulation and rehydration, although the use of anticoagulation in the setting of hemorrhage is somewhat controversial. If there is no hemorrhage, endovascular thrombolysis may be beneficial.

Case Conclusion   An emergent CT scan of the head was performed and revealed no evidence of hemorrhage. A magnetic resonance venogram was performed and confirmed thrombosis of the superior sagittal sinus. Heparin therapy and rehydration were initiated. The patient was seen by the endovascular service and endovascular thrombolysis was performed. Venous flow was restored. The patient gradually recovered full function, after a prolonged period of rehabilitation.

Thumbnail: Dural Venous Sinuses

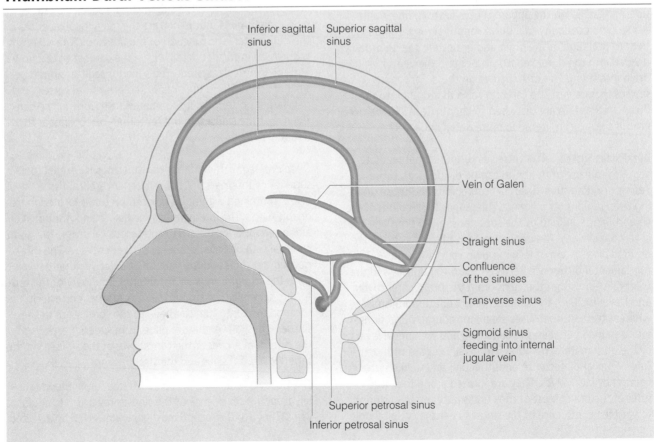

Key Points

▶ Cerebral veins and dural venous sinuses mediate venous drainage of the cerebrum.

▶ Venous drainage of the cerebrum can be divided broadly into superficial and deep regions.

▶ Dural sinus thrombosis occurs in the setting of hypercoagulability.

▶ The most common presenting symptom of sinus thrombosis is headache.

▶ The sinuses most likely to be affected by thrombosis are the superior sagittal and the transverse sinuses.

Questions

1. A 58-year-old woman presents to your office complaining of a severe headache that has been troubling her for the past week. Over the past 24 hours she has developed ringing in the right ear and severe positional vertigo. Which structure might be involved?
   A. Superior sagittal sinus
   B. Inferior sagittal sinus
   C. Transverse sinus
   D. Cavernous sinus
   E. Vein of Galen

2. A 23-year-old woman presents for evaluation of a severe headache that developed gradually over 5 days. She reports that this morning she found she is unable to walk because of weakness in both legs. What is the most likely vessel to be involved?
   A. Sigmoid sinus
   B. Transverse sinus
   C. Middle cerebral vein
   D. Superior sagittal sinus
   E. Vein of Rosenthal

3. A 68-year-old diabetic man presents to your office complaining of a severe head and eye pain on the right. He is proptotic on the right. Which structure might be involved?
   A. Superior sagittal sinus
   B. Inferior sagittal sinus
   C. Transverse sinus
   D. Cavernous sinus
   E. Vein of Galen

4. A 32-year-old female smoker who is taking oral contraceptives collapsed after the sudden onset of a headache. Her examination reveals UMN findings on the left. A CT scan of the head confirms hemorrhage on the right. A venous occlusion is suspected. In which space has the blood collected?
   A. Intraparenchymal
   B. Subarachnoid
   C. Subdural
   D. Epidural
   E. Intradural

HPI: VM is a 75-year-old right-handed woman who has been getting progressively more confused over the past 3 weeks. Her family reports that she is no longer able to care for herself. She was previously highly functioning, with no evidence of dementia. She is only minimally cooperative with your examination. She has poor comprehension and non-sensical speech. She does not appear to move her right side as well as her left, although formal power testing is not possible. She has an up-going toe on the right. When you ask family members about trauma history, they report that she did fall off of a chair while adjusting a painting last month. She struck her head at that time but did not lose consciousness. She declined a medical evaluation at that time.

Thought Questions

- What structures are responsible for her signs and symptoms?

- How are they anatomically related?

- What is their vascular supply?

- What is their venous drainage?

Basic Science Review and Discussion

This elderly patient has a subacute encephalopathy that has developed over several weeks. Although many metabolic or structural processes could be responsible, the hemiparesis and the history of head injury raise the possibility of a **subdural hemorrhage.** Subdural hemorrhages are divided into acute and chronic categories on the basis of their clinical features. **Acute subdural hemorrhages** must accumulate quickly to present acutely. They generally occur in the setting of more severe trauma and often are associated with other injuries such as subarachnoid hemorrhage, skull fracture, and cerebral contusion. **Chronic subdural hemorrhages** are more commonly encountered in the elderly. Brain volume loss resulting from generalized atrophy can expose **cerebral bridging veins** to more potential shearing forces during traumatic impacts. There is also more room for subdural hemorrhages to accumulate slowly over days or weeks before causing significant clinical impairment. The clinical manifestations vary but usually include **altered mental status** and **focal findings** related to the region of cortex being compromised.

Bridging Veins Many of the veins draining the cerebrum are contained within the subarachnoid space. **Bridging veins** emerge from the cerebral veins in the subarachnoid space and penetrate the **arachnoid mater** and inner layer of **dura mater** to reach **the dural venous sinuses.** They "bridge" the subdural space, a potential space, to reach their targets. These vessels are particularly vulnerable to **shearing forces** because they are relatively mobile near their origin and their dural end is relatively fixed. Shearing forces can be produced

even with relatively mild trauma, tearing these vessels. When these vessels are torn, blood accumulates within the subdural space. This causes a crescentic **subdural hemorrhage.** As the hemorrhage grows, the underlying cortex can be compressed, leading to focal neurologic deficits.

A subdural hemorrhage tracks easily between the dura mater and the arachnoid mater, following the contour of the brain. When viewed on axial (horizontal) imaging studies, subdural hemorrhages do not cross the midline, which is defined by the **falx cerebri** (an extension of the dura mater). This is in contrast to an **epidural hemorrhage,** which can cross the midline because it is superficial to the dura mater. Blood does not track easily through the epidural space and requires higher pressure to accumulate. In general, epidural hemorrhages are arterial (particularly middle meningeal artery) and subdural hemorrhages are venous. Subarachnoid hemorrhages are most often seen in the setting of trauma or aneurysm rupture.

Cerebral Veins

Superficial cerebral veins The **cerebral veins** can be divided into superficial and deep subgroups. Both groups drain into the dural venous sinus system. They are similar to the dural sinuses in that they do not have valves. The superficial veins drain the cerebral cortex and subcortical white matter. The **superior superficial cerebral veins** (about 10 of them) empty into the **superior and inferior sagittal sinuses. The inferior superficial cerebral** veins empty into the **cavernous, petrosal, and transverse sinuses.** Although the anatomy of the superficial cerebral veins can vary considerably, some can be prominent during the venous phase of cerebral angiograms. The **middle cerebral vein** parallels the middle cerebral artery. The **vein of Trolard** connects the middle cerebral vein to the superior sagittal sinus. The **vein of Labbé** connects the middle cerebral vein to the transverse sinus. These veins are illustrated later in this case (see Thumbnail: Cerebral Veins).

Deep cerebral veins The **deep cerebral veins** drain deep gray and deep white matter, including the thalamus, basal ganglia, and internal capsule. They also drain choroid plexus and periventricular regions. Many of these veins empty into the **internal cerebral veins.** The internal cerebral vein is located within the third ventricle, along the superior aspect of the thalamus. The two internal cerebral veins come together near the pineal gland to form the **great cerebral vein of Galen.** The basal vein of Rosenthal drains the ventral aspect of the cerebrum and joins the vein of Galen. The vein of Galen extends posteriorly to join with the inferior sagittal sinus and form the **straight sinus.**

Venous Drainage in the Posterior Fossa   Cerebellar veins can be grouped into lateral and median groups. Each group has superior and inferior veins. The superior lateral cerebellar veins empty into the superior petrosal sinuses. The inferior lateral cerebellar veins empty into the inferior petrosal sinuses. The superior median cerebellar vein empties into the great cerebral vein of Galen. The inferior median cerebellar vein empties into the straight sinus. Veins draining the midbrain and the ventral pons empty into the basal veins of Rosenthal. Veins draining the dorsal pons, the choroid plexus of the fourth ventricle, and the rostral medulla empty into the petrosal and sigmoid sinuses. Veins draining the caudal medulla empty into spinal veins.

Case Conclusion   VM was taken to radiology where an emergent CT scan of the head was performed. It revealed a crescentic fluid collection overlying the left cerebral hemisphere that was nearly isodense with brain parenchyma. Acute subdural blood is usually hyperintense on CT scan. The intensity gradually decreases, becoming isointense by 2 weeks and hypointense by 4 weeks, as the hematoma becomes liquefied. A neurosurgical consultation was requested for surgical drainage, after which the patient gradually recovered with intensive rehabilitation.

Thumbnail: Cerebral Veins

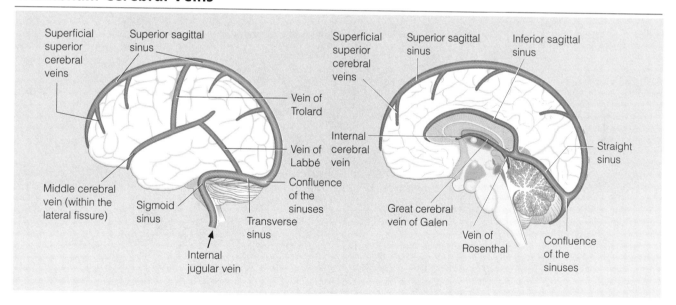

Key Points

- Bridging veins connect cerebral veins to dural venous sinuses.
- Tearing of bridging veins from shearing forces is the most common cause of subdural hemorrhage.
- Subdural hemorrhages can present either acutely or chronically.
- A subacute subdural hemorrhage may appear isointense to brain on CT scan and can easily be missed.

Questions

1. A 45-year-old assault victim was struck with a brick on the left side of the head and is now unresponsive. Which of the following vessels is most likely to have been injured?
   A. Middle cerebral vein
   B. Middle meningeal artery
   C. MCA
   D. Transverse sinus
   E. Superior sagittal sinus

2. A 26-year-old man had sudden onset of the worst headache of his life while straining on the toilet. Which of the following vessels is most likely involved?
   A. Middle cerebral vein
   B. Middle meningeal artery
   C. MCA
   D. Bridging vein
   E. Superior sagittal sinus

3. A 37-year-old man collapses while jogging during the summer. He is stuporous and has bilateral up-going toes. Which of the following vessels is most likely involved?
   A. Middle cerebral vein
   B. Middle meningeal artery
   C. MCA
   D. Bridging vein
   E. Superior sagittal sinus

4. A 46-year-old woman has been having a terrible headache that is constant and came on suddenly several weeks ago. It was initially associated with vertigo, but this has resolved. The headache does not have any classic migraine features and she has no previous history of such headaches. Which of the following vessels to you suspect to be involved?
   A. Vein of Galen
   B. Transverse sinus
   C. MCA
   D. Bridging vein
   E. Cavernous sinus

HPI: SD is a 57-year-old right-handed diabetic woman. She has been having upper respiratory symptoms for several weeks. Yesterday she developed a right-sided headache that has persisted. The pain was worst behind her right eye. When she awoke this morning, her right eye was red and painful. She is febrile.

PE: She has proptosis of the right eye and periorbital inflammation. She is unable to cooperate with testing of extraocular movement because of her severe pain; however, her gaze does not appear to be conjugate. She seems to have restricted movement of the right eye. The right pupil is larger than the left and does not react to light. She has ptosis on the right.

Thought Questions

- What structures are responsible for her signs and symptoms?

- How are they anatomically related?

- What is their vascular supply?

- What is their venous drainage?

Basic Science Review and Discussion

The past two cases have summarized venous drainage of the brain and brainstem. This case emphasizes the cavernous sinus. Although it is part of the dural venous sinus system, the **cavernous sinus** merits special attention because of its clinical importance. It is adjacent to several key structures, which define the clinical manifestations of cavernous sinus syndromes. Features of cavernous sinus disease can include disruption of extraocular movement, face and head pain, pupillary abnormalities, proptosis, periorbital inflammation, and conjunctival injection.

Cranial Nerves in the Cavernous Sinus   One can think of the **cavernous sinus** as a honeycomb of venous passages behind each orbit. The CNs that enter the orbit through the **superior orbital fissure** all pass through the cavernous sinus. These CNs include the nerves controlling eye movements (CN III, IV, and VI) and the **ophthalmic division of the trigeminal nerve.** All of them are located within the lateral wall of the cavernous sinus except for the sixth CN, which is located more centrally and close to the **carotid artery.** Because of its location, the sixth CN is often the first to be affected by disease of the cavernous sinus. The orientation of the CNs as they pass through the cavernous sinus is illustrated later in this case (see Thumbnail: Cavernous Sinus).

Disorders of the orbit, the superior orbital fissure, and the cavernous sinus can sometimes be difficult to distinguish because of their close relationship. They can all be associated with proptosis (bulging eye), eye pain, impaired eye movement, diplopia, and altered sensation over the upper face. It is important to remember, however, that the **maxillary branch of the trigeminal nerve** also passes through the cavernous sinus. It does not pass through the superior orbital fissure and is not contained within the orbit. Instead, the maxillary branch of the trigeminal nerve exits the skull through the **foramen rotundum.** The middle face is more likely to be affected with cavernous sinus disease for this reason, whereas it is spared in disorders of the superior orbital fissure and orbit. The optic nerve does not pass through the cavernous sinus and, therefore, is more likely to be involved in disorders affecting the orbital apex than in cavernous sinus disease.

Boundaries of the Cavernous Sinus   The medial wall of each cavernous sinus contains the **sphenoid air sinuses** and the **sella turcica,** containing the **pituitary gland.** The two cavernous sinuses are connected to each other by venous plexuses. The **anterior intercavernous sinus** is located immediately anterior to the sella turcica and pituitary gland, and the **posterior intercavernous sinus** is located posterior to these structures. The **carotid artery** passes through the cavernous sinus. Carotid artery disease, such as carotid dissection, can cause a cavernous sinus syndrome for this reason. Fistular connections between the carotid artery and venous system in this area can be associated with **orbital bruits.** The **superior and inferior petrosal sinuses** emerge from the posterior aspect of the cavernous sinuses. They empty into the **transverse and sigmoid sinuses,** respectively. As a general rule, more superficial regions of the cerebrum are drained by the superior sagittal sinus and the cavernous sinuses.

Case Conclusion   Empiric antibiotic and antifungal therapy were initiated. MRI studies confirmed inflammation in the region of the right cavernous sinus. Mucormycosis was confirmed by culture. Thrombosis of the cavernous sinus often occurs in the setting of sphenoid sinusitis. Cavernous sinus thrombosis is usually preceded by upper respiratory tract and sinusitis symptoms. This complication is more likely to occur in an immunocompromised state. Fungal sinusitis, particularly mucormycosis, is a cause of cavernous sinus thrombosis in diabetic patients. The initial symptoms of cavernous sinus thrombosis are often unilateral, although extension to the contralateral cavernous sinus is not uncommon. Cavernous sinus thrombosis is a medical emergency, requiring prompt intervention. Other causes of cavernous sinus syndrome include either local or metastatic tumors.

Thumbnail: Cavernous Sinus

Cross-section through Cavernous Sinus

Key Points

▶ The cavernous sinus is adjacent to the sphenoid air sinuses.

▶ The carotid artery passed through the cavernous sinus.

▶ The CNs mediating control of eye movement pass through the cavernous sinus.

▶ The ophthalmic and maxillary divisions of the trigeminal nerve pass through the cavernous sinus.

▶ The maxillary division of the trigeminal nerve is the only CN branch to pass through the cavernous sinus that does not enter the orbit or pass through the superior orbital fissure.

Questions

1. A 40-year-old woman presents with right eye pain and proptosis. She has no constitutional symptoms and no history of diabetes or thyroid disease. She has impaired extraocular movement of the right eye. What structure is involved?
   A. Right orbit
   B. Superior sagittal sinus
   C. Right cavernous sinus
   D. Right globe
   E. Right optic nerve

2. A 50-year-old man has right eye pain and proptosis. He does not have constitutional symptoms. He has impaired extraocular movement of the right eye. What structure is involved?
   A. Right third CN
   B. Right superior orbital fissure
   C. Right trochlear nerve
   D. Right abducens nerve
   E. Right optic nerve

3. A 46-year-old woman has bilateral proptosis and eye pain. She has a history of thyroid disease. What is the most likely affected structure?
   A. Orbit
   B. Cavernous sinus
   C. Superior orbital fissure
   D. Optic nerve
   E. Globe

4. You evaluate a patient with a suspected superior orbital fissure syndrome (Tolosa-Hunt syndrome). Which of the following functions is most likely to be spared?
   A. Pupillary constriction
   B. Upward gaze
   C. Lateral gaze
   D. Sensation below the eye
   E. Sensation above the eye

HPI: An 18-year-old male is brought to the ED by his college roommate after having a witnessed seizure. He is becoming arousable again but remains confused and combative. His speech is slurred and he spits at the paramedics as he is brought in. His roommate explains that he has had a sore throat for several days but was otherwise completely normal yesterday.

PMHx: Broken right clavicle as a child; otherwise negative.

He did not take any medications before this incident and his toxicology screen is negative for alcohol or illicit drugs.

PE: T 102.6°F   HR 136   BP 185/90   RR 28   SaO$_2$ 94% on room air

He responds to pain in all four extremities with what appears to be normal strength; reflexes are intact. He is uncooperative and does not follow commands, and his consciousness is diminished with the exception of combativeness when stimulated. His neck is rigid. He reflexively flexes his knees when his hips are flexed and claims that his neck hurts when the knee is extended.

Thought Questions

- What is the likely diagnosis?

- How are his symptoms explained by the process involved?

- What preventive measures should be taken at this point?

Basic Science Review and Discussion

The Meninges   The meninges are the three supportive and protective soft tissue layers that surround the CNS, which includes the brain and spinal cord. The relatively soft, gelatinous brain and spinal cord need a cushion to protect them from abrasion and shear forces with the activities of daily life. The surrounding skull and spine provide the first line of defense against compressive injury. Further shock absorption, support, and protection are provided by surrounding and suspending the brain and spinal cord in the meninges and CSF.

Three Layers of Meninges   The meninges are divided into three layers: two light layers collectively called the **leptomeninges,** which includes the **pia mater** ("soft mother") and *arachnoid* layer, and an outer fibrous layer called the **dura mater** ("hard mother").

The **pia mater** forms the innermost thin layer and is directly attached to the entire exterior of the brain and spinal cord. It acts to minimize abrasions or tearing of the CNS when subjected to trauma. It anchors the spinal cord in place via numerous **dentate ligaments,** which are attached to the arachnoid layer along the spinal cord. The pia also runs inferiorly beyond the conus medullaris to form the **filum terminale,** which is anchored to the outer meninges as they converge at spinal level S2.

The **arachnoid** forms the middle layer, which envelops the CSF. The space between the pia and arachnoid in which the

CSF circulates is accordingly called the **subarachnoid space.** CSF is reabsorbed in the **arachnoid granulations** of the arachnoid layer, which are evaginations of the arachnoid membrane through which CSF may flow into the superior sagittal venous sinus via a pressure gradient. Cerebral arteries and bridging veins are also located within the subarachnoid space. **Arachnoid trabeculations,** running from the pia to the arachnoid throughout the subarachnoid space, gently tether the brain in place.

The **dura mater** is the tough, fibrous outermost layer that anchors the meninges to the skull or paraspinal tissue, and is closely apposed to the arachnoid. It is composed in part of the actual periosteum of the skull and forms a supportive scaffolding for the brain, which is discussed in the subsequent "Structure" section. The space between the skull and dura, usually nonexistent, is called the **epidural space,** which becomes important when the dura is separated from the skull (usually from trauma). The space between the dura and arachnoid, which is also usually closed, is called the **subdural space,** which readily expands when blood or other fluid enters (also usually from trauma). The intracranial dura is innervated by CN V and spinal nerves C1–C3 and may be exquisitely sensitive to inflammation.

Peripheral Nerves   As CNs or spinal nerves exit the CNS, they are "coated" by the subarachnoid and dural layers, which form the perineurium or sheath of the peripheral nerve.

Structure   The fibrous dura forms several "shelves" to hold the cerebellar and cerebral hemispheres in place. These supportive dividers prevent excessive movement of the brain, but also cause compression and potentially herniation should expansion of the brain occur. They also contain the venous sinuses.

The dura eventrates into the medial longitudinal fissure of the brain, forming a midsagittal divider running anteroposterior within the skull called the **falx cerebri,** or "falx." The falx separates the cerebral hemispheres and contains the **superior sagittal venous sinus** (adjacent to the skull) and **inferior sagittal sinus** (along the deep aspect of the falx). Expansion of one of the cerebral hemispheres may force it to cross the midline under the falx, that is, **subfalcine herniation.**

A horizontal shelf of dura extends in the axial plane just inferior to the cerebrum, separating the occipital lobes from the cerebellum, called the **tentorium cerebellum. The transverse venous sinuses** run within the tentorium to the midsagittal **straight sinus,** where the falx and tentorium intersect. The presence of the tentorium creates a rigid "ceiling" in the posterior fossa, so small changes in cerebellar size may displace it inferiorly, causing cerebellar **tonsillar herniation** into the foramen magnum. The anterior aspects of the tentorium run under the uncus of the temporal lobe. Temporal lobe displacement secondary to mass effect may force it under the tentorium, causing **uncal herniation.**

The midsagittal plane of dura, which makes up the falx cerebri, extends inferior to the tentorium, at which point it is called the **falx cerebellum.**

Disease Processes of the Meninges The most lethal and fulminant disease specific to the meninges is infectious meningitis. Meningitis refers to meningeal inflammation, which may arise from viral ("aseptic"), bacterial, fungal, parasitic, malignant, or autoimmune causes. Meningitis generally involves seeding of the CSF with the pathogen from either **blood-borne spread** or direct spread, in the case of meningeal injury or sinusitis. The CSF serves as an ideal culture medium with only limited immune response available from adjacent blood vessels. As an infection takes hold, an inflammatory response follows with exudate of leukocytes (and RBCs) into the CSF and meningeal irritation, causing neck pain and stiffness. Patients' necks may become entirely rigid **(meningismus)** to guard against movement, as movement places tension on the already inflamed meninges. They may develop photophobia, headache, seizures, mental status changes and coma, fever, and sepsis, among other conditions. Two other physical findings are worth noting:

Kernig's sign: pain with flexing hip and extending knee (places traction on lumbar roots which is transmitted to meninges)

Brudzinski's sign: flexing the hip and knees with neck flexion (to relieve traction on meninges)

Bacterial meningitis Bacterial meningitis is among the most lethal of all known infections, although it is generally completely curable if treatment is started early. It is caused by three major organisms in the adult: *Haemophilus influenzae, Streptococcus pneumoniae,* and *Neisseria*

meningitidis. Listeria monocytogenes may infect children younger than 5 years or elderly patients, and *Escherichia coli* may infect immunocompromised patients.

Patients may present with a **prodrome** of sinusitis, respiratory tract infection, or otitis media with backache. Severe meningismus and photophobia usually follow. Acute bacterial meningitis should lead to deposition of a purulent PMN exudate within the subarachnoid space, usually most concentrated around the brainstem, which leads to edema and inflammation of the external brain, CNs, and penetrating arteries and veins, which can cause vasculitis and thrombosis. Ischemia, infarct, and seizures may develop.

CSF analysis correspondingly shows a **PMN pleocytosis with elevated protein** and **low glucose** levels because of the metabolic demands of the PMN cells. Gram stain and culture may reveal the bacteria and give further information about treatment, which must be started immediately. Untreated bacterial meningitis is lethal within hours to days.

Viral (aseptic) meningitis Viral or "aseptic" meningitis is named for the inability to grow a pathogen out of CSF culture, which otherwise shows elevated leukocytes consistent with meningitis. **Enterovirus** causes the majority of viral meningitis cases, with a seasonal peak in late summer. Other viruses include *Epstein-Barr virus (EBV),* mumps virus, *HSV-2* (HSV-1 tends to cause encephalitis), *lymphocytic choriomeningitis* (LCV, from rodent droppings), and *HIV.*

Patients may present with meningismus and photophobia but otherwise appear much more stable than those with bacterial meningitis.

CSF analysis generally shows a **lymphocytic pleocytosis with normal or high protein and normal glucose levels.** Viral culture or PCR may recover the infecting virus, but bacterial cultures remain bland. Patients generally do not require treatment and recover over several days.

Tuberculous meningitis Tuberculous meningitis has a more vasculitic component, causing ischemia and stroke of brain and spinal cord. *Mycobacterium tuberculosis* and *Mycobacterium bovis* are the causative organisms.

Presentation may be indistinguishable from bacterial meningitis, although hemiparesis from stroke are more common in tuberculous meningitis. It is seen mostly in adults, often years after primary TB infection. Onset may be acute or indolent over months.

CSF analysis generally shows **lymphocytic pleocytosis with elevated protein and low glucose levels.** *Acid-fast bacilli* may be seen on the CSF smear. Treatment is standard triple/quadruple antimycobacterial therapy in accordance to resistance patterns.

Syphilitic meningitis   Neurosyphilis usually causes asymptomatic meningitis, only detectable on lumbar puncture. In a minority of cases, meningismus and CN abnormalities will follow. This may resolve without treatment, allowing the later complications of neurosyphilis to ensue: meningovascular syphilis, optic atrophy, and tabes dorsalis.

CSF analysis shows **lymphocytic pleocytosis with elevated protein and low glucose levels.** CSF rapid plasma reagent (RPR) titer or dark-field microscopy may be used to demonstrate neurosyphilis. **Penicillin** remains the treatment of choice, preventing later complications of syphilis.

Fungal meningitis   Fungal meningitis usually presents indolently in **immunocompromised** patients. **Cryptococcal meningitis** is the most common entity, although *Candida, Nocardia,* and *Aspergillus* may cause meningitis. CSF generally **shows lymphocytic pleocytosis with elevated protein and low glucose levels.** Gram stain or culture may show the causative organism, with **India ink stain** confirming *Cryptococcus*. **Amphotericin B** is usually the treatment for fungal meningitis.

Carcinomatous meningitis   Infiltration of the CSF with malignant cells (usually lung, breast, and GI tract cancers) may cause meningitis. Back pain and radiculopathy are common. CSF shows an abundance of **abnormal cells,** which may be used to diagnose the primary tumor. Treatment relies on chemotherapy and radiation, although carcinomatous meningitis usually portends a grave prognosis.

Autoimmune meningitis   Sarcoid or systemic lupus erythematosus (SLE) may involve the meninges, causing possible CN abnormalities and CSF lymphocytic pleocytosis.

Parameningeal infection   Infection abutting the meninges, such as mastoiditis or epidural abscess, may give a lymphocytic pleocytosis. Organisms may not be present in the CSF, and protein and glucose levels may be normal.

Other Disease Processes of the Meninges

Epidural hematoma   Invasion of blood into the epidural space occurs after rupture of a meningeal artery, usually in the setting of trauma. The **middle meningeal artery** is particularly susceptible to shearing because it lies deep to the thin temporal bone, which is fractured relatively easily. Generally only arterial pressure may separate the fibrous dura to open the epidural space, causing epidural hematomas to be **"football shaped"** as the edges are slowly pried apart. If the epidural hematoma continues to expand, mass effect leading to cerebral herniation and death may occur if surgical decompression is not performed. Patients may be initially unconscious from a traumatic injury, wake up, and appear normal during the **"lucid interval,"** during which the epidural hematoma continues to expand. Once it causes adequate mass effect, consciousness is again impaired and the patient may become comatose.

Subdural hematoma   The subdural space, by contrast, is easily formed, and **bridging veins** penetrating the meninges may bleed into this space after blunt head trauma. This is most common in **elderly** patients with a history of **alcohol abuse** (bridging veins are more likely to tear as cerebral atrophy increases their "tethering"). Subdural hematomas are **crescentic** because arachnoid and dura come apart easily, spreading the subdural blood along the arc of the crescent. They may also cause mass effect, which may require surgical decompression.

Meningioma   The arachnoid (particularly the granulations) may give rise to benign calcified tumors called **meningiomas.** They very rarely invade adjacent tissues but may cause symptoms resulting from local mass effect. Nearly half involve the falx or frontal convexities. Pathology shows characteristic "whorls" of fibrous tissue and calcified **psammoma bodies.** Surgical removal is performed to eliminate unacceptable symptoms.

Case Conclusion   This patient was immediately treated with IV antibiotics empirically for suspected bacterial meningitis. Often vancomycin will be chosen to cover *S. pneumoniae,* with third- or fourth-generation cephalosporin added for coverage of *N. meningitidis* and *H. influenzae*. Ampicillin should be added if *Listeria* is suspected. After obtaining a normal head CT scan, a lumbar puncture was performed, which registered an elevated opening pressure. CSF Gram stain showed a significantly elevated WBC count with 98% PMN leukocytes and gram-negative coccobacilli consistent with *N. meningitidis* infection. The patient became afebrile with a normal neurologic examination 3 days after initiation of treatment; he was given 10 days of IV antibiotic therapy. Preventive single-dose ciprofloxacin was given to the patient's roommate, close contacts, and health care workers who were exposed to the patient's respiratory secretions.

Thumbnail: Meninges

Meningitis			
Type	**Symptoms**	**CSF studies**	**Treatment**
Bacterial	Fever/meningismus, confusion, seizures, coma	High polys, high protein, low glucose, Gram stain	Vancomycin + third-generation cephalosporin ± ampicillin (*Listeria*)
Viral	Meningismus, more benign	High lymphocytes, normal protein/glucose	Supportive
Tuberculous	More cranial neuropathies, strokes	Acid-fast smear Lymphocytic pleocytosis, elevated protein, low glucose	Antitubercular antibiotic therapy
Syphilitic	Often asymptomatic	CSF RPR	Penicillin
Fungal	More indolent, immunocompromised patients	India ink (Crypto)	Amphotericin B
Carcinomatous	Back pain, radiculopathy	Cytology	Radiation/chemotherapy
Autoimmune	Cranial neuropathies		Immunosuppression

Key Points

▶ The three layers of meninges—pia mater, arachnoid, and dura mater—support and protect the brain and the venous sinuses within the bony skull.

▶ Infectious meningitis is caused by a variety of organisms and must be diagnosed and treated rapidly in most cases. CSF analysis is usually sufficient to make the diagnosis.

▶ Other complications involving the meninges include epidural hematoma, subdural hematoma, and meningioma, all of which may require surgery if they cause mass effect.

Questions

1. An elderly patient is brought in for confusion by a stranger. You notice that the patient's neck is stiff and a fever of 101°F. Kernig's and Brudzinski's signs are present. What is the most appropriate next course of action?
   A. Start IV vancomycin/cefotaxime
   B. Obtain head CT scan
   C. Start IV vancomycin-cefotaxime-ampicillin
   D. Perform lumbar puncture
   E. Obtain plain neck films

2. A 68-year-old man is brought to the attention of his doctor because his wife says that his memory is poor and he has appeared vague and inattentive for the past 3 months. He is a retired physician but has difficulty giving his previous medical history when asked (it is notable for hypertension and benign prostatic hypertrophy). His wife mentions that he had a fall in the shower preceding this change, and he was able to recite esoteric medical facts in great detail before the fall occurred. What is the most likely cause of his mental status change?
   A. Meningioma
   B. Subdural hematoma
   C. Fungal meningitis
   D. Alzheimer's dementia
   E. Viral meningitis

3. A 16-year-old girl is attending a hockey game when she is struck on the head by a stray puck. Although she is initially arousable and complains of pain over her left temple where she was struck, she becomes progressively more somnolent and is rushed to the hospital. Upon arrival an hour later, she has become comatose. What would the head CT be expected to show?
   A. Left temporal skull fracture with cerebral contusion
   B. Left temporal skull fracture with a crescentic mass adjacent to brain with mass effect
   C. Left temporal skull fracture with football-shaped mass adjacent to brain with mass effect
   D. Left temporal skull fracture with calcified mass adjacent to brain with mass effect
   E. Intact skull with cerebral edema and mass effect

4. A 34-year-old patient with no previous medical history presents to his doctor's office with a complaint of stiff neck. He states that this began 5 days ago with headache and neck stiffness so bad that he could not move it, with fevers and chills. He says that this began to improve 2 days ago and he now has some residual neck stiffness and photophobia, but otherwise feels well. His examination is otherwise unremarkable and mental status is intact. He has no fever, has stable vital signs, and results of laboratory tests show no electrolyte or blood count abnormalities. What is the most appropriate course of action?
   A. Immediate IV vancomycin-cefotaxime
   B. Lumbar puncture for culture and cell count
   C. Head CT
   D. Observation
   E. Head MRI

Case 32

1. B
2. C
3. A
4. C

Case 33

1. A
2. B
3. B
4. A

Case 34

1. B
2. B
3. D
4. B

Case 35

1. C
2. D
3. D
4. A

Case 36

1. B
2. C
3. E
4. B

Case 37

1. A
2. B
3. A
4. D

Case 38

1. C
2. B
3. C
4. D

Part V

Neurophysiology and Neurotransmitters

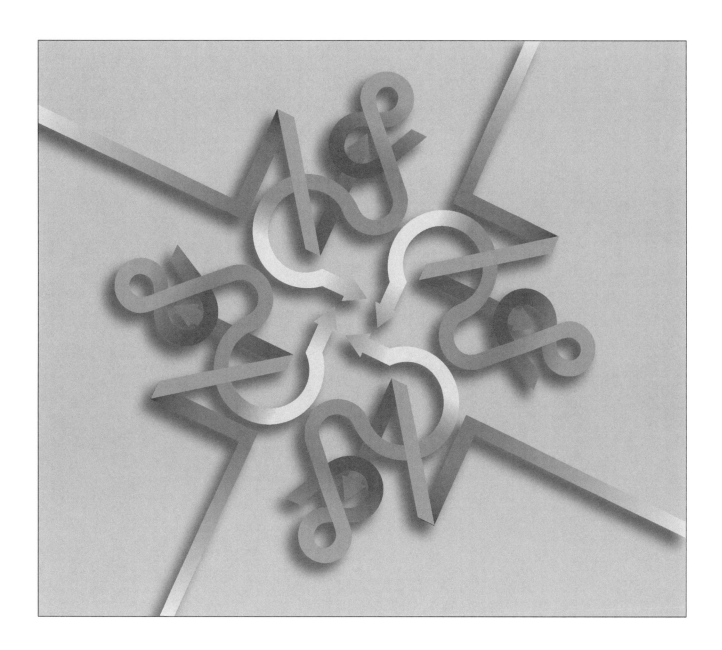

HPI: A 34-year-old social worker comes to your office complaining of periodic cramps in his legs, arms, and hands. He notes that at times he gets cramps so severe that he can see groups of muscles distorted while they contract uncontrollably. During these episodes, he is unable to willfully move the affected limb. This periodic paralysis usually lasts less than an hour but at times has lasted up to 6 hours. The patient denies pain or other symptoms along with these episodes. He specifically notes that he has good strength normally and hasn't seen any changes outside of these attacks. He reports he has experienced bouts of cramping all his life but has noticed an increase in frequency since he started a new jogging regimen. On questioning, he reports that his father experienced similar cramping episodes most of his life.

PE: He is generally well appearing. You note that by percussing the thenar eminence, you can elicit sustained muscle contraction.

Thought Questions

■ What single cellular structure could account for widespread neuronal dysfunction?

■ How do neurons maintain the necessary intercellular conditions?

■ What stimuli can change the flow of ions into and out of the cell?

Basic Science Review and Discussion

This patient presents with bouts of periodic paralysis and prolonged contraction of muscles, both after use and mechanical stimulation. These symptoms are definitive of a myotonia. Myotonias can result from a number of causes; in all cases, disorders of ion channels are the basis of symptoms.

Ion Channels   For neurons to function and fire action potentials, cells must have a mechanism for changing the intercellular environment quickly and specifically. Ion channels are openings in neuronal membranes that allow certain ions to pass through under given conditions. Ion channels are selective; each channel favors specific ions. This is possible because of the molecular structure of ion channels. Most channels are integral transmembrane proteins, spanning the membrane repeatedly. The composite structure of the transmembrane domains is a central charged pore. This creates an opening spanning the membrane, but the charge repels most ions from passing through. Furthermore, the structure of the central opening is highly specific, serving as a filter for ions based on shape and size. Many ion channels are relatively specific to one type of ion, such as Na^+ or K^+. Others are less specific, for example, allowing both Na^+ and K^+ in and out of the cell. In this way, the cell has a path that will allow the flow of only certain ions to change the intercellular environment.

Ion channels are further able to allow ion flow only under certain conditions. A well-studied example of this is voltage-gated channels. Some channel proteins have a structure that changes at different electrical voltages. At very negative voltage, for example, a protein may have a tertiary structure that is "closed"; it will not allow movement of ions. However, the same protein at a more positive voltage changes conformation and becomes "open." Voltage-gated channels specific for Na^+, K^+, Cl^-, and Ca^{2+} have been characterized in neurons. Likewise, some ion channels are ligand gated. These are generally single proteins with at least two domains: one channel pore and one binding site for a ligand. These proteins normally adopt a closed conformation, but when a specific ligand interacts with the binding domain, the tertiary structure of the entire protein is altered to an open conformation allowing ions to flow through. The binding domain can be on the intercellular or extracellular surface of the membrane, making the channel sensitive to either intercellular or extracellular signaling molecules. Through such mechanisms, channels are able to regulate the specific flow of ions into and out of the neuron according to environmental conditions (Figure 39-1).

Some ion channels are even further specialized. Some channel proteins have additional domains that under certain circumstances close off the inside of the channel. For example, some sodium channels are inactivated after prolonged depolarization. That is, the blocking domain changes configuration with prolonged depolarization, entering the center of the channel's pore. It remains in this configuration for a set time. As such, even if the external opening of the channel, the voltage gate, is open, Na^+ cannot pass through. The channel is in its inactivation stage until the blocking domain reverts to the open position. This mechanism acts in combination with the external voltage gate to finely regulate the flow of Na^+ into the neuron. At a certain voltage, the gate opens for sodium to flow into the cell, but only briefly, as the inactivation gate soon closes within the channel. Furthermore, because this inactivation cannot be reversed for a set time, the channel is in a state of absolute inactivation, meaning no conditions would cause it to open during a brief refractory period. There are many varieties of ion channels, each with a different combination of specificity for ions and sensitive to

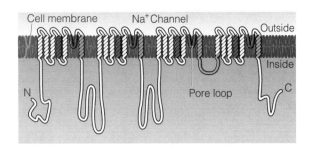

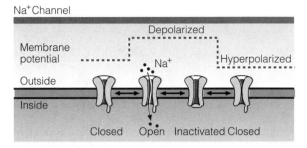

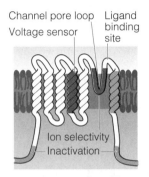

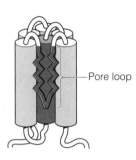

Figure 39-1 Ion channel structure. Most ion channels are composed of multiple subunit loops of a single protein, as shown. When these transmembrane loops come together, their three-dimensional structure forms a central pore, whose shape and charge selectively allow ions to flow through.

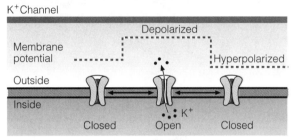

Figure 39-2 Function of voltage-gated sodium channels. When the surrounding membrane is depolarized, the central pore opens to allow ions to flow through. In certain sodium channels, after a period of depolarization, a special inactivation gate then closes to block ion flow. This stops ion flux regardless of the state of the central pore or the depolarization of surrounding membrane; the channels are inactivated. When the membrane potential becomes hyperpolarized, the central pore closes.

different environmental stimuli. This becomes useful in neuronal signaling and the transmission of action potentials. Without functional ion channels, nerves and muscle cells cannot fire signals or function normally (Figure 39-2).

Clinical Correlation Disorders that affect ion channels are sometimes referred to as **channelopathies.** Understanding of these diseases has increased dramatically as molecular techniques in research have improved over the past few decades. Ion channel disorders are now thought to underlie a number of syndromes, from cardiac disorders such as long QT syndrome to familial syndromes of periodic paralysis. In each case, the proposed pathology is a mutation in a gene coding for an ion channel. Alterations in specific ion channels cause deficits in signaling and function of cells throughout the body. While memorizing varieties of channelopathies and their related mutations is generally not necessary for the USMLE, one must understand the pathophysiology of ion channels.

Myotonia is prolonged muscle contraction, often in multiple locations. There are several inherited myotonias; most are now thought to be channelopathies. One well-understood myotonia has been traced to mutations in a single Na$^+$ channel gene (SCN4A). The mutation has been observed to cause delayed inactivation of the Na$^+$ channel at the sarcolemma. This means there is increased sodium flux, and the cell is hyperexcitable and contracts more than usual. Patients

report muscle stiffness or cramping as symptoms. Contraction can be elicited by either normal use, electrical stimulation, or mechanical stimulation (such as direct pressure). These cramps can have a duration ranging from minutes to days. Symptoms may be exacerbated by altered metabolic states, such as hyperkalemia and hypokalemia, as well as cold or exercise. Treatment aims to lessen symptoms and manage electrolyte balance to minimize attacks; muscles of respiration or swallowing are generally not affected. Another example also affecting SCN4A, voltage-gated sodium channels have a mutation that results in excessive inactivation. In these cases, periodic flaccid paralysis results, because inactivated channels are unable to allow sodium flux necessary for signaling. Patients report bouts of muscle weakness at times so severe that they cannot move their limbs. Still other channelopathies have been associated with mutations in genes for Cl$^-$ channels in muscle cells. In **myotonia congenita,** a mutation in the muscle chloride channel gene results in hyperexcitability, manifesting as stiffness and cramping in muscle. The disorder begins in childhood and is nonprogressive. Although certain gene defects have been well characterized through mouse knockouts and gene analysis, many other myotonias remain poorly defined or not associated with a known mutation. Research has just begun to tease out distinctions between various myotonias; understanding of ion channels in most cases has proven invaluable.

Case Conclusion   The patient's symptoms appear consistent with a lifelong myotonia. Electromyographic (EMG) studies support this diagnosis, showing sporadic prolonged contraction of muscle after brief electrical stimulation. Further history reveals that the patient's symptoms have not been progressive and have been directly correlated with his new early morning jogs. A better understanding of his "cramping" and the nonprogressive and nonlethal nature of most myotonias provides great relief to your patient. At his request, he schedules a visit with a genetic counselor to further trace the hereditary pattern of his myotonia and to ascertain whether he might have one of the known channelopathy mutations.

Thumbnail: Ion Channels

Examples of Important Ion Channels		
Channel	**Type**	**Compounds affecting channel (effect)**
Axonal Na^+ channel	Voltage gated	Tetrodotoxin (antagonist)
Axonal K^+ channel	Voltage gated	Dendrotoxin (antagonist)
Synaptic terminal Ca^{2+} channels	Voltage gated	—
Nicotinic Na^+ channel	Ligand gated	ACh (agonist)
$GABA_A$ Cl^- channel	Ligand gated	GABA (agonist)
Glycine Cl^- channel	Ligand gated	Glycine (agonist)

Key Points

▶ Ion channels allow specific ions to enter and leave a cell; they are **selective**.

▶ Voltage-gated and ligand-gated channels have structures that open or close only under certain conditions.

▶ Some channels have inactivation gates that absolutely prevent the flow of ions for a short time.

Questions

1. Tetrodotoxin is a natural toxin produced by certain puffer fish that acts by obstructing excitable Na^+ channels in somatic nerves. A patient presents to the ED after accidentally ingesting tetrodotoxin in a fish. Which of the following symptoms would be most likely?
   A. Convulsions of all extremities
   B. Increased urinary sodium level
   C. Weakness and paralysis of limbs
   D. A and C
   E. All of the above

2. Scorpions paralyze their prey by injecting a toxin that acts on Na^+ channels. These alpha toxins delay the inactivation of the Na^+ channels. Neuronal action potentials are altered, and movements of the prey are impaired. A person stung by a scorpion will experience, among other effects, impaired local signaling at the site of the wound. Which of the following effects occur at the level of the affected neuron?
   A. Increased flow of sodium and increased flow of potassium
   B. Increased flow of sodium and normal flow of potassium
   C. Decreased flow of sodium and decreased flow of potassium
   D. Decreased flow of sodium and normal flow of potassium
   E. No movement of sodium and normal flow of potassium

3. Strychnine is a competitive antagonist for glycine. What effect will strychnine poisoning have on glycine-associated channels?
   A. Remove channel selectivity
   B. Increase voltage threshold for pore opening
   C. Block ion channel pores
   D. Trigger inactivation gate closing
   E. Interfere with ligand-gate opening

4. Lidocaine blocks voltage-gated sodium channels. How does this lead to anesthesia when applied locally to a nerve fiber?
   A. Impair signaling at nicotinic receptors
   B. Raise the threshold for excitation
   C. Act as an agonist at $GABA_A$ channels
   D. Increase intracellular levels of sodium
   E. Prevent inactivation of channels

HPI: A 31-year-old computer programmer comes to your office complaining of numbness and painful tingling in his hands and feet bilaterally. These paresthesias began about a year ago and have gotten progressively worse. At first he thought his feet were just "cold," but he notices that the decreased sensation and "pins and needles" feeling has now progressed up to about knee level and has begun to affect sensation in his hands. The accompanying burning pain has become intense enough to disrupt his function at home and work and does not respond to the normal aspirin or NSAIDs he has tried. His medical history is significant for testing HIV positive 8 years ago, but he reports he has been fully compliant with his complex medication regimen. He has had few opportunistic infections, although all were in the past 2 years, as his CD4 count has decreased.

PE: You find decreased light-touch sensation in both his hands as compared with his arms, and almost no response to pinprick stimuli on the plantar surface of his feet. His deep tendon reflexes are absent in the ankles and diminished at the patella, but normal at the biceps and brachioradialis. He has mild strength impairment distally in the lower extremities but is otherwise normal.

Thought Questions

- How does the presentation of neuropathy differ from that of other lesions, such as stroke?

- How do nerves generate electrical signals?

- What allows electrical signals to travel along nerves?

- What factors can change or block these signals?

Basic Science Review and Discussion

This patient is describing symptoms of a polyneuropathy. To understand the presentation of sensorimotor polyneuropathy, one must be aware of the normal function of the axons affected, and the axon potentials that become disrupted.

Action Potentials The membrane of the neuronal axon is a barrier separating concentrations of ions such as potassium (K^+), sodium (Na^+), and chloride (Cl^-). These ions are present in the external environment and can enter the cell through selective channels (as previously described). They can also be removed from the cell via transporters, which use adenosine triphosphate (ATP) to pump ions such as sodium out of the cell. The most important of these is the Na^+-K^+ pump, which extrudes 3 Na^+ ions in exchange for 2 K^+ ions. In neurons, selective channels and transporters maintain a higher concentration of K^+ inside the cell than in the external environment and a higher concentration of Na^+ outside the cell than inside. Intracellular proteins, which cannot cross the cell membrane, also carry a net negative charge.

The unequal concentrations of these ions create chemical "gradients," sources of potential energy. The distribution of ions also creates a net electric charge. Because each ion carries a positive or negative charge, their unequal distribution builds up an electrical potential as the inside of the cell becomes more negatively (or positively) charged than the

outside. These forces combine to create one electrochemical potential between the inside and outside of the cell. When the cell is in steady state, this **membrane potential** is generally around −70 mV inside the cell.

When ion channels open in response to either neurotransmitter stimuli or electrical changes, the ions are free to flow down their gradients, doing electrical work. Sodium rushes into the cell, causing a massive reversal of charge as many of these positive ions enter the cell. This change in the membrane potential is called **depolarization,** as the polarization of charge is transiently reversed. This depolarization is the electrical signal that forms the basis of the **action potential.**

Depolarization brings the membrane potential toward zero; it makes it more positive and can even bring it above zero toward 40 mV. If the depolarization is large enough, it can open voltage-gated Na^+ channels in the membrane. This allows an even greater influx of sodium and perpetuates the rising membrane potential. When an initial depolarization is great enough to open voltage-gated channels and initiate this process, it is said to have reached "threshold."

The membrane potential does not remain depolarized indefinitely. The sodium channels close after about a millisecond, and voltage-gated K^+ channels open as greater depolarization occurs. This means that positively charged potassium rushes out of the cell, down its gradient, and no new sodium can enter, causing the membrane potential to again become negative. In fact, as the sodium channels remain closed and the positive charge leaves, the membrane becomes **hyperpolarized,** or more negative than usual for a few milliseconds. Transporters in the membrane act to bring the ion distribution back to steady state, and the cell quickly returns to its resting membrane potential. (See Thumbnail: Action Potentials, later in this case.)

Axonal Transmission This normal sequence creates a local, transient depolarization in the membrane. However, the change in ion concentration within the cell does affect the adjacent membrane, as does the spread of depolarization along the axon. As such, the first depolarization can bring the region of membrane next to it to threshold, causing a depolarization there. This can spread to the next adjacent region, and so forth, until the depolarization occurs at every place along the axon. When this occurs, it is said that an **action potential** has been generated and transmitted down the axon. Transient hyperpolarization after each depolarizing event usually ensures that action potentials travel only in one direction and don't regenerate in the same patch of membrane. Action potentials are very quick, and thus many can be fired down the same length of an axon in a second. This allows the nervous system to transmit many distinct signals very close together in time.

For an action potential to properly form, all the functional components of the axon must be intact. The initial signal from a neurotransmitter ligand or other stimulus must be received by the dendrites of the neuron. The ion channels of the axon hillock must be selective for only specific ions, and only open and close under proper conditions. Ion transporters must be intact and have a good source of ATP to maintain the normal ion gradient inside the axon. The membrane itself must be intact, with no "leaks" to disrupt the ion balance. Furthermore, the external environment must be correct to create the potential. In an environment with insufficient external sodium, for example, there would not be enough of a gradient to generate a depolarization beyond threshold. Conditions that alter any of these parts can cause disease that affects signaling to and from the brain.

Clinical Correlation **Axonal neuropathies** are diseases in which neuronal axons themselves are destroyed. (This is in contrast to demyelinating disorders, in which the axons remain relatively spared, but their myelin is destroyed.) As axons are destroyed, action potentials can no longer be generated, and sensory and motor signaling is disrupted. Furthermore, as action-potential generation is disrupted, many patients experience a burning, tingling pain along the course of the nerve. This **neuropathic pain** may not be relieved by traditional therapies and can be extremely intense. It has been suggested that incorrect firing of action potentials or the absence of action potentials is poorly interpreted by the brain, and the resulting perception is pain. When disease affect multiple neurons, it is referred to as a **polyneuropathy.** Most axonal polyneuropathies affect both sensory and motor function to some degree but usually preferentially disturb one depending on the specific disease. Numbness and tingling generally begin bilaterally in the feet and then progress up to the lower extremities and begin to affect the distal upper extremities because neuropathy is a length-dependent process. For this reason, the deficit is said to have a characteristic "stocking-and-glove" distribution. One of the most common causes of peripheral neuropathy is uncontrolled diabetes mellitus, which leads to severe permanent injury in thousands of patients each year. When diagnosing peripheral neuropathy, the pattern of deficit is key: stocking-and-glove distributions indicate polyneuropathy. In contrast, nerve injuries affect only one nerve distribution usually on one side, and injury to the root or cord follows a dermatomal pattern.

A common example of an axonal neuropathy is the distal, symmetric **sensorimotor polyneuropathy** often seen in patients with HIV infection. Up to 40% of patients who develop AIDS will also have peripheral neuropathy at some point in their disease. This neuropathy can develop at any point after HIV infection and does not solely affect suppressed patients with AIDS. The exact pathophysiology of this disease is unknown but in some patients may partially be due to vitamin deficiency or the neurotoxic effects of some drugs. It is thought that HIV itself does not directly cause the axonal injury. Usually, sensory symptoms appear first, and weakness is minor. The accompanying burning or tingling pain can be severe enough to cause marked disability. This disease is progressive, and no treatment is known to reverse or slow deterioration. However, a number of new pharmacologic treatments for neuropathic pain have been found effective for these patients; many respond to trials of antiepileptic or antidepressant drugs.

Case Conclusion You complete a thorough history and examination, which rule out many autoimmune, infectious, toxic, and metabolic causes of polyneuropathy. Given this patient's symptoms and history, you recognize this is most likely a sensorimotor polyneuropathy. You advise the patient that although this disease is generally progressive, you can help alleviate some of his pain. You prescribe regular dosing of gabapentin, an antiseizure drug that has been shown to have efficacy in neuropathic pain. Although this complicates an already intense drug regimen, the patient finds that within 2 weeks, his pain is significantly lessened and he is able to resume most of his daily activities.

Thumbnail: Action Potentials

Steps in Action Potential Generation

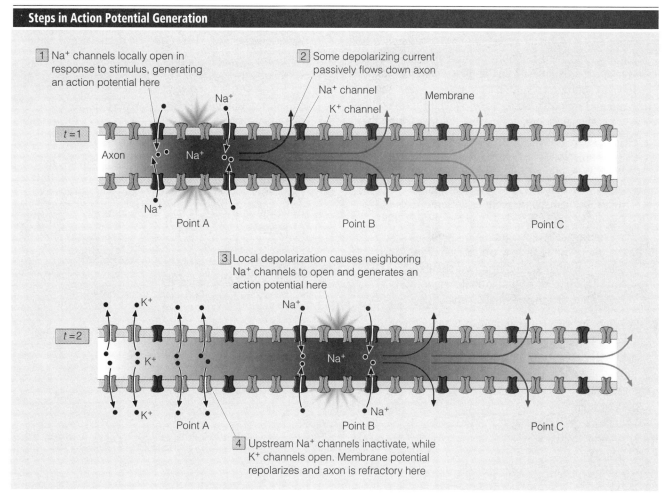

1 Na⁺ channels locally open in response to stimulus, generating an action potential here

2 Some depolarizing current passively flows down axon

Na⁺ channel

K⁺ channel

Membrane

t = 1

Axon   Na⁺   Na⁺

Na⁺

Point A   Point B   Point C

3 Local depolarization causes neighboring Na⁺ channels to open and generates an action potential here

t = 2

K⁺   Na⁺   Na⁺

K⁺

K⁺

Point A   Point B   Point C

4 Upstream Na⁺ channels inactivate, while K⁺ channels open. Membrane potential repolarizes and axon is refractory here

Key Points

▶ Neurons use depolarizing electrical signals called *action potentials* to communicate.

▶ Action potentials are generated by both electrical and chemical gradients.

▶ Most neurons have a resting membrane potential of about −70 mV and must be depolarized beyond a certain threshold to fire an action potential.

▶ For action potentials to travel, an axon must have intact membrane, ion channels, and ion transporters, along with the correct external environment.

▶ Damage to axons or their environment can cause neuropathy, in which sensation and motor function are impaired.

Questions

1. A swimmer comes to the ED after being stung by a sea anemone. He reports that he felt pain immediately after stepping on a spine, but now in addition to the swelling, he feels a new numbness and tingling where he was stung. In addition to causing local inflammation, some sea-creature stings release a toxin that blocks Na^+ channels on cell membranes. How could this toxin cause the new symptoms the swimmer is experiencing?

   A. Hyperpolarizing the resting axonal membrane, thus preventing action potential formation
   B. Hyperpolarizing the resting axonal membrane, thus causing many frequent action potentials
   C. Depolarizing the resting axonal membrane, thus preventing action-potential formation
   D. Depolarizing the resting axonal membrane, thus causing many frequent action potentials
   E. Not changing the resting axonal membrane, but preventing action potential formation

2. Flooding the external environment with which of the following would cause a decrease in (make less negative or slightly depolarize) the membrane potential of a normal neuron?

   A. Sodium
   B. Potassium
   C. Chlorine
   D. A and B
   E. B and C

3. If toxin severely depleted available ATP levels, what would be the most likely effect on axonal action potentials?

   A. No effect
   B. Inhibit action-potential firing
   C. Shorten the duration of action potentials
   D. Increase action-potential firing
   E. Lengthen the duration of action potentials

4. A researcher isolates a compound that increases the duration potassium channels remain open when triggered. What effect would this have on the action potential?

   A. Prevent action potentials
   B. Lower the depolarization threshold
   C. Lower the magnitude of depolarization
   D. Lower the resting potential
   E. Lengthen the hyperpolarization phase

HPI: A 32-year-old waitress presents to the ED complaining of double vision since the morning. She also reports on-and-off numbness of her foot this summer and is concerned she "might be having some kind of stroke." She cannot recall any specific event precipitating these symptoms, although she has been under more stress at work since she has been "more tired and clumsy lately." Three years ago, she had an episode of numbness of her other foot, but this spontaneously resolved after 1 week.

PE: You observe nystagmus and elicit heightened deep tendon reflexes in her left leg. She has slightly decreased strength in her left lower extremity, but no diminished sensation.

Thought Questions

- What is this woman's most likely diagnosis?

- How does axonal conduction normally occur?

- What properties affect the velocity of axonal conduction?

- What is the role of myelin in the CNS and peripheral nervous system (PNS)?

- What signs and symptoms would present if axonal conduction is impaired?

Basic Science Review and Discussion

This young woman with a variety of seemingly unrelated neurologic findings in her extremities and vision most likely has MS. The pathophysiology of MS is related to the transmission of the electrical signals along neurons; understanding of neuron and membrane function is critical to understanding this disease.

Action Potentials and Neuronal Function Nerves transmit electrical signals from one point in the body to another. Action potentials are generated at the **axon hillock,** where

the cell body meets the **axon,** a tubular elongated process. The signal must travel the full length of the axon, from hillock to the synaptic terminal, without degeneration. Although axons within the brain can be miniscule, those of spinal neurons are several feet long, transmitting impulses to the most distal points of our extremities.

The axonal membrane is a phospholipid bilayer containing voltage-gated ion channels that conduct impulses both passively and actively. Action potentials arise at the axon hillock and cause a depolarization of the surrounding membrane. This depolarization spreads to the portion of axon immediately downstream, which has a more negative charge. This spread is **passive;** it is due to the imbalance of charge and occurs without any facilitation by the axon. Once slightly downstream, the arriving depolarization causes voltage-gated ion channels to open and the action potential is regenerated. This is the **active propagation** of the signal; the action potential is regenerated by the flux of ions through membrane channels. The new action potential then passively spreads further downstream. The signal cannot return to the axon hillock because the ion channels upstream are immediately closed, in a refractory stage that prevents backward propagation. The entire process repeats until the action potential moves down the length of the axon (Figure 41-1).

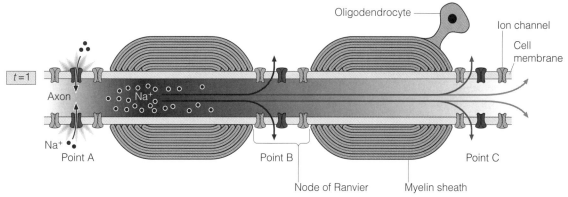

Figure 41-1 Action-potential propagation across neuronal membrane. The action potential begins at point A, where massive depolarization occurs. This charge travels passively down the membrane, which is insulated by a myelin sheath. At the node of Ranvier, where there is a gap in the myelin, the charge is regenerated as voltage-gated ion channels open and propagate the depolarization.

The velocity of an action potential is limited by the need to regenerate as it travels down the axon. Passive conduction alone is not sufficient for transmission. The axon membrane has inherent resistance, which wears down the charge of the impulse as it travels. Just as electricity flowing across uninsulated wire leaks out over distance, the magnitude of the depolarization "leaks" as it travels down stretches of axon. Furthermore, passive conduction is impeded by the bilayer structure of the axonal membrane. The space between the two conductive layers forms a capacitor; that is, for an action potential to move down the membrane, some voltage must serve to fully charge the space within the bilayer. This requirement also slows membrane conduction. (For the electrically inclined, the axon may be thought of as a resistor and a capacitor in parallel.) The result of these factors is that passive conduction cannot transmit an action potential down an entire axon. Therefore, the action potential must be actively regenerated as it moves. The cost of regeneration is conduction speed. The signal must "wait" to be regenerated at various points on the axon.

Because speed is essential in signal transmission, nerves have a few adaptations to recover the velocity of active propagation. First, increasing the numbers of ion channels ensures that action potentials will be regenerated quickly. Faster axons have greater **ion channel densities.** Second, increasing the **diameter** of the axon allows the charge to travel further without regeneration. (This increases the volume inside the axon, which transmits the impulse, relative to the membrane that impedes it.) Axons that have longer lengths are often thicker than their shorter counterparts. Finally, the best way to improve axonal conduction is to provide insulation to prevent charge from "leaking" out.

Myelin is a lipid-rich substance formed by **oligodendrocytes** in the CNS and **Schwann cells** in the PNS. It acts as an excellent insulator for axons, increasing the distance and speed with which an action potential may passively travel by minimizing the leak of charge. In the CNS, oligodendrocytes extend thin processes that wrap around axons, surrounding them in many layers of myelin. In the CNS, one oligodendrocyte can myelinate many different axons. One Schwann cell in the PNS also creates a myelin sheath, but for just one axon. Myelinated axons conduct charges quickly down their length to gaps in the myelin called **nodes of Ranvier.** At these unmyelinated nodes, clusters of ion channels regenerate the action potential, which in turn is conducted down the next segment of myelinated axon. The interspersed jumping of charges down myelinated segments with halting at regenerating nodes is called **saltatory conduction.** Myelin insulation greatly decreases the frequency with which the action potential must be regenerated, increasing its speed down the axon. Myelin greatly increases conduction velocity; although unmyelinated axons have a conduction velocity of about 2 m/second, myelinated axons can have a conduction velocity of up to 100 m/second. By far, myelination is the most important enhancement that allows signals to be conducted down nerve fibers.

Clinical Correlation   **MS** is progressive demyelination throughout the CNS that is thought to be autoimmune in origin. It is a relatively common disease, usually affecting young adults (ages 20 to 50 years) and occurring in women more often than men. Myelin insulation provided by oligodendrocytes is slowly destroyed and then is replaced by a glial scar. Conduction is impaired in affected axons; scarring can eventually block axonal conduction completely. The hallmark of MS is neurologic deficits that are **transitory and scattered** in location. In fact, the diagnosis of MS requires evidence of multiple lesions and more than one attack over time. Symptoms can appear after periods of infection or stress and tend to worsen with elevated body temperature. The most common complaints at presentation include paresthesia, weakness, abnormal gait, and visual loss. As demyelination periodically worsens and then remits, symptoms wax and wane. Most patients have relapses every few years. Although there is no fixed pattern to the demyelination, MRI often shows plaque formation in the periventricular white matter. In addition to MRI evidence, the diagnosis can be supported by CSF analysis; most affected patients have increased immunoglobulin G (IgG) levels in the CSF with oligoclonal bands on electrophoresis. (This fact also supports the proposed autoimmune basis for the disorder.) MS always follows a progressive course. The rate of decline varies from patient to patient though. Deterioration cannot be reversed, but worsening of disease can be slowed by regular interferon-β (IFN-β) injections.

In addition to MS, **Guillain-Barré syndrome** is a well-understood example of a demyelinating disease. Guillain-Barré is an acute, idiopathic demyelination of the PNS. Symptoms of weakness and eventual paralysis usually occur after resolution of an infectious illness, inoculation, or surgery. Weakness begins in the distal lower extremities and spreads upward. Immediate medical care is essential, as weakness can progress to paralysis of the muscles of respiration. If ventilation is maintained, the illness is self-limited. It generally resolves with no permanent sequelae.

Case Conclusion   CSF analysis demonstrates oligoclonal IgG bands on electrophoresis. MRI reveals multiple periventricular white matter plaques. You refer the patient to a neurologist, who confirms the diagnosis of MS. The neurologist gives the patient a guarded prognosis: Although her immediate symptoms will probably resolve, most patients develop some degree of disability within 10 years of diagnosis. Her young age and relatively mild symptoms are good prognostic signs. A course of weekly IM IFN-β injections is begun in hope of lengthening the interval before the next relapse. The patient also joins a support group, where she can learn more about MS and the experiences of others who share her illness.

Thumbnail: Membrane Properties

Property	Effect on conduction velocity
Density of ion channels	Increases
Diameter	Increases
Myelination	Increases

Key Points

▶ Axons actively propagate action potentials as they travel down nerves.

▶ Conduction velocity increases with increased membrane channel density and diameter.

▶ Myelin serves as an insulator for axons. In the CNS, myelin is supplied by oligodendrocytes; in the PNS, it is supplied by Schwann cells.

▶ In myelinated axons, action potentials travel passively through myelinated segments and are regenerated at the nodes of Ranvier.

▶ One oligodendrocyte can insulate many neurons in the CNS, but one Schwann cell insulates only one axon in the PNS.

Questions

1. Which of the following would most likely remain unaffected in a patient with MS?
   A. Oligodendrocyte structure
   B. Muscle strength
   C. Deep tendon reflexes
   D. Optic nerve function
   E. Schwann cell function

2. Which of the following nerves would be expected to have the greatest conduction velocity?
   A. An unmyelinated pain fiber, 30 cm long, 1 μm in diameter
   B. An unmyelinated interneuron, 5 mm long, 0.8 μm in diameter
   C. An unmyelinated interneuron, 1mm long, 0.2 μm in diameter
   D. A myelinated motor fiber, 20 cm long, 0.9 μm in diameter
   E. A myelinated sensory fiber, 10 cm long, 0.8 μm in diameter

3. Gliosis at the cell membrane would have which of the following effects?
   A. Enhance action-potential propagation by insulating axonal membrane
   B. Slow action-potential propagation by blocking passive movement of depolarization
   C. Enhance action-potential propagation by increasing the diameter of the axon
   D. Slow action-potential propagation by increasing the depositions of oligodendrocytes
   E. Enhance action-potential propagation by increasing the density of ion channels

4. A 26-year-old kindergarten teacher comes to the ED with rapidly increasing weakness. She notes that a few weeks ago, she felt "run down" with a flu, but over the past 2 days, she has become very weak; what began as tripping over her feet evolved to trouble with stairs and now she has difficulty with any walking. Her examination is notable for areflexia of the lower extremities. Which of the following structures is impaired in this patient?
   A. Axon hillock
   B. Nodes of Ranvier
   C. Axonal ion channels
   D. Oligodendrocytes
   E. Schwann cells

> **HPI:** A 73-year-old writer presents to your practice complaining of fatigue and general weakness of 5 months' duration. He notes his fatigue has gotten worse, and he now has trouble standing up or sitting up out of bed. He has stopped exercising since his fatigue began, although he has not gained any weight. He continues to drink socially and smoke five packs of cigarettes a week. The patient denies visual changes, but notes dry mouth and on questioning admits to recent-onset impotence.
>
> **PE:** You note bilateral proximal muscle weakness, especially of the lower limbs, as well as hypoactive deep tendon reflexes of all extremities.

Thought Questions

■ What clinical signs and symptoms distinguish neuromuscular junction disease from other nervous or muscular disorders?

■ How do action potentials lead to neurotransmitter release?

■ What defects at the presynaptic terminal could cause neuromuscular junction disease?

Basic Science Review and Discussion

This patient has a presentation typical of Lambert-Eaton syndrome. Lambert-Eaton myasthenia is an autoimmune syndrome affecting the neuromuscular junction (NMJ), most commonly seen in patients with an underlying malignancy. Understanding how a malignancy can cause diffuse weakness requires knowledge of the structure and function of the presynaptic terminal of the synapse.

Presynaptic Membrane Structure and Function Synapses between nerves allow the transmission of electrical signals from a presynaptic to a postsynaptic neuron. The most direct means of transmission is via a **gap junction,** in which a direct connection between the two neurons facilitates the spread of action potentials down a tract. More commonly, **chemical synapses** exist to allow signal transmission between neurons.

These synapses convert action potentials into chemical signals that diffuse across a physical gap, the synaptic cleft, to the postsynaptic neuron. Thus, a presynaptic ending, or terminal, must have a means to convert electrical signals into chemical signals. The classic example of a chemical synapse is the **NMJ,** where signals from the nerve are transmitted via ACh to the postsynaptic muscle endplate, resulting in muscle contraction. Chemical synapses have the advantage of allowing integration or amplification of signals, rather than the direct transmission of gap junctions.

The membrane of the presynaptic terminal contains many voltage-gated Ca^{2+} channels. Within the presynaptic termi-

nal are vesicles containing neurotransmitter. For a given neuron, the amount of neurotransmitter contained in each synaptic vesicle is approximately equal. Thus, transmitter is released in multiples of this amount: If each vesicle contains n molecules of transmitter, the total amount released into the synaptic cleft will be n multiplied by the number of vesicles emptying their contents. The type of transmitter and exact size of vesicle varies from neuron to neuron. After an action potential travels down an axon, it arrives at the presynaptic terminal. The depolarization causes the Ca^{2+} channel to open. Calcium may then flow into the cell, down its electrochemical gradient. The rapid influx and increased intracellular Ca^{2+} levels in turn cause the synaptic vesicles to fuse with the cell membrane, opening to pour their neurotransmitter contents into the synaptic cleft. The result is a chemical signal that can diffuse toward the postsynaptic neuron, without a gap junction. After each burst of exocytosis, the vesicles are recycled via endocytosis into the membrane to be refilled with transmitter. (See Thumbnail: Presynaptic Membrane, later in this case.)

Clinical Correlation: Lambert-Eaton Myasthenic Syndrome
Lambert-Eaton myasthenic syndrome is an acquired autoimmune disease in which auto-antibodies form against voltage-sensitive calcium channels, resulting in defective release of ACh at presynaptic nerve terminals. Because the presynaptic function is altered, there is decreased signaling to other nerves and to muscle. Clinically, patients develop fatigue and weakness of trunk muscles and the proximal muscles of the limbs. Lambert-Eaton syndrome most often occurs in patients with existing small cell carcinoma, although it may also occur in autoimmune disease. The syndrome may become evident before a tumor is detected. (Keep this in mind when presented with a patient with new proximal muscle weakness who also has risk factors for lung cancer!)

In addition to proximal muscle weakness, defective ACh release can cause diminished or absent deep tendon reflexes, as well as autonomic dysfunction (e.g., xerostomia, anhidrosis, orthostatic hypotension, and sexual dysfunction). Because the deficit in Lambert-Eaton syndrome is in channel activity allowing ACh release, weakness may be somewhat overcome by tetanic contraction. Repeated stimulation of the presynaptic terminal maximizes the number of remaining calcium channels open, whereas increasing intracellular calcium levels allows increased ACh release. Thus, although initial muscle responses may be weak, after repeated stimulation, the response may approach normal. Electrophysiologic testing reveals that this increased muscle response with repeated stimulation and is useful in distinguishing Lambert-Eaton syndrome from other neuromuscular diseases. Treatment of Lambert-Eaton myasthenic syndrome relies on immunosuppression to decrease auto-antibody formation, as well as plasmapheresis to decrease circulating antibody levels.

Case Conclusion   EMG studies show initially low muscle responses to nerve stimulation, but facilitated response with tetanic stimulation. Because of the high co-incidence of myasthenic syndrome with carcinoma, you order a chest scan. CT shows a 3-cm hilar lesion in the right lung; biopsy of the mass reveals small cell carcinoma. The patient is referred to oncology, to discuss surgical resection and chemotherapy of this newly discovered tumor.

Thumbnail: Presynaptic Membrane

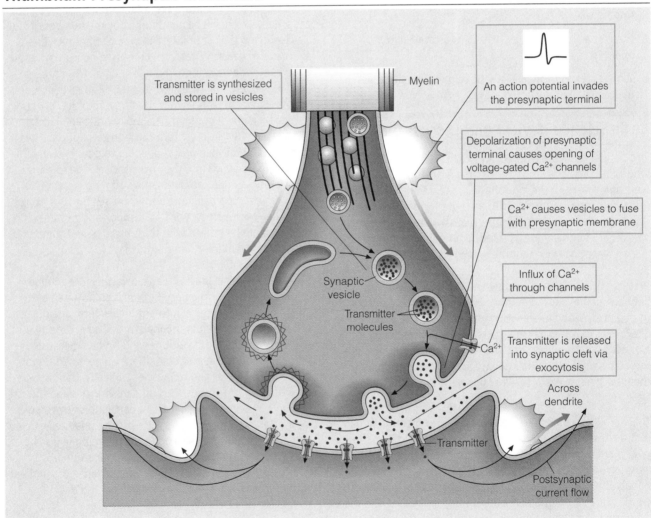

Key Points

▸ Most synapses are chemical synapses; they convert electrical signals into chemical signals that cross the synaptic cleft.

▸ Synaptic transmission is usually unidirectional; there is a presynaptic (upstream) and a postsynaptic (downstream) component.

▸ Neurotransmitter is released from vesicles containing relatively fixed quantities of chemical. As a result, the release of neurotransmitter is quantal.

▸ Presynaptic function is calcium dependent.

Questions

1. You see an 8-month-old girl in the ED who is suspected of having ingested food contaminated with *Clostridium botulinum.* After eating some homemade jam, she began to show symptoms of botulism. You recall that botulinum toxin acts at the presynaptic terminal, inactivating proteins involved in exocytosis. This manifests clinically as which of the following signs?
   A. Flaccid paralysis
   B. Hyper-reflexia
   C. Excessive salivation
   D. Spastic paralysis
   E. Crying and hyperventilation

2. Aminoglycoside drugs (e.g., gentamicin and streptomycin) can compete with calcium at the presynaptic terminal, sometimes causing or enhancing muscle paralysis. At which level would the aminoglycosides have their effect?
   A. Impair action-potential propagation at the presynaptic terminal
   B. Decrease amount of neurotransmitter in vesicles
   C. Inhibit the ion influx that normally allows exocytosis
   D. Inactivate neurotransmitter in the synaptic cleft
   E. Promote rapid endocytosis of synaptic vesicles before neurotransmitter is fully released into cleft

3. Reserpine is a drug that inhibits the transport of NE into vesicles at the presynaptic terminal. Which of the following would have the same effect at the synapse as reserpine?
   A. Stimulating NE synthesis
   B. Depolarizing the presynaptic terminal
   C. Blocking presynaptic Ca^{2+} channel function
   D. Stimulating vesicle fusion with the membrane
   E. Promoting exocytosis

4. Repeated presynaptic depolarization could result in greater neurotransmitter release by which mechanism?
   A. Increased numbers of vesicles fusing with the membrane
   B. Larger vesicles fusing with the membrane
   C. Vesicle fusion of a longer duration
   D. A and C
   E. All of the above

HPI: A 44-year-old office manager is referred to your neurology clinic by her primary care physician, who observed ptosis and mild nystagmus at her last visit. The patient reports increasing fatigue over the last few months and has considered switching to part-time work because she "can never make it through the day anymore." Even though her only flu this year was several months ago, she describes persistently "getting tired more easily: By 3 P.M., I can't stand looking at my computer screen for another minute."

PE: You elicit mild nystagmus and note ptosis, greater in the left eye than the right. When you ask the patient to maintain an upward gaze, this ptosis worsens notably. Facial sensation is normal, but you observe mild facial muscle weakness. Deep tendon reflexes are normal, and strength and sensation of the extremities are within normal limits.

Thought Questions

- What is this patient's most likely diagnosis?
- What effect does ACh normally have at the NMJ?
- How does neurotransmitter release usually lead to postsynaptic action potentials?
- How can the events at the synapse be altered by drugs to change postsynaptic effects?

Basic Science Review and Discussion

In this patient with increasing fatigue over the past few months and neurologic findings of nystagmus and ptosis, particularly with worsening of ptosis upon maintained gaze, myasthenia gravis should be considered. The pathophysiology of myasthenia gravis is related to ACh and its function.

Acetylcholine Neurotransmitter released into the synaptic cleft is a chemical signal that can diffuse toward the postsynaptic neuron. However, for transmission to be complete, this chemical signal must be converted back into an electrical signal. The classic illustration of this process includes the events at the NMJ. After ACh is released from the presynaptic membrane into the synaptic cleft, it diffuses toward the postsynaptic membrane of the muscle fiber. There, ACh receptors bind the transmitter. These receptors are attached to ion channels; the entire unit at the NMJ is called a **nicotinic ACh receptor**. This is an example of a **ligand-gated ion channel**. When ACh binds to its receptor, the protein changes conformation and directly opens the ion channel, allowing an influx of Na^+ and an efflux of K^+. The net result is depolarization at the postsynaptic membrane, an area called the **endplate** of the muscle fiber. Each molecule of ACh that binds with a receptor opens an ion channel, producing a **miniature endplate potential (MEPP)**. If enough ACh binds to enough receptors, the potentials from many MEPPs are summed into one larger depolarization, an **endplate potential (EPP)**. This depolarization, in turn, is large enough to open voltage-gated ion channels, which generate an action potential. The action potential travels across the muscle fiber, triggering calcium release and resulting in muscle contraction. The chemical signal of ACh has been converted to an electrical signal at the postsynaptic membrane. The unit then "resets" by clearing out ACh from the synaptic cleft. Acetylcholinesterase is an enzyme in the synaptic cleft that degrades ACh to acetate and choline. These breakdown products reenter the presynaptic cell, where they are recycled into ACh. The presence of acetylcholinesterase ensures that the effect at the NMJ is limited; synaptic activity is transitory rather than permanent (Figure 43-1).

Postsynaptic Membrane Although the example of the NMJ is well understood, the exact events at the postsynaptic membrane vary throughout the nervous system. Postsynaptic receptors vary in structure and in their effects on neurons. For example, not all cholinergic synapses work through ligand-gated ion channels. Muscarinic ACh receptors instead are bound to G-proteins, which activate second messengers. When ACh in the synaptic cleft binds with a muscarinic receptor, an enzyme cascade is triggered, with varying final results depending on the specific type of cascade triggered. These second-messenger receptors are sometimes called **metabotropic** receptors (as opposed to directly **ionotropic** receptors). In some cases, the second messengers cause the opening of Na^+ channels or closing of K^+ channels, resulting in a depolarization much like that at the endplate. This brings the postsynaptic neuron closer to threshold; it is now in an "excited" state where action-potential generation is facilitated. The general term for a potential of this type is **EPSP**. A series of EPSPs (either repeatedly from the same presynaptic input or at once from several presynaptic synapses) can sum to push the neuron past threshold and fire an action potential. In other instances, the second messenger leads to the opening of K^+ or Cl^- channels or the closing of Na^+ channels. In this case, the result at the postsynaptic membrane is a hyperpolarization, moving the cell further from threshold. Because the cell is now further from the threshold required to generate an action potential, these potentials are called **IPSPs**.

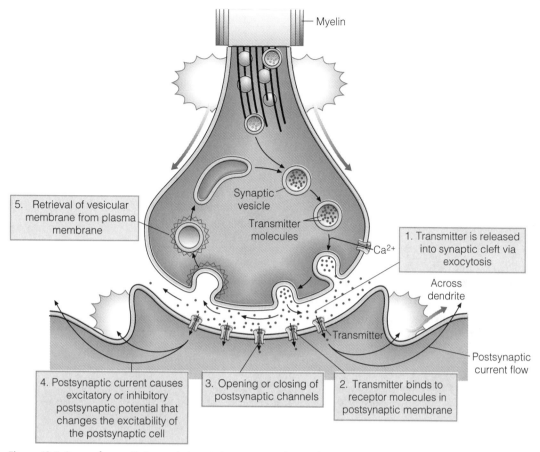

Figure 43-1 Steps of synaptic transmission at the postsynaptic membrane.

Various combinations exist in which a given transmitter activates either a metabotropic or ionotropic receptor, eliciting either an EPSP or an IPSP. Any neurotransmitter can have either excitatory or inhibitory effects depending on the structure of its receptor. Nonetheless, certain receptors predominate in the nervous system, and so neurotransmitters can have a generally excitatory or inhibitory effect. (For example, glutamate is largely excitatory, whereas GABA is usually inhibitory.)

These effects can occur simultaneously at one postsynaptic neuron, which allows integration of multiple incoming signals. If the EPSPs outweigh the IPSPs at a postsynaptic membrane, an action potential results. Likewise, IPSPs can counteract excitatory input from upstream neurons. In this way, multiple synapses on one neuron can be processed to result in one event, the firing (or nonfiring) of an action potential.

Just as there are many different receptor types, there are various methods by which neurotransmitter is cleared from the synaptic cleft. Some synapses employ enzymatic degradation, like **acetylcholinesterase,** to break down neurotransmitter. Others use transporter pumps to bring the neurotransmitter back into the presynaptic terminal or into surrounding glial cells. All rely on simple diffusion to some

degree. These mechanisms are popular targets for pharmaceutical therapy; by prolonging neurotransmitter release in the synaptic cleft, they increase its activity. Examples of such drugs are selective serotonin reuptake inhibitors (SSRIs) (e.g., fluoxetine), which block reuptake pumps, or monoamine oxidase inhibitors (MAOIs) (e.g., phenelzine), which prevent degradation of catecholamines. Eventually, though, neurotransmitter is removed from the synaptic cleft and the signaling process can start over.

Clinical Correlation   **Myasthenia gravis** is an autoimmune disorder that attacks the NMJ. Auto-antibodies to nicotinic ACh receptors block signaling; ACh release in the synaptic cleft thus has less effect on the postsynaptic membrane. The disease most often affects cranial muscles, such as the extraocular muscles and those innervated by CN VII. The resulting symptom is fatigable weakness, that is, muscle weakness that worsens with sustained contraction and improves after rest. The diagnosis is classically confirmed by a **Tensilon (or edrophonium) test.** Tensilon is an acetylcholinesterase inhibitor; it counters the enzyme that normally degrades ACh in the synaptic cleft. In a patient with myasthenia gravis, Tensilon administration lengthens the life of ACh in the synapse, which allows increased effect at the postsynaptic membrane and thus improved strength and immediate relief from symptoms. Likewise, long-term treatment usually involves regular administration of an anticholinesterase drug. The origin of the auto-antibodies in myasthenia gravis is unclear, but there is a high incidence of comorbidity in the thymus. Therefore, each patient should be evaluated for thymoma, and thymectomy may be performed in an effort to lessen symptoms. Likewise, because symptoms are mediated through auto-antibodies, steroid treatment to inhibit immune function can alleviate symptoms of myasthenia gravis. Generally, myasthenia gravis is progressive, although the course may involve lengthy periods of maintenance without remission of symptoms.

Case Conclusion   A Tensilon test in the office produces dramatic improvement in the ptosis, as well as complete cessation of nystagmus. Facial musculature shows increased strength. The patient is begun on a regular schedule of anticholinesterase drugs, which allow her to resume her prior activities. Although a CT shows no thymic mass, the patient elects thymectomy, which leads to an almost total remission of her symptoms. She understands she is not "cured" of her disease, but her symptoms remain minimal after surgery and with her new drug regimen.

Thumbnail: Acetylcholine and Postsynaptic Membrane

Postsynaptic Receptors		
Receptor type	**Ionotropic**	**Metabotropic**
Works via . . .	Ligand-gated ion channels	G-proteins and second messengers
Speed	Faster	Slower
Example of excitatory receptor	Nicotinic ACh receptor at NMJ	M_1 muscarinic ACh receptors in the autonomic nervous system
Example of inhibitory receptor	$GABA_A$ receptors in the brain	$GABA_B$ receptors in the brain

Key Points

▶ ACh in the NMJ directly opens ligand-gated ion channels, causing a depolarization of the endplate (EPP).

▶ A sufficient number of depolarizations at the postsynaptic membrane (EPSPs) can drive a neuronal membrane past threshold and generate an action potential.

▶ Hyperpolarizations (IPSPs) drive the cell further from threshold, preventing action-potential generation.

▶ Postsynaptic receptors either can be ligand-gated ion channels (ionotropic) or affect channels via a second messenger (metabotropic).

▶ The effects of a neurotransmitter on the postsynaptic membrane are determined by the properties of the specific receptor on that membrane, not by the neurotransmitter itself.

▶ Neurotransmitter effects can be enhanced by drugs that prolong their time in the synaptic cleft.

Questions

1. Dopamine is an example of a neurotransmitter that has both excitatory and inhibitory effects in the CNS. Dopamine can have an excitatory effect on a given post-synaptic neuron in the striatum, but an inhibitory effect on a postsynaptic neuron in the cortex. The best explanation for this is which of the following?
   A. More dopaminergic vesicles are released at the striatal synapse than at the cortical synapse.
   B. The receptors on the striatal neuron are ionotropic, and the cortical receptors are metabotropic.
   C. The receptors on the striatal neuron have a higher affinity for dopamine than those of the cortical neuron.
   D. The ion channels affected in the striatal postsynaptic neuron are different from those in the cortical cell.
   E. The receptors at the striatal membrane have greater dopaminergic activation because of lower levels of enzymatic degradation.

2. A spinal interneuron integrates signals from two presynaptic inputs. One input has an excitatory effect via glutamate release, and the other has an inhibitory effect via glycine release. When the excitatory presynaptic neuron fires alone, glutamate release leads to an action potential in the postsynaptic neuron. When both presynaptic neurons are fired simultaneously, the postsynaptic membrane is inhibited; it does not fire an action potential. How does glycine negate the otherwise excitatory effect of glutamate on this cell?
   A. Glycine blocks glutamate release at the presynaptic membrane.
   B. Glycine binds to glutamate, rendering it unable to bind to postsynaptic receptors.
   C. Glycine competes with glutamate for the same receptors on the postsynaptic membrane.
   D. Glycine binds to different receptors on the postsynaptic membrane, affecting ion channels.
   E. Glycine activates the pump on the presynaptic membrane, which removes glutamate from the synaptic cleft.

3. Some nerve gases are potent acetylcholinesterase inhibitors. Through what mechanism do they have their effect?
   A. Inhibiting the release of ACh, thus blocking signaling
   B. Acting as antagonists at postsynaptic ACh receptors, thus blocking signaling
   C. Inhibiting postsynaptic G-protein signaling pathways
   D. Inhibiting the synthesis of signaling neurotransmitter
   E. Increasing ACh available in the synaptic cleft

4. Fluoxetine, sertraline, and paroxetine are all examples of SSRIs. How do these drugs increase activity at the synapse?
   A. Acting as agonists at the postsynaptic membrane
   B. Increasing vesicle fusion at the presynaptic membrane
   C. Inhibiting transporters on the postsynaptic membrane
   D. Directly depolarizing the postsynaptic membrane
   E. Inhibiting transporters on the presynaptic membrane

HPI: A 65-year-old retired professor comes to your practice complaining of difficulty "getting around," gradually increasing for more than 1 year. On observation, you see he has difficulty standing and is slow to begin walking. He walks slowly, taking very small short steps.

PE: You note rigidity on examination. The patient sits quietly throughout the examination, continually making small, repetitive movements of his hands and fingers. Although he states he is very distressed by his symptoms, he remains almost completely without facial expression during his visit.

Thought Questions

- What is the most likely diagnosis of this patient?
- What is the possible cause of and which areas of the CNS are affected by this disorder?
- How is dopamine synthesized?
- Where else in the body does dopamine act?

Basic Science Review and Discussion

This gentleman's most likely diagnosis is Parkinson's disease (PD). His gait, with small, short steps, diminished extremity movements, and limited facial expression are all classic findings. The physiology of the neurotransmitter dopamine is intimately involved in this disease, so understanding its biochemistry, receptors, and actions is important in understanding and treating **PD**.

Dopamine Dopamine is a catecholamine neurotransmitter that acts both in the brain and outside the CNS. All the catecholamines (dopamine, NE, epinephrine) are synthesized via a common pathway from the amino acid phenylalanine, which is also the precursor to melanin and thyroxine (T_4) synthesis. The dopamine synthesis pathway is important both as a frequent topic in Step 1 questions and as a target for drug therapy in PD, where there is a deficit of dopamine (Figure 44-1).

Dopamine acts primarily on five types of receptors, D_1 to D_5. All are seven-transmembrane segment G-protein receptors. These receptors are found on tissues throughout the body, including the renal vasculature, anterior pituitary, and the GI tract. In the brain, dopamine acts in the basal ganglia, limbic system, and cortex, affecting mood, reward pathways, cognition, and movement. Drugs such as amphetamine and cocaine produce euphoria and motor agitation by increasing dopaminergic activity in the brain. In the basal ganglia, D_1 has an excitatory effect on adenylate cyclase postsynaptically, whereas D_2 has an inhibitory effect on adenylate cyclase both presynaptically and postsynaptically. Although dopamine is found throughout, 80% of the brain's dopamine is found in the substantia nigra.

The **substantia nigra** is a nucleus at the base of the midbrain composed of two parts, the **substantia nigra pars compacta** and the **substantia nigra pars reticulata**. The cells of the nucleus have high concentrations of melanin and thus have a dark appearance to the naked eye. (Hence, the name, which is Latin for "dark substance.") The substantia nigra compacta projects dopaminergic axons to the striatum, where dopamine acts on both D_1 and D_2 receptors in the caudate and putamen. The overall effect of increased dopamine from the substantia nigra is increased motor activity.

In the normal brain, the dopaminergic axons from the substantia nigra have a net excitatory effect on the striatum, which in turn inhibits the internal segment of the globus

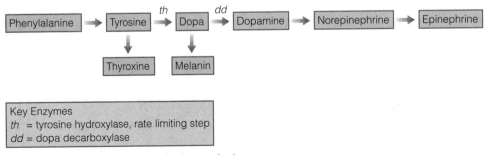

Figure 44-1 Dopamine and catecholamine synthesis.

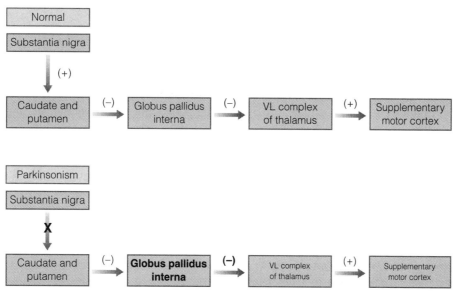

Figure 44-2 Normal motor pathways are altered in Parkinson's disease by a lack of dopaminergic input from the substantia nigra; the result is increased inhibition by the globus pallidus and decreased motor output. For simplicity, only the direct pathway is depicted.

pallidus via the direct pathway. This dampens the effect of the internal segment of the globus pallidus, which otherwise acts to inhibit the excitatory stimulation of the ventrolateral thalamus, on motor cortex. If the substantia nigra is not functioning, there is less excitement to the striatum, and thus less inhibition of the internal segment of the **globus pallidus.** The globus pallidus is then free to inhibit the ventrolateral thalamus, and end-motor activity is decreased as a result of excessive indirect pathway activity (Figure 44-2). "Short-circuiting" the indirect pathway by deep brain stimulation of the subthalamic nucleus has proven to be a good symptomatic treatment for PD. The direct and indirect pathways are discussed further in Case 11.

Clinical Correlation Parkinsonism is a syndrome defined by a collection of motor deficits such as "cogwheel" **rigidity,** resting "pill-rolling" or "head-nodding" **tremor, bradykinesia,** difficulty initiating movement, stooped posture, diminished facial expression ("Parkinson's mask"), and festinating gait. This syndrome is found after damage to the substantia nigra or its connections to the striatum. The substantia nigra may be damaged after exposure to certain drugs or toxins, such as dopamine antagonists, 1-methyl-4-phenyl-1,2,5,6-tetrahydropyridine (MPTP), or manganese; during an acute viral encephalitis, although this has become exceedingly rare; or due to ischemia in atherosclerotic disease. In each of these cases, parkinsonism may occur (Figure 44-3).

Although parkinsonism is a clinical syndrome with a number of possible causes, **PD** is the most common. Idiopathic PD occurs later in life, when degeneration of the dopaminergic cells of the substantia nigra causes an overall deficit of

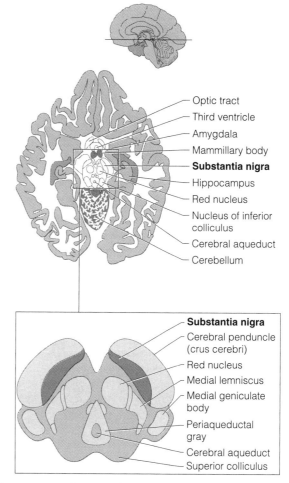

Figure 44-3 Axial section of brain at level of midbrain. Note the location of substantia nigra in relation to the cerebral peduncles, red nucleus, and tegmentum of midbrain.

dopamine in the basal ganglia. For symptoms to be present, there must be a loss of at least 80% of the cells of the substantia nigra. On microscopic examination, the remaining neurons can show Lewy bodies, which are dense deposits of filament inside the neuronal body. The cause of these deposits and of neuronal degeneration is unclear. Untreated, PD will progress, with symptoms worsening until death. About 15% to 30% of patients also develop dementia, usually attributed to Lewy body deposits in the cortex. Although there is no cure for PD, a number of therapies attempt to correct the dopamine deficiency and relieve

symptoms. Action on D_2 receptors has been shown to be particularly important, although some benefit can be gained by action on D_1 receptors as well. Drug therapy includes **levodopa (L-dopa),** a form of dopa that can cross the blood-brain barrier and be converted to dopamine. Other useful drugs are dopamine agonists and MAOIs. Although these may allow dramatic improvement when initiated, there is often a "wearing off" of the drug's effect and responsiveness may be lost completely. In severe cases, surgery may also be employed, as described above.

Case Conclusion   The patient underwent neuropsychiatric testing and was found to have no signs of dementia. Drug therapy was initiated, consisting of oral L-dopa daily. The patient began physical therapy to maximize his mobility. This resulted in significant improvement, and after 1 month, the patient was able to walk relatively well with a cane. The patient was advised that this gain may be temporary and was informed that future options may include addition of other drugs to his regimen or possibly surgical intervention.

Thumbnail: Dopamine and Substantia Nigra

Dopamine Receptors

Type of receptor	Primary location	Effect on cyclic adenosine monophosphate (cAMP)
D_1	Striatum, vascular tissue	↑
D_2	Throughout brain, smooth muscle, presynaptic nerve terminals	↓
D_3	Limbic system, cortex	↓
D_4	Limbic system, cortex, cardiovascular muscle	↓
D_5	Cortex, hippocampus, renal vasculature	↑

Key Points

▶ Dopamine is a catecholamine; its synthesis is limited by the conversion of tyrosine to dopa, dopamine's immediate precursor.

▶ In the basal ganglia, the net effect of dopamine is to promote movement.

▶ The substantia nigra is located in the midbrain; although the dark pigment distinguishes the nucleus in normal specimens, the region can be completely pale in cases of PD with severe neuronal loss. Thus, to identify the substantia nigra, know the characteristic color **and** the relative location of the nucleus in the midbrain.

▶ Parkinsonism is a syndrome characterized by rigidity, difficulty initiating movements, resting tremor, slow movement, diminished facial expression, and shuffling gait. It may occur after any type of damage to the substantia nigra.

▶ Idiopathic PD is the most common cause of parkinsonism.

Questions

1. A 26-year-old chef with schizophrenia has been admitted to the inpatient psychiatry service after her second florid episode in a year. Her physician prescribes chlorpromazine and alprazolam to be taken immediately. At the urging of her family, the patient also resumes taking the haloperidol she was prescribed by another doctor after her earlier episodes. After a week in the hospital, her nurses notice a resting "head-nod" tremor, as well as slowness in movements. Her facial expression is also markedly diminished. A review of medication reveals she is taking high doses of two antipsychotics, which are considered the cause of her parkinsonism. The haloperidol is discontinued and L-dopa begun to alleviate symptoms. Which of the following enzymes catalyzes the rate-limiting step required for L-dopa to be converted to dopamine in the brain?

   A. Phenylalanine hydroxylase
   B. Tyrosine hydroxylase
   C. Dopa decarboxylase
   D. Monoamine oxidase A
   E. Monoamine oxidase B

2. MPTP is a toxin that can be unintentionally synthesized in the illicit manufacturing of opioid drugs . MPTP is selectively taken up by the dopaminergic neurons of the substantia nigra, where its active form causes neuronal death. Cases have been reported of opioid users self-administering MPTP contaminate and developing a severe acute-onset PD. A patient developing this type of toxin-mediated PD will have symptoms resulting from altered activity in which set of brain areas?

   A. Substantia nigra reticulata, caudate, putamen, cerebellum
   B. Substantia nigra reticulata, striatum, internal segment of the globus pallidus, motor cortex
   C. Substantia nigra reticulata, putamen, ventrolateral thalamus, motor cortex
   D. Substantia nigra compacta, striatum, internal segment of the globus pallidus, ventrolateral thalamus
   E. Substantia nigra compacta, striatum, internal segment of the globus pallidus, cerebellum

3. Which of the following is an identified cause of parkinsonism?

   A. Viral encephalitis
   B. Head trauma
   C. Ischemia
   D. All of the above
   E. None of the above

4. Which structures lie directly adjacent to the substantia nigra?

   A. Cerebral peduncle
   B. Red nucleus
   C. Cerebral aqueduct
   D. A and C
   E. All of the above

HPI: A 25-year-old paralegal comes to your family practice office complaining of months of fatigue. She is also bothered by occasional headaches and sporadic stomach and back pain. She reports difficulty sleeping: she wakes early every morning and is unable to fall back asleep. On questioning, the patient reports she has also lost about 20 pounds over the past 8 months, since moving across the country to begin her new job. She looks at the floor throughout the conversation, maintaining a flat affect with little positive expression. She does not have friends or family in the area and finds it difficult to come up with any interests or activities she enjoys as recreation.

PE: Normal, not revealing any obvious pathology.

Thought Questions

- How can major depression present?
- Which neurotransmitters have been implicated in depression?
- How is serotonin formed?
- Where does serotonin act?

Basic Science Review and Discussion

This patient comes to her physician with multiple vague physical complaints, including fatigue and insomnia. Such a presentation is very common of cases of major depression.

Because understanding the action of serotonin is useful in the diagnosis and treatment of depression, we begin with a discussion of its biochemistry and physiology.

Serotonin Serotonin, or 5-hydroxytryptamine **(5-HT),** is an indolamine neurotransmitter. Serotonin is synthesized from the amino acid tryptophan (also the precursor of niacin and melatonin). Its major metabolite is 5-hydroxyindole acetic acid (5-HIAA) (Figure 45-1).

Serotonin receptors are found throughout the body; there are more than 12 receptor subtypes. Some play important roles in pain and local inflammation after tissue damage. Others are important in local signaling in the GI tract. In fact, more than 80% of the body's serotonin is in the enterochromaffin cells of the intestine. In the brain, serotonergic neurons are mainly located in the **nucleus raphe.** This is a vertical cluster of neurons in the pons and upper midbrain that sends projections both up throughout the brain and downward into the spinal cord. Serotonin acts primarily on the 5-HT$_1$, 5-HT$_2$, and 5-HT$_3$ subsets of receptors in the CNS.

The projections of the nucleus raphe have been implicated in control of pain, nausea, sleep, and mood. The **descending analgesia circuit** of the midbrain and spinal cord is a hierarchic system that can suppress ascending pain signals. The circuit begins in the midbrain, where the periaqueductal gray is activated by endorphin release. When activated, projections from the periaqueductal gray stimulate the nucleus raphe. In turn, the projections of the nucleus raphe release more serotonin in the dorsolateral spinal cord. There, serotonin inhibits pain signals and mediates release of enkephalins. This decreases the transmission of pain signaling before it can reach the brain. This circuit is thought to be one mechanism by which extreme emotion or physical stress can modulate the sensation of pain.

Other circuits that require serotonin are not as well understood. For example, the nucleus raphe is known to be a part of the **reticular formation,** a dispersed mesh of neurons that control sleep patterns via inputs to the thalamus. It has been observed that increased serotonin activity in the reticular formation is correlated with slow-wave (non-REM) sleep. Furthermore, decreased serotonin activity is required to "turn on" REM sleep. The exact mechanism, though, is unclear. Likewise, serotonin is known to be important in controls of nausea through 5-HT$_3$ receptors on the gut and in the brainstem. Particularly, serotonin acting at specific areas of the medulla is thought to underlie nausea and vomiting in response to noxious stimuli. The interplay between signals from the GI tract and the **medullary vomiting center,** though, is unclear. Finally, serotonin levels are known to have a profound effect on mood. However, much remains unknown about how exactly mood is controlled.

Clinical Correlation **Major depressive disorder** is very common; it affects 10% to 20% of individuals at some point during their life. Patients experience fatigue, anhedonia, and a loss of interest in formerly motivating activities. A

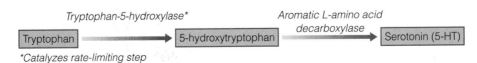

Figure 45-1 Serotonin is synthesized in a series of steps from its precursor tryptophan.

sense of hopelessness is a common feature, and suicidal ideation may result. Although some spend more time eating or sleeping, most depressed persons experience a loss of appetite and insomnia. Classically, depressed individuals sleep less, have less slow-wave sleep, and wake early in the morning. The exact pathophysiology of depression is unclear, but a number of theories have been suggested. The **amine hypothesis** is based on the known effects of drugs that act at amine synapses. Drugs that block the release of NE and serotonin have been found to induce depression in some patients. Likewise, drugs that inhibit monoamine degradation or reuptake have been found to ameliorate symptoms of depression. In normal persons, drugs that increase amine transmitter activity cause a sense of euphoria or symptoms of mania. This evidence has been proposed to suggest that decreased levels of NE and serotonin in the brain cause depression and insomnia, whereas increased levels cause mania. A variation of the amine hypothesis is based on more recent findings that drugs that affect only serotonin, such as SSRIs, can also give relief from depression with a much lower incidence of side effects. The **permissive serotonin hypothesis** proposes that dysfunction of serotonin allows altered catecholamine levels to cause changes in mood. That is, alterations in serotonin levels are required for abnormal catecholamine levels to affect mood. Current research aims at elucidating the exact relationship between serotonin, catecholamines, and mood disorders.

Pharmaceutical agents that increase functional serotonin levels have been proven effective in many cases of depression. In addition to SSRIs, MAOIs and tricyclic antidepressants (TCAs) increase the time serotonin lasts in the synaptic cleft. Drugs that act directly on 5-HT receptors have not been widely employed in depression but have found other applications. Sumatriptan is a 5-HT$_{1D}$ agonist that acts at receptors on the cerebral and meningeal vasculature. By directly stimulating these receptors, it provides immediate relief from migraine headaches for many patients. Ondansetron is a 5-HT$_3$ antagonist that is a powerful antinauseant and antiemetic. Its effects at the medullary vomiting center have been extremely helpful to patients undergoing chemotherapy. Although the primary application of serotonin-affecting drugs is in mood disorders, other applications are of significant importance as well.

> **Case Conclusion**   With further discussion, the patient admits she has been feeling sad and even hopeless lately. At times she feels guilty or worthless for no particular reason, but she denies contemplating suicide. You suggest that her symptoms could be a part of a larger case of depression. She reluctantly agrees and accepts your recommendation to visit a psychologist for a trial of cognitive-behavioral therapy with antidepressant medication. With this combination of treatment, more than two thirds of patients can expect significant remission of symptoms.

Thumbnail: Serotonin and Nucleus Raphe

Important 5-HT Receptors in the CNS			
Receptor subtype	**Location**	**Receptor type**	**Effect**
5-HT$_{1A}$	Nucleus raphe, hippocampus	Metabotropic	Inhibition
5-HT$_{1D}$	Cerebral and meningeal vessels	Metabotropic	Vasoconstriction
5-HT$_2$	Cortex, striatum	Metabotropic	Excitation
5-HT$_3$	Medullary vomiting center (a.k.a., area postrema)	Ionotropic	Excitation

Key Points

▶ Serotonin is an amine neurotransmitter synthesized from tryptophan.

▶ Serotonin acts throughout the body in pain, inflammation, and GI tract function.

▶ In the brain, serotonin-containing neurons are found mainly in the nucleus raphe and send projections throughout the CNS.

▶ Serotonin is active in descending inhibition of pain in the spinal cord, sleep and wakefulness, and mood.

Questions

1. Serotonergic projections from the nucleus raphe act on neurons in the spinal cord and dorsal root ganglia as part of the descending analgesia circuit. This activation of 5-HT receptors in the spinal cord has which of the following effects on ion channels?

   A. Increase postsynaptic K^+ conduction
   B. Decrease postsynaptic K^+ conduction
   C. Increase postsynaptic Na^+ conduction
   D. Decrease postsynaptic Cl^- conduction
   E. Increase presynaptic Ca^{2+} conduction

2. Which of the following receive serotonergic projections from the nucleus raphe?

   A. Reticular formation
   B. Enterochromaffin cells
   C. Descending analgesia circuit
   D. A and C
   E. All of the above

3. A strong serotonin agonist that acts in the area postrema of the medulla would most likely have which of the following effects?

   A. Elevate mood
   B. Cause vasodilation
   C. Cause headache
   D. Promote vomiting
   E. Descending analgesia

4. The pontine reticular formation regulates sleep patterns mainly through direct inputs to which brain region?

   A. Periaqueductal gray
   B. Thalamus
   C. Nucleus raphe
   D. Hippocampus
   E. Cerebral cortex

> **HPI:** A 36-year-old homemaker is referred to your psychiatry practice for feelings of persistent anxiety. She describes constantly feeling worried, "even when things are going fine." She often has difficulty falling asleep and at times even suffers attacks of acute anxiety, during which she experiences palpitations, dizziness, and shortness of breath with a sense of impending doom lasting about 15 minutes. She reports that she has had anxiety since her twenties, but that she never sought any treatment. Over the past few years, her symptoms have worsened and have begun to seriously affect her marriage.

Thought Questions

- What neurotransmitters regulate awareness and excitement?

- Where does NE act in the body?

- How is NE synthesized?

- Where are most of the brain's noradrenergic neurons found, and what do they do?

Basic Science Review and Discussion

This patient describes insomnia and pervasive anxiety, symptoms of a generalized anxiety disorder, complicated by anxiety attacks. Anxiety disorders are thought to involve a heightened state of arousal, which has been linked to dysregulation of NE in the brain. Understanding anxiety disorders and new possible treatments requires knowledge of NE and related circuits in the brain.

Norepinephrine NE is a catecholamine neurotransmitter synthesized (like all catecholamines) from tyrosine. It is also a precursor of epinephrine. Vanillylmandelic acid (VMA) is a metabolite of catecholamine breakdown that can be measured in urine to assess catecholamine levels in the body (Figure 46-1).

Peripherally, NE acts on postganglionic synapses in the sympathetic nervous system. There are four subtypes of receptors: α_1, α_2, β_1, and β_2. The "1" subtype of each is excitatory, and the "2" subtype is inhibitory.

The α_2-receptor provides an example of direct negative feedback in the nervous system. These receptors can be found on the presynaptic terminal at noradrenergic synapses. Here, in addition to binding at the postsynaptic

terminal, some of the NE released into the synaptic cleft binds with the α_2-receptor on the presynaptic terminal. This causes the amount of NE subsequently released from the terminal to decrease. Because these receptors bind transmitter released from their own terminal, they are also called **auto-receptors.**

Most noradrenergic neurons in the brain are found in the **locus ceruleus** of the upper brainstem and in the lateral tegmental area of the reticular formation. The locus ceruleus has the highest concentration of noradrenergic cells in the body. It sends a particularly large number of projections to the amygdala and hippocampus, where NE release is thought to mediate emotion and memory formation.

As previously discussed, NE is known to have a profound effect on mood. The amine hypothesis proposes that along with serotonin and dopamine levels, low NE levels in the brain are responsible for depression. Antidepressant drugs such as MAOIs and TCAs have some of their effect by increasing the effects of NE at the synapse.

Noradrenergic inputs are also important in the reticular formation, which controls sleep, awareness, and arousal. (For this reason, it has been referred to as the **reticular activating system.**) NE release from the locus ceruleus to the reticular formation has been shown to "shut off" REM sleep. Likewise, heightened NE levels are correlated with increased arousal and wakefulness. Although the exact mechanism is unclear, NE is clearly crucial in arousal and sleep.

Drugs such as amphetamines and cocaine, which increase functional levels of catecholamines, demonstrate the global effects of NE on the nervous system. Decreased drive for sleep and heightened arousal and anxiety have been associated with these drugs. Likewise, as the amine hypothesis would predict, these drugs can have a euphoric effect or lead to a manic state.

Dopamine β-hydroxylase

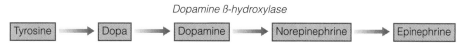

Figure 46-1 Steps in norepinephrine synthesis. Norepinephrine is produced from a series of reactions beginning with tyrosine. Note the enzyme dopamine β-hydroxylase catalyzes the conversion of dopamine to norepinephrine. Norepinephrine can be further metabolized to epinephrine.

Clinical Correlation **Generalized anxiety disorder** is ongoing worry with insomnia, tension, or irritability lasting more than 6 months. It may present with or without **panic attacks,** which are episodes of acute anxiety that usually include somatic symptoms such as palpitations, nausea, shortness of breath, sweating, and dizziness or vertigo. Often patients with panic attacks are treated for acute cardiovascular distress because of the similarity of presentation. Although psychological factors can contribute, anxiety disorders have been shown to have biologic components as well. One theory proposes that anxiety is the result of dysregulation of the locus ceruleus. Normally, α_2-receptors provide presynaptic feedback inhibition to noradrenergic neurons. It has been suggested that an impairment in this feedback results in excessive NE release from the locus ceruleus, and thus overactivation of the reticular formation and the autonomic system. Support for this hypothesis includes the finding that clonidine, an α_2 partial agonist, can relieve anxiety in some patients. Likewise, β-blockers have been used to prevent isolated episodes of anxiety, such as stage fright. Additionally, it has been suggested that paroxysmal discharges from the locus ceruleus are responsible for acute panic attacks. Direct stimulation of the locus ceruleus produces feelings of anxiety, palpitations, and other signs and symptoms similar to those seen in panic attacks. Whether the locus ceruleus is the root of the pathology in these cases or altered secondary to an underlying pathology is unknown.

Treatment of generalized anxiety disorder includes behavioral therapy to help identify stressors and learn relaxation techniques. TCAs and SSRIs have both been proven effective in anxiety disorders as well. Anxiolytics may be prescribed for acute anxiety, but the long-term use of benzodiazepines for insomnia is discouraged because of their addictive potential.

Case Conclusion The patient begins individual psychotherapy, which helps her address many of her current sources of anxiety and learn ways to prevent and cope with her panic attacks. She begins a low-dose TCA, which gives her partial relief from her symptoms while she begins therapy. The reprieve from worry makes a significant difference in her relationship; after 6 months of treatment, she feels "almost totally new."

Thumbnail: Norepinephrine and Locus Ceruleus

Norepinephrine Receptors			
Receptor subtype	**Location**	**Type**	**Effect**
α_1	Throughout brain	Metabotropic	Excitatory
α_2	Presynaptic terminals	Metabotropic	Inhibitory/negative feedback
β_1	Throughout brain	Metabotropic	Excitatory
β_2	Throughout brain	Metabotropic	Inhibitory

Key Points

▶ NE is a catecholamine, synthesized from tyrosine.

▶ NE receptors are prevalent throughout the ANS.

▶ The highest concentration of NE in the brain is in the locus ceruleus.

▶ The α_2-receptor is a well-documented example of an auto-receptor providing negative feedback at the synapse.

▶ NE plays a role in the regulation of sleep, arousal, and mood.

Questions

1. Which of the following has been shown to reverse the effects of noradrenergic antidepressants?
   A. Ingestion of cocaine
   B. Ingestion of a low-tyrosine diet
   C. Ingestion of a low-tryptophan diet
   D. Ingestion of amphetamines
   E. Ingestion of MAOIs

2. A clinical trial shows that administration of clonidine (which is an agonist at α_2-receptors) immediately after traumatic events decreases the incidence of post-traumatic stress disorder in victims and witnesses. Through what mechanism might clonidine have this effect?
   A. Decreasing the amount of NE released
   B. Increasing available NE in the synaptic cleft by blocking reuptake
   C. Stimulating postsynaptic NE receptors
   D. Decreasing NE breakdown in the synaptic cleft
   E. Increasing NE synthesis

3. A patient is undergoing a work-up for a pheochromocytoma, an endocrine neoplasm that can profoundly alter a patient's physiology through secretion of excess catecholamines, including NE. Urine tests showing increased levels of which of the following would be consistent with pheochromocytoma?
   A. 5-HIAA
   B. Epinephrine
   C. Tyrosine
   D. VMA
   E. Dopamine

4. An immunohistologic stain serves as a marker for noradrenergic neurons. Such a stain would bind most selectively to which of the following regions?
   A. Nucleus raphe
   B. Substantia nigra
   C. Periaqueductal gray
   D. Red nucleus
   E. Locus ceruleus

HPI: A 20-year-old laborer comes to the ED in status epilepticus. He began seizing while at work and did not stop during the 30-minute ambulance ride to the hospital. Upon arrival, his wife informs you that he has had epilepsy since childhood, but until 2 years ago, it was controlled by medication. Since then, he has been unable to afford regular refills on his prescription and has been having more frequent and severe seizures. This episode is the most severe she has seen to date. You are unable to perform a complete examination, as the patient continues to undergo convulsions.

Thought Questions

- What neurotransmitters are implicated in seizures?

- What receptors do they act on, and what are their effects?

- Why does seizure activity tend to get worse if not controlled by medication?

- How do antiepileptic drugs help control seizures?

Basic Science Review and Discussion

This patient is experiencing a continuous series of seizures known as *status epilepticus.* Seizures can result from a number of factors, such as toxins, trauma, and metabolic disturbance. In epilepsy, however, patients experience repeated seizures that cannot be attributed to outside causes. One hypothesis for why these seizures occur is that they are triggered by an imbalance of excitatory and inhibitory neurotransmitters. Understanding these neurotransmitters and their functions in the brain is critical for understanding current methods of seizure treatment.

Glutamate   Glutamate is the primary excitatory neurotransmitter in the brain. It is an acidic amino acid synthesized from glutamine in the presynaptic terminal. Glutamate is found throughout the CNS and is not localized to any one part of the brain. It can be either recycled to glutamine in glial cells by glutamine synthase or further metabolized to form GABA (Figure 47-1).

Glutamate acts on several subtypes of receptors, including *N*-methyl D-aspartate (NMDA), α-amino-3-hydroxyl-5-methyl-4-isoxazole-propionate (AMPA), kainite, and metabotropic receptors. The latter three are sometimes collectively called the *non-NMDA receptors.* As the terminology indicates, the NMDA receptor is particularly notable and has been the focus of much research. The **NMDA receptor** (an agonist) is a direct ionotropic receptor with a special feature. It not only requires a chemical ligand to open its ion channel, but it also must be depolarized. In the resting state, a Mg^{2+} ion blocks the channel, preventing ion flux. With excitation, either from another neuron or from repeated stimulation from a single presynaptic input, the depolarized membrane repels Mg^{2+} from the receptor. In this state, the ligand (glutamate) is free to bind with the receptor and the channel can fully open to allow an EPSP and influx of calcium. The EPSP creates an excitatory signal, and the calcium triggers a second-messenger cascade. This cascade can cause modification of the receptor or signals back to the presynaptic terminal, all strengthening the connection at the synapse. In other words, when the NMDA receptor detects a combination of events (simultaneous depolarization and glutamate release), it has a short-term excitatory response and it undergoes long-term changes to strengthen the neural connection. This basic mechanism is thought to be the basis of such phenomena as **conditioning** and **learning,** in which repeated simultaneous stimuli lead to a strengthening of neuronal connections. Extensive work examining NMDA agonist and antagonist effects in conditioning supports this hypothesis.

Although glutamate is absolutely essential for brain function, too much glutamate can be toxic to neurons. Animal models have shown that glutamate may mediate some of the damage in prolonged seizures or ischemic events. When blood flow to brain tissue is impaired, mechanisms of normal glutamate uptake stop. Glutamate then accumulates in the synaptic cleft. (Likewise, in uncontrolled seizures, glutamate can be released in quantities much larger than can be taken up by surrounding astrocytes.) The high concentration of glutamate triggers a huge influx of calcium into postsynaptic cells. This extremely high calcium concentration, in turn, can initiate apoptosis or even necrosis of neurons. Thus, although small amounts of glutamate are excitatory to neurons, excessive glutamate causes **excitotoxicity.** Glutamate excitotoxicity has been implicated as a cause of cell death in a number of disorders, including stroke, HD, and epilepsy.

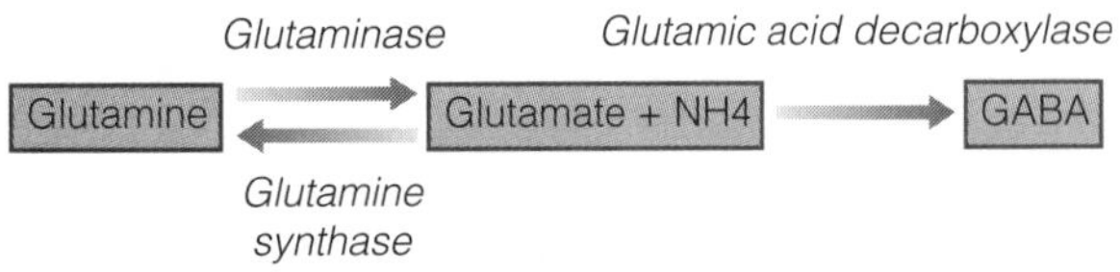

Figure 47-1 GABA synthesis. Glutamine is the amino acid precursor, which is metabolized by the enzyme glutaminase to glutamate. Glutamic acid decarboxylase catalyzes conversion of glutamate to GABA.

GABA GABA is the primary inhibitory neurotransmitter in the brain. It is a neutral amino acid that is synthesized from glutamate. GABA receptors can be found throughout the cerebrum and cerebellum, as well as in the spinal cord. GABA is cleared from the synaptic cleft by GABA aminotransferase, as well as reuptake pumps.

GABA acts on the $GABA_A$ and $GABA_B$ receptors. $GABA_A$ receptors directly open Cl^- channels on postsynaptic membranes, causing Cl^- influx, hyperpolarization, and thus IPSPs. $GABA_B$ receptors are found on presynaptic terminals, where they act to decrease neurotransmitter release. Both have net inhibitory effects.

The inhibitory effects of GABA are important in maintaining balance in the brain. Drugs such as anxiolytics and some "tranquilizers" take advantage of GABA's inhibitory effects. Benzodiazepines act at GABA receptors to increase the frequency with which the Cl^- channel opens in response to stimuli. Barbiturates act to increase the duration the Cl^- channel remains open. Both serve to enhance the inhibitory effect of GABA. As such, they are useful as anxiolytics, in seizure control, to decrease perception of pain, and as muscle relaxants.

Clinical Correlation Epilepsy is a condition of repeated seizures that cannot be attributed to any other cause, such as trauma or infection. About 1% of the population has epilepsy. It has been suggested that one cause of seizure is uncontrolled excitatory activity; there is too much glutamatergic action in the brain. Likewise, it has been posited that GABA normally provides an inhibitory balance to stem glutamate activity, and that in seizures a dysfunction of GABA allows excitatory impulses to run wild.

Kindling is the term used to describe spreading excitement in the brain, usually mediated by glutamate. Some seizures begin in a very small localized portion of the brain. As they continue unchecked, however, the excitatory impulse spreads to neighboring areas of the brain, forming and strengthening excitatory connections between neurons. Eventually, what began as a small focus of hyperactivity can spread to uncontrolled excitatory impulses across the entire cortex. Because of this phenomenon, seizure control is particularly crucial. It is necessary to prevent seizures not only because of their immediate negative effects, but also to prevent kindling and the spread of seizure activity to larger regions of the brain.

Some antiseizure drugs attempt to counteract the glutamate hyperactivity by enhancing the inhibitory effect of GABA. Diazepam (Valium) is among the benzodiazepines that have proven effective for breaking the constant seizures of status epilepticus. Likewise, some antiseizure drugs such as tiagabine and vigabatrin derive part of their antiseizure effects by blocking GABA aminotransferase. This allows GABA to have a greater effect in the synaptic cleft, increasing its inhibitory effect. Hopefully, this inhibition is sufficient to oppose excitatory seizure activity.

Case Conclusion The patient is treated with diazepam to stop his immediate seizures. As he stabilizes, the diazepam is decreased and his regular maintenance medications restarted. The patient is initially confused as he recovers but slowly regains normal mental status and function. He undergoes an EEG, which shows some increased seizure activity when compared with previous EEG studies done at the same hospital. After a short hospitalization, the patient is discharged home with a new supply of antiepileptic medication and a plan for careful follow-up to ensure that he does not go without his preventive medicines again.

Thumbnail: Glutamate and GABA

Glutamate receptors		
Subtype	**Mechanism**	**Effect**
NMDA	Increased cation conductance, allows Ca^{2+} influx	Immediate excitation (EPSP), slow increase in long-term excitation
AMPA	Increased cation conductance	EPSP
Kainate	Increased cation conductance	EPSP
Metabotropic	Presynaptic: inhibits calcium influx; postsynaptic: increases K^+ efflux	Inhibitory, IPSP
GABA receptors		
Subtype	**Mechanism**	**Effect**
$GABA_A$	Opens postsynaptic Cl^- channels	Inhibitory
$GABA_B$	Inhibits presynaptic neurotransmitter release	Inhibitory

Key Points

▶ Glutamate is the most prevalent excitatory neurotransmitter in the brain.

▶ The NMDA glutamate receptor is important in modifying neuronal response with experience, thought to underlie learning.

▶ In extreme concentrations, glutamate can be excitotoxic to neurons.

▶ GABA is the major inhibitory neurotransmitter in the brain.

▶ GABA acts on two types of receptors, $GABA_A$ and $GABA_B$

Questions

1. Ketamine is a drug that selectively blocks NMDA receptors. Which of the following is an expected effect of administering ketamine to a patient?

A. Lowered seizure threshold
B. Excitotoxicity
C. Increased GABA formation
D. Increased pain sensation
E. Impaired memory formation

2. A patient is brought to the ED stuporous and with depressed respiration after taking an unknown quantity of benzodiazepines with one fifth of vodka. He is very difficult to arouse and is only mildly responsive to pain. His severe respiratory depression has resulted in dangerously high carbon dioxide levels. By what mechanism do benzodiazepines act on the CNS to cause the symptoms observed?

A. Increasing the number of IPSPs
B. Increasing Ca^{2+} entry to cortical neurons
C. Acting as antagonists at glutamate receptors
D. Inciting excitotoxicity
E. Inhibiting GABA uptake

3. Which of the following is the amino acid precursor of the most prevalent excitatory neurotransmitter in the brain?

A. Glutamate
B. Glutamine
C. Aminobutyric acid
D. Tyrosine
E. Tryptophan

4. Which of the following has been implicated as a cause of cell death in stroke, HD, and epilepsy?

A. Glutamate excitotoxicity
B. Glutamate deficiency
C. GABA excitotoxicity
D. GABA deficiency
E. Kindling

HPI: A 27-year-old woman is brought to the ED with her 3-year-old daughter after a motor vehicle accident in which their compact sedan completely overturned. Paramedics arrived on the scene to find the woman had not only freed herself from the vehicle, but also the child from her car seat. The patient complained of no pain or injuries at the time but in the subsequent hours since the accident has begun to experience severe pain throughout her body. Examination and subsequent imaging reveal the woman has a fractured femur, shattered patella, and two fractured ribs, along with multiple lacerations and contusions. As she awaits treatment for her injuries, she is given an opiate analgesic, which results in significant immediate pain relief.

Thought Questions

- What neurotransmitters are required for the perception of pain?

- What circuits and neurotransmitters might delay or lessen perception of pain?

- What endogenous peptides act as analgesics?

- What is the relationship between opioids and opiates?

Basic Science Review and Discussion

Pain is a complex phenomenon resulting from a combination of sensory stimulation, emotion, and psychological factors. In this patient, pain was completely unnoticed in the immediate aftermath of trauma but became more severe when she was moved to safety. The alleviation of pain is often central to patient care; in this patient, a narcotic was required to provide relief. Although pain can have a profound impact on a patient's well-being, the underlying mechanisms remain only partially understood. Research has elucidated that **peptide neurotransmitters** are essential in the signaling and relief of pain in the CNS.

Substance P   **Substance P** is an 11-amino acid peptide that has been clearly shown to act in pain signaling. When a harmful or painful stimuli affects the periphery, specialized fibers send signals to the CNS that can be perceived as pain. One subset of these fibers, C fibers, rely heavily on substance P to send such signals. When noxious stimuli activate C fibers, they release substance P locally to initiate neurogenic inflammation. Locally, substance P causes vasodilation, mast cell degranulation, and attracts leukocytes. Pain fibers also fire action potentials and release neurotransmitter in the CNS. Substance P is released from primary afferent neurons onto neurons in the dorsal horn. Here, its release with other **cotransmitters,** such as glutamate, initiates "pain" signals to be transmitted toward the thalamus and cortex. Substance P not only has been found to act in pain transmission in the dorsal root ganglia but also has been implicated in movement control through release in the substantia nigra

and striatum, where GABA serves as a cotransmitter. More remains to be understood about substance P in these circuits. Although substance P may also be important in movement initiation and related disorders, its best-understood role is that of pain signaling in the CNS.

Opioid Neurotransmitters   Just as the CNS relies on substance P to initiate and maintain pain signaling, the opioids are peptides acting in the CNS to decrease pain signaling and produce analgesia.

The term *opiate* originally referred to analgesic and euphoric drugs derived from the opium poppy. The term *opioid* was originally applied to synthetic chemicals that mimicked the effects of opiates but has come to refer to any of the peptides (synthetic or endogenous) that bind opiate receptors in the CNS and produce pain relief. Endogenous opioids act on opiate receptors to decrease the transmission of pain signals and inhibit substance P release to lessen the overall perception of pain. Their action has been implicated as part of the **descending analgesia circuit** of the periaqueductal gray, which uses serotonin as a major transmitter.

Opiate receptors have their highest concentration in the periaqueductal gray and the dorsal horn. When bound by ligand, opiate receptors on the presynaptic membrane of pain fibers decrease the influx of Ca^{2+}. This inhibits the release of neurotransmitter, thus blocking signal transmission. Furthermore, postsynaptic opiate receptors can trigger an influx of K^+, resulting in an IPSP that further inhibits pain signaling. The opioid receptors are classified as μ, δ, and κ, each with different affinities for specific opioids. Of these, the μ-receptor is thought to produce the most profound analgesia and euphoria.

There are more than 20 endogenous opioid peptides, divided into three groups. The most powerful opioids are the **endorphins.** This group of peptide neurotransmitters acts primarily in the periaqueductal gray of the brain, where they create significant analgesia. Among the most powerful endorphin is β-endorphin, an analgesic with potency 48 times that of morphine. The **enkephalins** are the most widely distributed and abundant opioids in the CNS. They have their highest concentration in the globus pallidus but also act throughout the brain and spinal cord. **Dynorphins** are the third group of opioids, which are distributed as widely as the enkephalins. They are weak agonists at opiate receptors but have some analgesic effect.

Each of the opioids is the product of a larger precursor molecule. These larger molecules are broken down by tissue-specific enzymes to create specific peptides for that tissue. Endorphins are derived from the precursor **prepro-opiomelanocortin (POMC)**. POMC is processed within tissue to form opioids β-endorphin, met-enkephalin, as well as ACTH and MSH. Preproenkephalin and preprodynorphin are other precursor molecules, broken down into met- and leu-enkephalin and dynorphin A and B, respectively.

Clinical Correlation   The extreme efficacy of opioids in analgesia is thought, along with serotonin in the descending analgesia pathway, to underlie the phenomena of delayed or inhibited pain perception. Persons who experience otherwise painful stimuli in extraordinary emotional or psychological circumstances often report no initial perception of pain. This is suggested to result from the descending analgesia circuit producing a massive release of opioids that impair pain signaling. As the person's environment changes,

the analgesia pathway decreases its firing and substance P is no longer opposed in transmitting pain signals to the brain.

The extreme efficacy of opioids in providing analgesia is mirrored by the power of exogenous **opiate agonists** that can be used for pain control. Drugs commonly referred to as *narcotics* (e.g., morphine and hydromorphone) have the medicinal benefit of powerful analgesia. These agonists can be given systemically, acting on opiate receptors both to activate the descending analgesia circuit and to act locally in the spinal cord. When given locally at the dorsal root or spinal cord, opiates can produce a powerful local analgesia by inhibiting substance P release. Unfortunately, some of the most powerful opiates, such as morphine and heroin, also have some addictive potential. In addition to analgesia, narcotics induce a euphoria that can provoke their repeated abuse and eventual dependence. Although some patients (particularly those with a history of substance abuse) may be at risk for dependence, it is important to recognize that the vast majority who receive opiate analgesics never become addicted. Although the stigma of narcotics might make some physicians and patients reluctant to employ opiate analgesics, they often provide safe effective pain control for people who would otherwise be severely impaired.

Case Conclusion   After the patient's fractures are reduced, she requires several days in the hospital to recover. She is initially hesitant to take opiates for pain relief but agrees to morphine patient-controlled analgesia (PCA) her first day after surgery. With minimal medication, she is able to control her worst pain. Upon discharge, she receives oral oxycodone to take as needed for pain. This allows her to resume her normal daily activities, including caring for her daughter. Within 2 months, she is again active, and no longer requires prescription medication for pain.

Thumbnail: Peptide Neurotransmitters

Note that each peptide can act on more than one receptor type.

Peptide neurotransmitter	Effect of action	Primary receptor	Primary location in CNS
Substance P	Pain	Substance P receptors	Primary afferents, spinal cord, striatum
Endorphins	Strong analgesia, euphoria	μ opiate receptor	Brain
Enkephalins	Analgesia	δ opiate receptor	Brain, dorsal root
Dynorphins	Analgesia	κ opiate receptor	Brain, dorsal root

Key Points

▸ Pain transmission relies heavily on the peptide neurotransmitter substance P.

▸ The descending analgesia circuit can modulate the transmission of pain signals and the perception of pain.

▸ Opioids are substances that act on opiate receptors in the CNS as powerful analgesics.

▸ Endorphins and enkephalins are the peptide opioids that provide greatest pain relief.

▸ Although all opiate receptors contribute to analgesia, the μ-receptor evokes the strongest euphoria and analgesia.

Questions

1. Naloxone is an antagonist that acts mainly at the μ-receptor. Which of the following patients would most likely be treated with naloxone?

A. A patient experiencing severe localized pain needing a spinal analgesic

B. A patient with severe generalized pain requiring an intravenous analgesic

C. A patient with localized neurogenic inflammation

D. A patient requiring long-term pain control with oral medication

E. A patient with respiratory depression from heroin overdose

2. Which of the following substances is an endogenous opioid?

A. POMC

B. Substance P

C. Morphine

D. Dynorphin

E. Naloxone

3. Capsaicin is a substance that is sometimes used to treat pain in cases of shingles (postherpetic neuralgia). Through which of the following mechanisms does capsaicin relieve pain?

A. Causes vasodilation

B. Promotes mast cell degranulation

C. Attracts leukocytes

D. Acts as a cotransmitter with substance P

E. Depletes substance P from sensory nerve endings

4. POMC is metabolized by tissue-specific enzymes into all of which of the following substances?

A. Met-enkephalin, leu-enkephalin, β-endorphin

B. ACTH, MSH, leu-enkephalin

C. β-endorphin, met-enkephalin, ACTH

D. MSH, dynorphin A, dynorphin B

E. Leu-enkephalin, dynorphin A, dynorphin B

Case 39

1. C
2. B
3. E
4. B

Case 40

1. E
2. E
3. B
4. E

Case 41

1. E
2. D
3. B
4. E

Case 42

1. A
2. C
3. C
4. A

Case 43

1. D
2. D
3. E
4. E

Case 44

1. C
2. D
3. D
4. A

Case 45

1. A
2. D
3. D
4. B

Case 46

1. B
2. A
3. D
4. E

Case 47

1. E
2. A
3. B
4. A

Case 48

1. E
2. D
3. E
4. C

Answers

Case 1

1. C The left MCA supplies the cortical areas mediating each of the functions listed except for control of the lower extremity. Although it is not uncommon to see lower extremity weakness in the context of an MCA infarction, this is due to involvement of subcortical white matter pathways rather than cortex. The cortical area controlling lower extremity function is located predominantly on the medial aspect of the frontal lobe. This area receives its vascular supply from the ACA.

2. B The frontal eye fields (Brodmann's area 8) mediate voluntary saccades and exert a tonic influence driving the direction of gaze to the contralateral side. When the frontal eye fields in the two hemispheres are both functional normally, the direction of gaze is balanced. If one side becomes relatively hyperactive, as with an ipsilateral seizure (transiently increased ipsilateral function) or contralateral structural process (loss of function on contralateral side), gaze is driven to the contralateral side. Eye deviation and head turning away from the seizure focus is called **versive behavior** and implicates involvement of the frontal eye field. Parietal seizures can also be associated with versive behavior, although this can be either ipsilateral or contralateral. Temporal lobe seizures can spread to frontal and parietal areas causing late versive behavior. For this reason, versive behavior is only helpful in localization if it occurs early in the seizure. The oculomotor nuclear group is located in the midbrain and is not associated with seizure genesis.

3. B Loss of the frontal eye field on the right resulting from a structural process such as stroke or tumor would result in relative imbalance of gaze control. In this patient, the preserved left frontal eye field would drive gaze to the right.

4. C An ideomotor apraxia is characterized by the inability to follow motor commands or imitate movements that can otherwise be performed spontaneously. It suggests a lesion involving the dominant premotor cortex, dominant inferior parietal lobule, or anterior corpus callosum.

Case 2

1. B This patient is exhibiting "echolalia," the automatic repetition of auditory input. In extreme examples, the patient may also mimic other perceived sounds. This is often seen in the setting of transcortical sensory aphasia. Essentially this is receptive (Wernicke's-like) aphasia with intact repetition. Given his ability to repeat, the peri-sylvian structure must all be spared. The dominant (left) hemisphere would be affected in this right-handed patient. Note that this patient also makes paraphasic errors. In **semantic paraphasic errors,** words with related meanings are substituted, such as saying "bus" instead of "train." In **phonemic paraphasic errors,** parts of words are substituted, such as saying "bar" instead of "car." **Neologisms** are novel nonsense words.

2. D Again, language deficits would be associated with the dominant left hemisphere. The peri-sylvian language structures are primarily supplied by the MCA. Compromise of the MCA-PCA border zone would be most likely to result in a transcortical aphasia. Compromise of the PCA would be associated with a visual fields deficit, although language impairment could also occur. Compromise of the MCA-ACA territory would be associated with a transcortical motor aphasia.

3. A This patient has alexia (he cannot read, not even his own handwriting) without agraphia (he can still write). Patients with this problem usually have a lesion involving the dominant visual cortex and the splenium of the corpus callosum. Their nondominant visual cortex is able to "read" but that information cannot get to the dominant side for language processing. The frontal cortex and therefore the ability to plan and execute written language are preserved. These patients are able to write but cannot read their own writing (many physicians seem to have this problem).

4. E This patient does not have aphasia. Dysarthria is often confused for a primary language problem. Note, however, that he has normal language production, comprehension, and repetition. The information provided does not strictly localize his problem. Dysarthria is a manifestation of lower CN dysfunction but can also be seen in various global and metabolic processes. Given the apparently new confusion, one might suspect a more global hypoperfusion. Given the history, a cardiac event is most likely.

Case 3

1. D The combination of bilateral leg weakness and incontinence localizes the lesion to the medial aspect of the frontal and prefrontal cortex. A meningioma arising from the falx cerebri in this area could explain the described symptoms. A lateralized lesion would not be expected to cause bilateral disease. Dorsolateral and orbitofrontal prefrontal lesions have more profound clinical manifestations, as discussed previously. A lesion in the area of the pineal gland would not be expected to manifest in this way. An important clinical correlation for pineal tumors is compression of the tectum causing Parinaud's syndrome (limitation of upgaze, near-light pupillary dissociation, convergence-retraction nystagmus).

2. B The dorsomedial nucleus is the main thalamic relay station for limbic information on its way to the frontal and prefrontal cortex. This pathway used to be lesioned deliberately in cases of psychosis and chronic pain to take advantage of the associated apathy as a means of pain control. The anterior nucleus of the thalamus is involved in limbic pathways but does not have a major projection to the frontal lobe. The ventral posterior nucleus of the thalamus relays somatosensory information to the primary somatosensory cortex. The ventral lateral nucleus of the thalamus relays information from the basal ganglia and cerebellum to the motor cortex. The MGN of the thalamus relays auditory information to the primary auditory cortex in the transverse gyrus of Heschl.

3. D Gait disturbance, incontinence, and confusion are the three principle features of NPH. Remember that these patients are wacky, wobbly, and wet. The frontal release signs listed in the other choices may also be seen, but they are not part of the classic triad.

4. B Orbitofrontal lesions tend to be associated with impulsive behavior and disruption of normal mood and affect. The other behavioral problems are associated with dorsolateral prefrontal lesions.

Case 4

1. C The supramarginal gyrus and angular gyrus together make up the inferior parietal lobule. This is the location of the major association cortex, where multimodal information is integrated. This area also corresponds to Brodmann's areas 39 and 40. The postcentral gyrus contains the primary somatosensory cortex. The parietal operculum contains the secondary somatosensory cortex. The superior parietal lobule (Brodmann's areas 5 and 7) contains supplementary and associative somatosensory cortical areas.

2. A The hallmark of cortical sensory loss is that primary sensory modalities remain intact, whereas integrative sensory function is lost. Stereognosis, graphesthesia, and extinction are tests that assess integrative cortical sensory function. The remaining functions listed represent primary sensory modalities and should be intact in cortical sensory loss.

3. B Constructional apraxia is a manifestation of nondominant inferior parietal lobule injury. This patient has a lesion in the dominant hemisphere. The remaining symptoms could all be seen with lesions of the dominant inferior parietal lobule. This collection of symptoms is also called Gerstmann's syndrome.

4. C Somatosensory information from the contralateral half of the body reaches the primary somatosensory cortex via the ventroposterolateral nucleus of the thalamus. Information from the face is relayed by the ventral posteromedial nucleus of the thalamus. The dorsomedial nucleus is involved with prefrontal cortex function. A facial nerve palsy would be associated with facial weakness. The most common manifestation of trigeminal dysfunction is trigeminal neuralgia.

Case 5

1. C Homonymous visual field defects (field cuts) are localized posterior to the optic chiasm. Lesions involving the optic tracts, LGN, or occipital cortex result in homonymous hemianopias. However, the optic radiations are much more diffuse and difficult to disrupt with a single lesion. Lesions of the optic radiations cause homonymous quadrantanopia. Temporal lobe lesions can injure the fibers of Meyer's loop, which carry information corresponding to the upper portion of the visual field (and lower retina), resulting in a homonymous superior quadrantanopia. Meyer's loop can extend almost all the way to the temporal pole. The optic radiations that carry information from the lower portion of the visual field (and upper retina) project directly posterior from the LGN to the visual cortex, passing through the parietal cortex. Parietal cortex lesions can be associated with homonymous inferior quadrantanopia. Quadrantanopia can also be seen with partial lesions of the visual cortex.

2. B The inferior temporal cortex is associated with the analysis of form and color. Stimulation of this area, as with a seizure, can be associated with visual hallucinations. The posterior parietal cortex is involved in the processing depth perception and motion. The occipitotemporal junction is involved in face recognition. The angular gyrus is involved with the visual recognition of objects. The calcarine cortex contains the primary visual cortex. Stimulation of this area is associated with flashes of light, not formed images.

3. D V1 corresponds to the primary visual cortex. Stimulation of this area is perceived as flashes of light. V2 and V3 correspond to secondary visual cortex and the processing of simple forms. V3 is associated with the processing of complex forms. V4 is associated with the processing of color information. V5 is involved in processing information regarding the motion of objects. Lesions in this area can be associated with illusions of motion.

4. E Discussed with previous answer.

Case 6

1. D Meyer's loop carries the optic radiations responsible for vision form the contralateral superior quadrant of the visual field. These fibers loop anteriorly, in some cases nearly to the temporal pole. Contralateral superior homonymous quadrantanopia is a known potential complication of this type of surgery. More limited procedures, like selective amygdalohippocampectomy, are less likely to cause this complication. The other structures listed would not be associated with visual field deficits.

2. E Neocortex in this region should be relatively spared by the procedure. The other cortical types are found primarily in the medial temporal lobe. The hippocampal formation and piriform cortex (primary olfactory cortex) are made of allocortex. The parahippocampal cortex and the entorhinal cortex are made of mesocortex.

3. A Lesions involving the primary auditory cortex may manifest as difficulty localizing sounds in space. The superior temporal gyrus contains both primary and higher order auditory cortices. The remaining lateral aspects of the temporal lobe are concerned with visual processing. The medial temporal lobe is involved in limbic circuitry.

4. C The arcuate fasciculus connects Wernicke's area to Broca's area. Lesions of this fiber tract are characterized by the inability to repeat. A superior homonymous quadrantanopsia would be seen with lesions of Meyer's loop. A homonymous hemianopsia would be associated with lesions of the optic tract, LGN, or primary visual cortex. The inability to localize sounds in space is associated with auditory cortex injury. Poor language comprehension implicates Wernicke's area.

Case 7

1. D Altered mentation in the setting of alcoholism should always raise concern for the possibility of Wernicke-Korsakoff syndrome. In fact, thiamine should be administered empirically to all patients who present with altered mentation of unclear etiology. This condition is associated with atrophy of the mammillary bodies. The other structures can be associated with the described symptoms but are less likely to be atrophic in this setting. The nucleus basalis of Meynert is a group of cholinergic neurons located near the junction of the septum pellucidum and the basal forebrain. It projects widely to other brain regions and has been implicated in memory function.

2. B The most vulnerable portion of the hippocampal formation is Sommer's sector, also called the **CA1 field.** All four hippocampal fields are contained within Ammon's horn, so this is also technically correct but less precise. The CA1 field is at the border between the pes hippocampus and the subiculum. The CA4 field is relatively resistant to injury. It is located at the border between the pes hippocampus and the dentate gyrus. The entorhinal cortex is part of the parahippocampal gyrus.

3. E Short-term memory is mediated by the frontal lobe. The remaining choices all represent variants of long-term memory. Their function has been linked to the temporal lobes, limbic system, and basal forebrain.

4. D The cingulate gyrus coordinates the emotional content of limbic function with decision-making processes in the frontal lobes. Hyperactivity in this area has been implicated in Tourette's syndrome.

Case 8

1. C Altered mentation in the setting of alcoholism should always raise concern for the possibility of Wernicke-Korsakoff syndrome. This is a syndrome resulting from thiamine deficiency in the diet, most commonly seen in the setting of alcoholism. Atrophy of the mammillary bodies is the most commonly sited anatomic finding. Hypertrophy of the pituitary gland would be associated with hormonal abnormalities. The most common clinical association for an enlarged pituitary gland is pregnancy. This can be so prominent as to cause visual field deficits related to compression of the optic chiasm (bitemporal visual field deficits). The other choices are not commonly encountered.

2. B The syndrome that is described is gelastic epilepsy. It is most commonly associated with bouts of uncontrolled and mirthless laughter. The most commonly encountered anatomic disturbance in these cases is a hamartoma in the hypothalamus. These seizures can be difficult to treat and surgical resection is controversial. The remaining structures are more commonly associated with seizures but less likely to be associated with this kind of seizure. Their role in epilepsy is discussed in Case 7.

3. D Temperature regulation is mediated by the posterior hypothalamus. The other functions are all mediated by the anterior hypothalamus and would be expected to be disrupted by lesions in this area.

4. A The control of appetite has been associated with the middle hypothalamic regions, including the tuberal and lateral areas. All of the other processes are associated with the posterior hypo-

thalamus and would be expected to be disrupted by lesions in this area.

Case 9

1. D Ischemic damage would cause a decrease in all the hormones released from the anterior pituitary, including ACTH, FSH, LH, TSH, and prolactin. Decreased ACTH would manifest as a decrease in cortisol, whereas lowered TSH levels would cause decreased T_4 secretion. ADH is released by the posterior pituitary and would not be affected in Sheehan's syndrome.

2. D The patient has a pituitary adenoma composed of acidophilic cells, so the tumor must have arisen from lactotrophs or somatotrophs. A GH-secreting adenoma would cause symptoms of acromegaly and glucose intolerance (answer D). Basophilic cells in ACTH-secreting adenoma would cause symptoms of hypercortisolism, such as altered fat distribution, diabetes, and hypertension (answer A). A TSH-secreting adenoma could cause symptoms of hyperthyroidism and appear basophilic on histology (answer B). Although prolactinoma does consist of acidophilic cells and can cause headache, it would be expected to cause galactorrhea and amenorrhea, not impairment of lactation or menorrhagia (answer C). Finally, inability to concentrate urine would be seen in diabetes insipidus, caused by decreased ADH secretion from the posterior pituitary (answer E).

3. A TSH, LH, and FSH all share the same α subunit. ACTH and MSH have a similar precursor, POMC, but are not related structurally to TSH, LH, and FSH (answers B through E).

4. D Vasopressin is another name for ADH. ADH is normally secreted by cells of the posterior lobe receiving projections from the supraoptic hypothalamus. It regulates fluid balance and urine concentration. Acidophilic cells of the anterior lobe secrete prolactin and GH (answer A). Basophilic cells of the anterior lobe secrete FSH, LH, ACTH, and TSH (answer B). The region of the posterior lobe with inputs from the paraventricular hypothalamus secretes oxytocin (answer C). No part of the posterior lobe receives signals through the portal venous system (answer E).

Case 10

1. E Postganglionic sympathetic innervation to the head enters the skull along the carotid arteries. Any carotid artery injury can be associated with ipsilateral sympathetic dysfunction. Elimination of the sympathetic tone on the left, as in this case, would result in unopposed parasympathetic function and relative pupillary constriction on the same side (miosis on the left). A carotid artery dissection can be associated with an ipsilateral Horner's syndrome (miosis, anhydrosis, ptosis).

2. B Postganglionic parasympathetic innervation to the eye travels along the surface of the third CN. Compression of this nerve by an extrinsic mass would be associated with ipsilateral parasympathetic dysfunction. Elimination of the parasympathetic tone, as in this case, would result in unopposed sympathetic function and relative pupillary dilation on the same side (mydriasis on the right).

3. B The syndrome described in this case is Hirschsprung's disease, or congenital megacolon. It is associated with a lack of parasympathetic neurons within the enteric ganglia of a segment of colon. This results in hypomotility of that segment of colon and associated fecal retention. Colostomy and resection or bypass of the affected segment are potential therapies.

4. E Of the given choices, the most likely neurons to have been affected are preganglionic parasympathetic neurons in the sacral spinal cord. These neurons help mediate erectile function. The cranial portion of the parasympathetic system does not innervate the reproductive organs. The sympathetic system mediates ejaculatory function and uterine relaxation in females, rather than erectile function.

Case 11

1. B Ballismus is the result of a lesion to the subthalamic nucleus. The subthalamic nucleus normally supplies excitatory input to the globus pallidus. Therefore, a lesion causing ballismus would decrease excitatory input to the globus pallidus.

2. A The striatum (caudate and putamen) normally inhibit the globus pallidus. In HD, striatal degeneration causes disinhibition of the globus pallidus. Note that the basal ganglia do not directly project onto the cortex or spinal cord (answers C through E).

3. B As illustrated in the circuit (Figure 11-1), the only part of the basal ganglia system to directly send projections to the cortex is the thalamus. The striatum receives input from the cortex, and the globus pallidus and substantia nigra send projections to the thalamus, which are then relayed to the cortex (answers A and C).

4. B The putamen and the caudate nucleus form the striatum. Of the two, the putamen is more lateral. The other structures listed are not parts of the striatum (answers C through E).

Case 12

1. E The lack of leg involvement suggests a lesion outside of the thalamus, with the cortex being a likely source (his presentation is suggestive of a left cortical infarct involving both the motor and sensory strips, as well as Wernicke's area, which are all adjacent to one another). Right thalamic infarct would cause left-sided symptoms, a simple parietal infarct would not be expected to cause weakness, and a left thalamic infarct or neoplasm would be likely to involve the leg. In addition, neoplasms usually have a more gradual onset of symptoms.

2. C Her hemianesthesia and neglect affecting the entire left side are suggestive of a right thalamic infarct. Her ability to move to command suggests that she has retained motor function, ruling out a sensorimotor picture, but she has developed a fairly dense **neglect** of the left side, which prevents her from using it easily, resulting in her falls. This picture is similar to a parietal lobe infarct, but cortical strokes do not generally involve the leg. The left thalamus, of course, would cause right-sided symptoms.

3. E Given weakness and anesthesia of the face and arm, without knowledge of the lower extremity, an MCA infarct cannot be distinguished from a thalamic process, that is, the lower extremity involvement is paramount in making this distinction. Because both motor and sensory function is involved, the frontal lobe or parietal lobe alone cannot explain her problem. An MCA infarct is possible because this could cause an infarct involving both the frontal and parietal lobes involving the face and arm, and a sensorimotor stroke involving the thalamus is also a possibility here (the lower extremity would also be involved as well).

4. D This presentation is suggestive of a receptive aphasia (ability to produce nonsensical speech with impaired comprehension) consisted with a Wernicke's aphasia (not listed) or a thalamic aphasia (usually from left-sided involvement). This patient's ability to improve with attention is also suggestive of a thalamic aphasia. The thalamus is more likely to spontaneously hemorrhage than the cortex, which may result in headache, although a headache is very nonspecific. This presentation is not consistent with Broca's aphasia, in which speech would be stunted and comprehension spared. The posterolateral frontal lobe contains Broca's area, so this answer is similar to answer A. Finally, the parietal lobe is not associated with aphasia.

Case 13

1. E Alcohol-related cerebellar degeneration is the most common acquired cause of ataxia. Of course, some degree of ataxia can be commonly encountered in the acutely inebriated. Alcoholic ataxia related to cerebellar degeneration is generally encountered in patients with a long-standing history of alcoholism. It is most common in the middle to late decades of life. In these patients, the truncal ataxia is usually more prominent than the limb ataxia. This is because the cerebellar vermis is particularly vulnerable to alcoholic degeneration. The other structures listed may also be affected, though less prominently.

2. A Eye movements are mediated by the vestibulocerebellum. This consists primarily of the flocculonodular lobe and fastigial nuclei. The remaining nuclei listed are more involved with coordination of axial and extremity movements.

3. B Most of the ventral cerebellum is supplied by PICA, which exits from the basilar artery at its caudal end.

4. B Of the presented choices, the Chiari malformations are the only ones with prominent herniation of the cerebellar tonsils as a principle feature. The syrinx of the spinal cord makes this a Chiari II malformation.

Case 14

1. D Dorsal horn lesions affect all sensory systems within the corresponding ipsilateral dermatome, because dorsal column, spinothalamic, and spinocerebellar fibers all enter at the dorsal horn. Thus, this patient should have complete loss of sensation, including fine touch, vibration, pain, temperature, and proprioception (conscious and unconscious). This is suggested by the case presentation, where ipsilateral pain/temperature loss is noted at the site of the lesion at the left T10 dermatome.

2. C This patient's diffuse loss of sensation, particularly a sensory ataxia (difficulty walking due to inability to sense joint position) and positive Romberg's sign suggest dorsal column dysfunction with apparent sparing of the motor and spinothalamic systems. In addition, absent pupillary response to light suggests an Argyll-Robertson pupil (sometimes remembered as "like a prostitute, the pupil accommodates but does not respond to light") consistent with neurosyphilis. Overall, the sensory ataxia is suggestive of tabes dorsalis. Peripheral neuropathies generally are not this dramatic; syringomyelia should present with pain or lack of sensation to pain with intact proprioception. Subacute combined systems degeneration may cause weakness and should not affect pupillary reflexes; Brown-Séquard's syndrome would cause unilateral plegia and fine sensory loss.

3. B This patient's presentation is suggestive of syringomyelia, with a "capelike" distribution of lack of sensation to pain and characteristic burning pain in the arms. She is also shown to have an Arnold-Chiari malformation with downward-displaced cerebellar tonsils, which is not prerequisite for a syrinx. Foraminal stenosis would be expected to give shooting radicular pain, which would not affect the torso in the cervical spine. Diffuse demyelination (MS) would be expected to have more widespread symptoms, and cord compression would give sensory loss and weakness below the level of the lesion with possible bowel/bladder incontinence. A normal scan is possible for peripheral neuropathies, which usually affect the feet and hands before the torso.

4. A This patient's lack of sensation appears to fit a "glove-and-stocking" distribution most consistent with peripheral neuropathy. A homeless patient with a possible history of alcohol abuse may develop neuropathy secondary to alcohol itself, as well as nutritional deficiencies: folate, B_{12}, or other B vitamins, in addition to other possibilities, such as diabetes. Subacute combined systems degeneration would be expected to have motor involvement and be more widespread. Syringomyelia usually affects the cervical cord, which does not localize to the distal extremities. Tabes dorsalis should be more widespread and potentially more profound. MS should also have a more diffuse, unpredictable pattern and may cause weakness.

Case 15

1. C This patient has LMN findings in the upper extremity and UMN findings in the lower extremity. This pattern implicates the cervical spinal cord, where the LMNs for the upper extremity are located. UMNs destined for the lower extremity pass through this area and are affected. Potential causes include traumatic, vascular, neoplastic, infectious, and inflammatory causes.

2. E This patient's clinical picture is consistent with motor neuron disease, such as ALS. In its classic form, this is a motor neuron disease that affects both LMNs and UMNs. The remaining options would be associated with diminished reflexes.

3. E A previous history of demyelinating disease in another CNS region supports the diagnosis of MS. A clinical history of optic neuritis, however, should raise the suspicion for Devic's disease. This inflammatory condition is localized to the spinal cord and optic nerves. It is considered a distinct entity, rather than a subtype of MS because the mechanism of injury does not remain limited to white matter. These lesions involve both gray and white matter very aggressively. This is thought to be mediated via involvement of CNS vasculature. These patients generally respond poorly to conventional steroid management, and early aggressive intervention, such as plasma exchange, has been advocated by some.

4. D Brisk reflexes, pathologic reflexes (such as the Babinski's response), and eventual spasticity are the results of injury to UMNs and associated descending pathways. There is relative increase of sensory impact on alpha motoneuron function and increased alpha motoneuron activity, but these effects are secondary to the lack of regulatory input from higher centers.

Case 16

1. B C7 radiculopathy. The constellation of neck pain and pain radiating in a dermatomal pattern is typical for a radiculopathy, with both C7 and C8 radiculopathies (C7 is more common) being likely to affect the fingers (C6 might affect the thumb, but dermatomes vary slightly among different individuals). Patients with stenosis of the spinal canal are more likely to develop radiculopathies as well. Triceps involvement also suggests C7 or C8 radicular involvement. Radial nerve injury could cause triceps weakness but is unlikely to cause neck pain. C6 will not involve the triceps, and neither will the musculocutaneous nerve. Cord compression may cause pain, but less likely to be shooting pain; it might also cause weakness of the arm(s) and leg(s) and possible bowel/bladder incontinence.

2. E Left dorsal S1 nerve root transection. It appears that only a dorsal nerve root is affected, as the patient only has a sensory deficit, making a peripheral nerve injury or ventral nerve root unlikely. The sole of the foot is generally confined to the S1 dermatome. The S1 dermatome generally also involves the lateral aspect of the foot and may involve part of the back of the lower extremity.

3. B Left L5 radiculopathy. Extensor hallucis longus (EHL) involvement is specific to the L5 myotome, which makes it a useful physical finding. In addition, the L5 dermatome usually involves the dorsal foot, as seen with this patient, and the shooting leg pain may be consistent with a radiculopathy (sciatica, which is discussed later, often involves the back of the leg). An L4 radiculopathy would not involve the EHL, nor would S1 or S2 (these would be expected to affect the ankle jerk and plantar flexion). A lumbar myelopathy would likely involve more myotomes/dermatomes throughout the lower lumbar and sacral nerves, and might present with bowel or bladder symptoms.

4. E Myelopathy is the best explanation due to the stool incontinence seen with this patient. The stool incontinence seen with jarring impact is particularly worrisome for unstable spine fracture with loose bone compressing the cord with each bump, making stable transport and immediate surgery crucial to minimize permanent spinal cord injury. Bowel incontinence may arise from compression at any point above the sacral cord, and the reduced pinprick at and below the kneecaps suggests cord compression/myelopathy localized to L4 with some preservation of spinal cord function (otherwise complete anesthesia would result). Radiculopathy or lumbar spinal nerve transection alone would not cause bowel incontinence, and L4 nerve transection would cause total anesthesia over the L4 dermatome (over the kneecaps). High cervical cord transection would result in quadriplegia and possibly respiratory paralysis.

Case 17

1. E This lesion is outside the brachial plexus, specifically involving the intercostobrachial nerve (T2), which is often victimized by mastectomies due to its vulnerable location in the superficial axilla. It supplies sensation to the medial upper arm, whereas the T1 root supplies the medial forearm, in addition to some of the intrinsic hand muscles. Thoracic outlet syndrome generally is not caused by surgery alone and generally does not present with simple sensory loss in the absence of pain. Lower plexus injuries often occur as a result of positioning of the arm during surgery but would present with more widespread weakness and sensory loss, as would upper plexus lesions.

2. B This is a classic description of a long thoracic nerve palsy, resulting in serratus anterior weakness and inability to abduct the arm above the shoulder. The serratus anterior muscle stabilizes the scapula during abduction, which is necessary for the deltoid muscle to continue contracting against the scapula and to elevate the arm above the shoulder. Serratus anterior injury thus results in winging of the scapula when the arm is lifted to the level of the shoulder. A C5 root injury would be expected to have sensory loss, whereas the thoracodorsal nerve palsy would affect the latissimus dorsi muscle (inability to extend the shoulder). Suprascapular nerve palsy would weaken initial abduction but has no role raising the arm above the head. Upper plexus lesions would affect elbow flexion and shoulder abduction.

3. C Weakness of initiating shoulder abduction is classic for suprascapular nerve injury. As the arm is raised higher, the deltoid muscle may compensate and the arm may be raised above the head if the long thoracic nerve may rotate the scapula. Also, the prominence of the shoulder blade is also suggestive of chronic suprascapular nerve injury leading to infraspinatus and supraspinatus muscle atrophy. An upper plexus injury would also cause elbow flexion weakness and anesthesia, whereas a lower plexus lesion would not involve the shoulder. Long thoracic nerve injury would result in winging of the scapula. C7 radiculopathy does not involve the shoulder (C5, C6).

4. D Upper brachial plexus injury. Traction of the upper extremity during childbirth is a classic cause of upper brachial plexus injury, as opposed to forced abduction for a lower plexus injury. Upper plexus injuries typically result in C5–C6 dysfunction with lateral upper extremity anesthesia and deltoid and biceps weakness. An axillary nerve injury would not affect the biceps or cause lateral

arm anesthesia. A C5 radiculopathy could cause diminished strength in the biceps and deltoids but should not result in paresis. Brachial neuritis is atypical in the newborn and should be less focal in presentation (i.e., involving other aspects of the arm or both arms).

Case 18

1. B Elderly patients with neck pain and degenerative changes in the spine often develop cervical radiculopathy secondary to compression of nerve roots from bone spurs and flattening of the intervertebral disks. This results in dermatomal anesthesia (the C5 dermatome runs along the anterolateral arm towards the thumb), frequent neck pain due to the arthritic changes, and myotomal weakness (biceps and deltoid are innervated by C5, C6). C5 radiculopathies are also known to cause referred pain to the scapular region (perhaps similar to how diaphragmatic pain also refers to this area, which is also innervated by C5). The median nerve does none of these things. The axillary nerve does not serve the biceps. Musculocutaneous injury could cause biceps weakness, and possibly anterior arm anesthesia, but not deltoid weakness. An upper brachial plexus injury could present in similar fashion but would be likely to involve more widespread weakness and/or anesthesia; it is also unlikely to present spontaneously without any trauma.

2. C With such a confusing array of findings, it is worthwhile to take each physical finding one at a time to find certain things that you can "hang your hat on," that is, that definitively demonstrate a particular type of injury. The inability to extend the wrist (waiter's tip) is consistent only with radial nerve injury, which is associated with fractures of the humeral shaft, presumably by shearing the radial nerve as it courses around the humerus. Ulnar nerve injury is associated with elbow dislocation, and is the cause of this patient's ulnar claw. Finally, the presence of thenar atrophy can only be consistent with *chronic* carpal tunnel syndrome, as muscular atrophy takes weeks to develop.

3. C Deltoid weakness with shoulder anesthesia is characteristic of axillary nerve injury, which may occur secondary to shoulder dislocation (the axillary nerve may be torn due to its proximity to the glenohumeral fossa). A C6 radiculopathy may cause shoulder weakness, but C6 anesthesia will run down the lateral upper extremity to the thumb. Radiculopathy also usually causes sharp shooting radicular pain. C4 radiculopathy will not affect the shoulder and causes pain above the clavicle. Musculocutaneous nerve injury will cause biceps weakness and anterior arm anesthesia. Radial nerve injury will cause triceps and posterior forearm compartment weakness and anesthesia of the dorsal upper extremity (including the hand).

4. A The nerve running within a groove around the humerus (the spiral or radial groove) is the radial nerve. Nerve injury at the level of the groove will result in denervation of the finger extensors of the forearm and posterior forearm anesthesia (triceps function may be spared because it is innervated proximally to the lesion). Finger flexion and anterior forearm sensation (median nerve) should be unaffected, so thumb adduction and palmar sensation should also be intact (median nerve in carpal tunnel). The ulnar nerve should be unaffected (ulnar claw and hand weakness), as well as the musculocutaneous nerve (elbow flexion and lateral forearm sensation).

Case 19

1. D Lumbar disk prolapse at the L2–L3 level is the best explanation for this patient's cauda equina syndrome (no UMN signs, pain, saddle anesthesia). The cauda equina is fullest at this level, because the spinal cord tapers off around the L1–L2 vertebral level. The patient's story is abrupt onset, making a disk prolapse more likely than the presence of a mass. Spinal stenosis may cause sacral pain and weakness, but it would not present abruptly. Compression fracture without cord involvement would only present with localized pain. Finally, spondylolisthesis at the S2–S3 level would only affect the S3 nerves, which would not affect the backs of the legs (S1–S2 dermatomes).

2. E All of the listed lesions may present with ankle areflexia. Spinal shock secondary to acute cord transection may result in areflexia inferior to the level of the lesion. Cauda equina syndrome generally causes ankle areflexia secondary to LMN involvement (S1 and S2). Conus medullaris syndrome may cause hyperreflexia if restricted to the cord but will cause areflexia if the adjacent spinal roots are involved. Finally, the ankle reflexes normally diminish with age and their isolated absence may be a benign finding in the elderly patient.

3. D This patient's presentation of saddle anesthesia, foot weakness, and bladder overflow with fecal incontinence suggests a problem in the conus medullaris. However, the prominence of the autonomic signs with minimal sensorimotor deficit makes a compressive lesion less likely, particularly in a patient with known MS who is at risk for spontaneous demyelination throughout the brain and spinal cord. The cauda equina is unlikely as it should present with areflexia, as would peripheral neuropathy (which is unlikely to present with prominent autonomic signs). Lumbar disk prolapse would compress the ventral cord, causing a greater degree of motor weakness, whereas ALS (Lou Gehrig's disease) affects motor fibers only.

4. A This patient is presenting with apparent motor weakness only and areflexia (although it is true that ankle jerks may normally be lost with age); he has no sensory or autonomic deficits. This makes the conus medullaris or cauda equina less likely, as they would typically present with motor, sensory, and possibly autonomic dysfunction (in addition to areflexia being atypical for the conus). A peripheral neuropathy should always present with sensory deficit if a motor deficit is present, as would subacute combined systems degeneration. The diagnosis of ALS (Lou Gehrig's disease), which exclusively affects motor fibers, is most likely.

Case 20

1. D This woman is demonstrating the classic signs of a upper lumbosacral plexopathy, including (most importantly) thigh adductor weakness. This is the key element that allows distinction from a pure femoral nerve palsy, which would not affect adduction (gov-

erned by the obturator nerve). Lumbosacral neuritis can generally only be diagnosed in the absence of an obvious source of mechanical compression. The lateral femoral cutaneous nerve has no motor function, ruling it out. Cauda equina syndrome would involve both lower extremities and would compromise strength of the entire leg, as well as possibly affecting bowel/bladder function.

2. D The history and examination of a chronic paresthesia over the bilateral lateral thighs is typical for lateral femoral cutaneous neuropathy (a.k.a., meralgia). The lack of anterior thigh or motor involvement makes an upper lumbosacral plexopathy or femoral nerve injury unlikely. Lumbosacral neuritis would be expected to have more diffuse symptoms and a more acute course. It is also typical for symptoms to worsen with weight gain, so it is possible that his symptoms may improve if he loses weight in light of his obesity.

3. B Right lower lumbosacral neuropathy would result in hamstring, ankle, and foot weakness, which would explain her problem, as well as anesthesia of the posterior and distal lower extremity. A sciatic nerve injury might present similarly. This neuropathy has likely occurred from mechanical compression due to expansion of her tumor. Both femoral nerve compression and upper lumbosacral plexopathy would affect quadriceps and hip flexion, not the posterior lower extremity muscles. The lateral femoral cutaneous nerve has no motor component, and the obturator nerve affects hip adduction.

4. C The lateral femoral cutaneous nerve runs underneath the inguinal ligament and would result in lateral upper thigh numbness if it were transected. Femoral nerve transection would give paralysis of hip flexion and the quadriceps, which would also be seen in an upper lumbosacral plexopathy. General anesthesia should not result in localized sensory loss. Obturator nerve transection would result in thigh adductor weakness and medial thigh anesthesia.

Case 21

1. E Right obturator and common peroneal nerve injury. The obturator nerve, which governs adductor function and the ability to cross one's leg, is susceptible to compression against the bony pelvis during vaginal delivery. Inability to dorsiflex the foot is the hallmark of a foot-drop. Foot-drop may be seen after general or epidural anesthesia, usually due to compression of the common peroneal nerve against a bed rail or other part of the bed. Sciatica would possibly involve the hamstrings, but not the thigh adductors; it generally does not result in foot-drop. The femoral nerve innervates the quadriceps and would cause weakness of knee extension.

2. B Left S1 radiculopathy. S1 radiculopathy is suggested by the pain along the back of the leg (S1 dermatome) in conjunction with absent ankle jerk and weakness of plantar flexion. Sciatica could present in a similar pattern; however, the onset of symptoms after lifting is more likely to precipitate radiculopathy, often via disk herniation. Common peroneal nerve injury would present with foot-drop (dorsiflexor weakness), not plantar flexion weakness.

Tarsal tunnel syndrome involves only the sole of the foot. Femoral nerve palsy would be restricted to the thigh and quadriceps muscles.

3. E Traumatic injury to the head of the fibula causes compression injury to the common peroneal nerve, which may result in a transient foot-drop: a fact known and exploited by police and other personnel when necessary. The common peroneal nerve passes over the head of the fibula, making it susceptible to compression injury. Tibial nerve injury does not cause foot-drop. Sciatica is not generally caused by trauma, neither does it cause isolated foot-drop. A fibular head fracture alone would not cause a foot-drop but would cause localized pain lasting more than a few hours. The femoral nerve is nowhere near the fibular head, nor would it cause foot-drop.

4. A The pattern of thigh anesthesia, hip flexor weakness, and quadriceps weakness is suggestive of femoral nerve dysfunction. The femoral nerve is particularly susceptible to compression from retroperitoneal processes because it runs along the bony pelvis near the iliopsoas muscle, which affords little space to move. The sciatic nerve is not susceptible to retroperitoneal compression and does not innervate the hip flexors. The obturator nerve may be compressed within the pelvis, but it would cause thigh adductor weakness. Hematomas generally do not cause radiculopathies because the nerve root is surrounded by the bony spine, which is protective in this case.

Case 22

1. B Noxious olfactory stimuli are detected by free nerve endings of the trigeminal nerve. The olfactory nerve mediated the response to volatile molecules, which become dissolved in the olfactory mucous and interact with relatively specific receptors. The other nerves listed do not have a prominent presence in the nasal mucosa.

2. A The most vulnerable portion of the olfactory system is the olfactory nerve. Fibers of the olfactory nerve pass through perforations in the cribriform plate of the skull. They are relatively fixed in this position. They are susceptible to shear injury in this location. Fractures of the skull also can affect the cribriform plate, severing the olfactory nerve fibers. The remaining structures can be affected, but this is less common.

3. C Primary olfactory neurons turn over on a monthly basis. This is unusual for neurons.

4. D The described features are most consistent with temporal lobe epilepsy. It is important to note, however, that different seizure features can overlap, so the clinical manifestation by itself does not exclude the involvement of other cortical areas.

Case 23

1. C A single lesion cannot explain all of the clinical findings. Monocular involvement in this case implicates the left optic nerve

or globe. The abnormal reflex findings suggest a UMN lesion involving either the left side of the spinal cord or a right-sided lesion above the pyramidal decussation. A midbrain lesion would not cause a visual field defect. Neurologic symptoms separated by space and time are a clinical hallmark of MS. This diagnosis could be confirmed by evidence of demyelinating white matter lesions on MRI of the brain and spinal cord. Demyelination also could be confirmed by laboratory analysis of the CSF.

2. D Meyer's loop describes the inferior-most optic radiations, which carry information from the upper quadrant of the contralateral visual field. On leaving the LGN, these fibers course anteriorly and superiorly around the temporal horn of the lateral ventricle, passing within a few centimeters of the temporal pole before turning toward the visual cortex. Contralateral quadrantanopia is a potential complication of temporal lobectomy.

3. D The pituitary gland can become significantly enlarged during pregnancy. This can sometimes result in compression of the optic chiasm, which would be expected to cause bitemporal (peripheral) visual symptoms. Pituitary tumor would be an important consideration. An electrical disturbance of the visual cortex could present in this manner, although there is no history of either seizure or migraine. Also, a large portion of the visual cortex is devoted to central vision. An electrical disturbance originating in the visual cortex would be less likely to remain isolated in the peripheral visual field. An optic tract lesion on one side would produce contralateral symptoms. Simultaneous bilateral optic tract lesions would be unusual.

4. A The patient has described amaurosis fugax, transient obstruction of blood flow through the ophthalmic artery. This is often an embolic event, which would be consistent with his medical history. Retinal ischemia is usually hemispheric, rather than involving the whole eye. Optic chiasm lesions cause heteronymous (bitemporal) visual disturbance. Optic tract and visual cortex deficits cause homonymous defects (perceived similarly in both eyes).

Case 24

1. C Sudden onset of a "worst headache ever" should raise the suspicion of subarachnoid hemorrhage. A sentinel bleed from an aneurysm could present this way in advance of an aneurysm rupture. Immediate medical attention, including CT scan of the head and if negative a lumbar puncture to assess for blood is needed. The clinical findings are consistent with compression of the left third CN. The most likely site of compression for this nerve would be by an aneurysm extending from the PCom on the left. The other locations would not be as likely to affect pupillary function on the left.

2. C The clinical findings implicate involvement of the cavernous sinus. The third, fourth, and sixth CNs all pass through the cavernous sinus. The first and second branches of the trigeminal nerve, conveying sensory information from the upper face, also pass through the cavernous sinus. An orbital process would be expected to spare facial sensation. The pituitary is a midline structure, not likely to impinge on the oculomotor nerve. Proptosis and injection are not associated with brainstem infarction and additional brainstem findings would have been expected. Meningitis would not be expected to localize to one eye. Immunosuppressed individuals, such as diabetics, are particularly at risk for mucormycosis sinusitis, leading to cavernous sinus thrombosis. The prognosis is guarded in general and death is very likely in the absence of treatment.

3. B Light-near dissociation describes pupils that constrict with accommodative vergence (looking at near objects) but fail to constrict in response to light (also called an Argyll-Robertson pupil). When this is encountered in the setting of limited upward gaze and convergence-retraction nystagmus, a compressive midbrain tectal lesion should be suspected. Also known as Parinaud's syndrome, this condition is seen more often on examinations than in the clinic. The most frequently tested lesion to cause this syndrome is a pineal tumor. The pituitary gland is not relevant in this case. Adie's tonic pupil is a benign condition in which light-near dissociation is the most prominent finding. Light-near dissociation can also be seen in the setting of bilateral afferent pupillary defects and in chronic neuropathies. In both cases, bilateral lesions need to be present.

4. E Patients with trochlear nerve palsies often complain of vertical diplopia and difficulty walking down stairs. The superior oblique muscle on the affected side is paralyzed and the eye is extorted (rotated outward). By tilting their head to the unaffected side, these patients use intorsion of the intact eye to compensate for excessive extorsion on the affected side. Their diplopia resolves when they tilt their head toward the intact side. This patient tilts his head to the right, suggesting a left superior oblique lesion. Trauma, diabetes, and idiopathic etiologies are common associations.

Case 25

1. B The presentation is a classic example of Parinaud's syndrome, involving the midbrain tectum. Given the insidious onset, a slow-growing tumor should be considered. The pineal gland is located immediately superior to the superior colliculi. Pinealomas can grow such that they compress the dorsal midbrain and can be associated with Parinaud's syndrome. Most of the remaining locations would be associated with third nerve palsies, which this patient does not have. The horizontal gaze center is located in the PPRF, near the abducens nucleus in the pons. Lesions in this area cause horizontal gaze palsies, rather than vertical gaze disturbance.

2. E This patient has PD, most prominently affecting the substantia nigra on the right. This disorder is associated with extrapyramidal motor deficits, like the ones described. Lesions of the corticospinal tract, which is contained within the cerebral peduncles, are usually associated with weakness in the acute phase. Chronically, these patients develop spasticity rather than rigidity and tremor. Disorders of the midbrain tectum would be expected to produce eye findings, as in the previous question. Disruption of the superior cerebellar peduncles would be expected to produce ataxia and tremor that is more prominent with action. PD is discussed further within the context of dopamine systems and the basal ganglia.

3. D Restriction of upward gaze suggests compression of the dorsal midbrain (midbrain tectum), particularly in this age-group. The combination of restricted upward gaze, nystagmus with apparent retraction of the eyes on attempted convergence, and light-near dissociation (pupils constrict on accommodation but not to light) is called Parinaud's syndrome. Pineal tumors can present in this way. They are more commonly encountered in younger patients. Pontine lesions are associated with horizontal eye movement problems, not vertical ones. Ventral midbrain processes would be expected to present with third nerve deficits and hemiparesis. Medullary syndromes are associated with vestibular problems and lower CN deficits (dysarthria, dysphagia).

4. D The patient tells you he had an old thalamic hemorrhage. This is often associated with contralateral hemianesthesia. His right-sided sensory loss is most likely related to that event. Thus, his left-sided hemiparesis is the new symptom. Although it can be localized to any part of the corticospinal tract, it is most likely related to a cerebral process on the right. One might be tempted to localize these crossed findings to the brainstem. However, a ventral midbrain process would most likely be associated with third nerve deficits and dorsolateral medullary process would not be associated with hemiparesis. A hemispinal cord lesion could result in crossed sensory and motor findings, but the sensory findings would also be crossed (ipsilateral vibratory and proprioceptive loss with contralateral pain and temperature loss). A spinal cord lesion also would manifest with a clinical level above which function is spared. A cerebellar process could manifest as weakness initially, but this would be ipsilateral to the lesion.

Case 26

1. B This patient most likely has SUNCT (short-lasting, unilateral, neuralgiform headaches with conjunctival injection and tearing). This syndrome is often associated with rhinorrhea and forehead sweating. The ophthalmic division of the trigeminal nerve is most commonly involved. Attacks last only seconds to a few minutes but can occur multiple times per day or even multiple times per hour. The syndrome is less responsive to treatment than trigeminal neuralgia. Sinus disease would not relapse and remit so abruptly. Involvement of the trigeminal ganglion would likely not be restricted to only one division of the trigeminal nerve. Involvement of the ophthalmic artery would compromise vision. Involvement of the ciliary ganglion would likely involve pupillary abnormalities.

2. C Right facial sensory disturbance localizes to the right trigeminal nerve, nucleus or tract. Left extremity sensory disturbance localizes to the ascending spinothalamic systems, which decussate in the medulla. The findings are consistent with a small lesion, likely a lacunar infarction, in the right dorsal pontine tegmentum involving the trigeminal nucleus and nearby medial lemniscus.

3. D This patient has a Bell palsy on the left. The seventh CN (facial) is affected. This nerve mediates motor control to the face. Innervation to the upper face has bi-hemispheric representation. The fact that both upper and lower face are affected suggests an LMN lesion. This is likely a peripheral lesion. A central lesion would spare motor function in the upper face. Branches of the trigeminal nerve briefly carry taste from the anterior two thirds of the tongue, but these fibers pass to the facial nerve via the chorda tympani nerve. The facial nerve does not mediate any other sensory function. However, patients with Bell's palsy often complain of subjectively altered sensation on the affected side. The physiologic basis for this is not clear.

4. C This patient also has Bell's palsy. The masseter muscle is spared, as are all of the muscles of mastication. These muscles are innervated by the trigeminal nerve, not the facial nerve. The levator palpebrae muscle also is spared because it is innervated by the third CN (oculomotor). Patients with peripheral seventh nerve palsies have facial weakness and difficulty closing their eyes (instead of ptosis).

Case 27

1. A This constellation of symptoms is the precise deficiency that would occur with complete compromise of CN VII. This would involve the motor, sensory, and secretory fibers, resulting in hemifacial palsy, loss of taste (from the fibers coming from the chorda tympani), hyperacusis (from loss of stapedius function), and loss of the sensory and secretory functions. All of these findings will be ipsilateral to the involved facial nerve. Lower facial palsy occurs when the UMNs (corticobulbar fibers) are compromised, such as in the case of stroke.

2. D The taste of the anterior two thirds of the tongue is governed by fibers that run along CN V, then diverge to form the chorda tympani (which runs in the middle ear), joins CN VII in the facial canal, and then diverges to the nucleus solitarius in the brainstem. The chorda tympani is thus susceptible to middle ear processes, and otitis media may result in chorda tympani dysfunction. Stroke, which involves the motor cortex without involving sensation, would not be expected to involve taste. The areas of the cortex that are associated with taste are not entirely clear. Bell's palsy is unlikely in a patient with only a left-sided *lower* facial droop.

3. D Ablation of the motor fibers of the facial nerve within the parotid gland will result in hemifacial palsy only, because the other fibers of the facial nerve have already diverged at that point. In contrast, a Bell's palsy involves the facial nerve within the facial canal, affecting autonomic fibers governing salivation, taste fibers, and the nerve to stapedius whose compromise leads to hyperacusis. Facial sensation is governed by the trigeminal nerve and should not be affected by the facial nerve in any circumstance.

4. A Lacrimation during a salivary stimulus in a patient with previous facial nerve injury (due to Bell's palsy or other causes) is the syndrome of crocodile tears. This is believed to occur because of inappropriate regeneration of facial nerve fibers along the wrong tracts, so fibers that should innervate salivary glands grow into the lacrimal glands. This may also occur with motor fibers, leading to facial twitching or hemifacial spasm when the patient attempts to smile or otherwise use the face, known as *synkinesis*. A recurrent Bell's palsy would not necessarily be different from a first episode of Bell's palsy, and conjunctivitis will give persistent lacrimation, as

would a hyperlacrimation syndrome. Crocodile tears and synkinesis are considered abnormal outcomes, so they are not a prodrome of normal recoveries.

Case 28

1. D In a patient with known MS, one would have to assume the symptoms are related to demyelination until proven otherwise. Although large demyelinating lesions can impinge on adjacent gray matter, this patient does not seem to have a large brainstem lesion, which would likely be associated with other symptoms. Thus, involvement of the cochlear or superior olivary nuclei is not likely. Lesions in the lateral lemniscus or trapezoid body are central to the cochlear nuclei in the auditory pathways and thus would not be associated with unilateral hearing loss. A demyelinating lesion in the lateral pons could involve fascicles of the eighth nerve before they reach the cochlear nuclei.

2. A This patient has a conductive hearing loss. Excessive buildup of cerumen can cause conductive hearing loss. All of the other choices are more likely to be associated with sensorineural hearing loss.

3. E Ménière's disease is associated with attacks of severe vertigo and decreased hearing. Vomiting, tinnitus, and fullness in the ears are also common associations. Symptoms are usually more prominent on one side. This condition is associated with increased endolymph pressure and distended semicircular canals. The cause of this syndrome is not known, but altered ionic flow is suspected and supported by the benefit some patients derive from dietary salt restriction. Shunting of the endolymphatic space can spare hearing in some cases.

4. D This patient has the classic features of Bell's palsy (seventh CN palsy). Hyperacusis can be seen in this condition because of involvement of the nerve to the stapedius muscle on the affected side. A slow-growing mass lesion would be less likely to cause an abrupt onset of symptoms.

Case 29

1. A In a patient with known MS, one would have to assume the symptoms are related to demyelination until proven otherwise. Although large demyelinating lesions can impinge on adjacent gray matter, this patient does not seem to have a large brainstem lesion. A white matter tract must be involved. The combined presence of tinnitus and vertigo implicated the eighth nerve, but MS is a central disease. A demyelinating lesion involving the lateral pons could involve fascicles of the eighth nerve before they reach the vestibular and cochlear nuclei.

2. D This patient has benign positional vertigo. A careful work-up is needed to exclude other deficits. Rotational vertigo is most often related to disorders of the semicircular canals. A central etiology is less likely to cause episodic events with no other deficits. If the eighth nerve were involved, one might see associated hearing deficits. BPV can be easily treated in some cases with canalith repositioning maneuvers.

3. **A** Of the given choices, the left pons is most likely to be affected. The absence of a VOR on the left suggests either an inner ear problem on the left or a pontine problem on the left. A pontine lesion is more likely given the level of consciousness. The patient has a normal VOR on the right. Midbrain lesions would not be expected to affect the VOR.

4. **D** Aminoglycosides are ototoxic, causing potentially permanent hearing loss and/or vestibular impairment in a dose-dependent manner. The toxicity affects the hair cells directly. The other listed structures are not affected.

Case 30

1. **C** Of the given choices, a left-sided Horner syndrome caused by involvement of the ipsilateral sympathetic pathways projecting from the hypothalamus to the intermediolateral cell columns of the spinal cord is most likely. This is a lateral pontine syndrome, most likely caused by infarction of the left AICA or other long circumferential branches. The relatively ventromedial corticospinal tract is spared. Tongue deviation would require involvement of either the corticospinal tract or the hypoglossal nucleus or nerve in the medulla. "Down-and-out" eye deviation implicates the oculomotor nerve or nucleus in the midbrain. Furthermore, all of these motor structures are close to the midline and would most likely be spared in a lateral syndrome.

2. **D** A right one-and-a-half syndrome is described. Involvement of the right sixth nerve nucleus disrupts function of the right lateral rectus. The left lateral rectus is intact, so the left sixth nerve nucleus cannot be involved. Both eyes have impaired adduction on horizontal gaze with intact adduction on vergence (reading). In this syndrome, a single lesion has to affect the ipsilateral sixth nerve nucleus, fibers from that nucleus destined for the contralateral MLF, and the ipsilateral MLF. The only horizontal gaze movement left intact is lateral gaze in the eye contralateral to the lesion.

3. **A** Pontine lacunar infarctions are most likely to be the result of thrombosis of small pontine penetrating branches from the basilar artery. The basilar artery runs along the inferior surface of the pons.

4. **D** The trochlear nerve is located at the junction of the midbrain and the pons. Its fibers do not pass through the body of the pons before exiting the brainstem. The remaining nerves either have their nuclei contained within the pons or have fascicles passing through the body of the pons.

Case 31

1. **D** The tongue deviates toward the side of an LMN lesion but away from the side of a UMN lesion. Both of the described deficits localize to the left ventral medulla. A left MCA stroke would be expected to cause right tongue deviation and right-sided weakness. It might also be associated with a degree of language deficit.

2. **B** All taste sensation projects to the nucleus solitarius. Taste from the anterior two thirds of the tongue is conveyed by CN VII. Taste from the posterior one third of the tongue is conveyed by

CN IX. Taste from the pharynx is conveyed by CN X. The latter is only a minor contributor to taste sensation.

3. **C** The patient has weakness in all four limbs. Bilateral cerebral disease would not be a likely explanation. Therefore, the posterior circulation needs to be considered. Brainstem involvement is unlikely because there are no other brainstem symptoms reported. Quadriparesis with facial sparing implicates a spinal cord process. The anterior spinal artery originates from the distal vertebral arteries. Embolization of this vessel during the procedure is the most likely interpretation.

4. **C** The patient has left-sided hemiparesis and the tongue also deviates to the left, suggesting left tongue weakness. A medullary process would be expected to give crossed finding (UMN weakness in the extremities and LMN weakness in the tongue). Of the choices given, the internal capsule is the most likely location for this patient's lesion.

Case 32

1. **B** Noncommunicating hydrocephalus results from an obstruction within the ventricular system, such as a brain tumor. HD can result in increased ventricle size through cell loss in the basal ganglia, but there is no obstruction within the ventricles (answer A). Likewise, meningeal adhesions can cause a communicating hydrocephalus by interfering with CSF flow in the subarachnoid space, but this does not block flow within the ventricles (answer C).

2. **C** The normal CSF pressure on lumbar puncture suggests this is a normal-pressure hydrocephalus. Frequent causes of normal-pressure hydrocephalus are subarachnoid scarring or fibrosis after meningitis or remote subarachnoid hemorrhage. The lumbar CSF pressure can be normal because the ventricles dilate as CSF builds up. Pseudotumor cerebri is characterized by increased CSF pressure, which manifests both on lumbar puncture and as papilledema (answer A). Mass lesions, such as cerebral tumors, are also more likely to manifest with increased CSF pressure as measured by lumbar puncture; by displacing a volume of CSF with their bulk, they increase overall pressure (answer B).

3. **A** Review the diagram of CSF flow to understand the relationship of the involved anatomy. A mass lesion at this level would most likely compress the cerebral aqueduct of Sylvius, resulting in dilation of all structures before it in the CSF path. Thus, the lateral and third ventricles would be dilated (answers A and D). However, the fourth ventricle (answer B) would be inferior to the lesion and thus not dilated (answer C). Likewise, the foramen of Magendie lies inferior to the fourth ventricle and would not dilate (answer B).

4. **C** The ependyma lining the ventricles is characterized by tight junctions between its cells. These tight junctions maintain the integrity of the barrier between the blood and CSF. The choroid plexus is the tissue that secretes CSF in the ventricles but is not the primary component of the blood-CSF barrier (answer A). Likewise, modified cilia are the structures that facilitate secretion of CSF, but not primarily the barrier between blood and CSF (answer B). Arachnoid villi and arachnoid granulations are structures that

facilitate the reabsorption of CSF into the blood; they are not the major structure creating a blood-CSF barrier.

Case 33

1. A This patient's symptoms appear to localize to Wernicke's area and the left motor strip. The patient is able to produce speech that is not understandable (word salad) and is unable to understand speech (receptive aphasia). The right-sided lower facial droop and arm weakness are consistent with left motor strip involvement. A brainstem infarct would not cause aphasia; facial nucleus involvement causes **lower** and **upper** facial droop and dysarthria. Broca's area infarct would cause a Broca's aphasia, with inability to form words. Left ACA infarct would affect the leg and spare the face and arm. Finally, right-sided lesions would cause left-sided symptoms and very rarely cause aphasias.

2. B Although the process causing this patient's expressive aphasia is not inherently clear, this is the only answer that localizes the infarct to Broca's area in the posterior frontal lobe of the dominant hemisphere, the correct location. A stroke such as this one in an otherwise healthy patient is often from a paradoxical embolus of some kind in the presence of a patent foramen ovale, with use of oral contraceptives and smoking as risk factors. A temporal lobe infarct might cause a receptive, not an expressive, aphasia. A frontal lobe hemorrhage or carotid occlusion is possible in the setting of paradoxical thromboembolus in this patient, but her symptoms localize to the left side, not the right. Septic emboli are not likely, and parietal lesions are not generally associated with aphasias.

3. B This gentleman appears to be experiencing acute retinal artery occlusion, with abrupt and total inability to see out of the affected eye due to retinal ischemia. A pale retina due to absence of blood flow confirms the diagnosis. If this spontaneously remits, then it is **amaurosis fugax** (transient monocular blindness caused by temporary retinal artery occlusion), which signifies unstable carotid atherosclerotic disease and possible impending stroke. A disrupted plaque fragment from the ICA temporarily occludes the ophthalmic artery, causing retinal ischemia. Ocular migraines are controversial and are associated with monocular visual disturbances, not total visual loss. Occipital lobe infarcts will affect one visual **field**, but not the vision of one eye. Elevated ICP may cause papilledema but will not cause abrupt monocular blindness.

4. A Diffuse weakness affecting the entire leg without respect to peripheral nerve territories is best explained by medial frontal lobe infarct, which would be caused by ACA occlusion (and not the MCA, which serves the motor strip of the face and arm). The ACoA joins the two anterior cerebral arteries and would not cause a stroke unless the ACA relied on it for blood flow due to more proximal occlusion. A pelvic mass would usually affect one nerve, would likely affect sensation, and would likely cause edema. Deep venous thrombosis should not cause weakness per se.

Case 34

1. B Weakness is not a prominent feature of the lateral medullary (Wallenberg's) syndrome. The motor pathways are spared because

they are supplied by paramedian branches from both vertebral arteries. One would expect to see an ipsilateral Horner syndrome in the context of a lateral medullary infarction. Loss of pain and temperature would, on the other hand, be seen contralateral to the lesion. Additional findings would include ipsilateral ataxia from involvement of the cerebellar peduncles, dysarthria and dysphagia from involvement of the lower CNs, vertigo and nystagmus from involvement of the vestibular nuclei, ipsilateral altered facial sensation from involvement of the trigeminal nucleus, and impaired taste from involvement of the solitary nucleus. Most commonly, the clinical picture does not include all of the features of the classic syndrome.

2. B Complete sensory loss to all modalities in half of the body usually can be localized above the brainstem, or in the rostral brainstem. More caudal lesions are likely to result in crossed sensory findings involving the face on one side and the contralateral body. They are also likely to be seen in association with other findings. Isolated thalamic injury can result in complete sensory loss with no other associated findings. Most of the thalamus derives its blood supply from branches of the PCA and PCoA. Cortical involvement would be less likely to lead to this because the vascular territory for the regions representing the face and arm is different from that representing the leg. Involvement of the internal capsule often results in hemiparesis.

3. D A hemianopia, or "field cut," is associated with disruption of the visual pathway posterior to the optic chiasm. A complete hemianopia, as opposed to involvement of just one quadrant, indicates that the visual cortex is affected contralateral to the perceived deficit. In this case, the vascular territory most likely to have been affected is that of the PCA on the left.

4. B The only objective finding on examination implicates the cerebellum. The lesion would have to be on the same side as the deficit. The right PICA is the only choice that could affect the cerebellum in isolation on that side. Although one would not expect prominent weakness with a lateral medullary or cerebellar process (for the reasons outlined earlier), subtle weakness can be associated with cerebellar lesions. It is also not unusual for large cerebellar lesions to manifest with relatively mild clinical symptoms. The MCA is also a good choice here but would be expected to result in some degree of objective weakness and language impairment because we are told the stroke is large.

Case 35

1. C Thrombosis of the transverse sinus can extend inferiorly to involve the sigmoid sinus and vessels that empty into it. The labyrinthine structures are drained by the labyrinthine vein. Blood flows from this vein into the inferior petrosal sinus, then into the sigmoid sinus. The neurologic deficits associated with sinus thrombosis depend on the region being drained. Although this patient's headache is relatively nonspecific, new onset of vertigo and hearing loss need to be evaluated. The combination of vertigo and hearing loss suggests a peripheral lesion involving the eighth CN or the labyrinthine structures. Thrombosis of the other vessels listed would not be expected to produce vertigo or hearing deficits.

2. D Because of its location in the midline, thrombosis of the superior sagittal sinus can present with bilateral motor cortex deficits involving the legs. Remember that the motor cortex is topographically organized as a homunculus. The regions of cortex controlling lower extremity function are located medially, along the midline, whereas the regions controlling the upper extremities and face are more lateral. Thus, a single midline lesion can cause bilateral lower extremity deficits. The other vessels listed are paired vessels, located on either side of the midline. Involvement of any one of these vessels would not be expected to cause bilateral deficits. This question, together with the case at the beginning of this chapter, highlights the broad clinical range with which sinus thrombosis can present.

3. D Cavernous sinus thrombosis is associated with proptosis and pain involving the eye, the orbit, and the head on one side. It often presents unilaterally but can spread to involve both sides. Diabetic patients are relatively immunocompromised and susceptible to fungal infections. The combination of fungal infection, diabetes, and cavernous sinus thrombosis is a clinical emergency. Outcome without treatment is often poor. It is frequently tested for this reason. This topic is covered in greater detail in Case 37.

4. A Hemorrhage resulting from venous occlusion occurs with the brain parenchyma first. Extension into the subarachnoid space can be seen with superficial parenchymal bleeding as a secondary event. Venous hemorrhage would not be as commonly associated bleeding in the other spaces listed.

Case 36

1. B Epidural hemorrhage can present with sudden alteration of consciousness following trauma to the temporal portion of the skull. The underlying middle meningeal artery is adherent to the internal surface of the skull in this area. It can easily be damaged by trauma to the side of the head. Trauma to the head can also result in acute subdural hemorrhage, but this is usually related to tearing of bridging veins, rather than the vessels listed. The dural venous sinus are contained within the dura mater ("tough mother") and are less likely to be affected by the described trauma.

2. C "Sudden onset of worst headache of life" are key words that should always bring to mind subarachnoid hemorrhage. This is particularly true in the setting of straining behaviors, which increase ICP. Subarachnoid bleeding is often related to aneurysms emerging from cerebral arteries. The other vessels listed would not be as likely to be associated with the described symptoms. Sentinal bleeds, which may precede an aneurysmal rupture, can present in this way. A CT scan of the head and, if negative, lumbar puncture are needed to evaluate for the presence of subarachnoid blood.

3. E A potential explanation for this patient's clinical presentation would be a dural venous sinus thrombosis related to dehydration. When this occurs, the large sinuses are most likely to be affected. The superior sagittal sinus is involved. Impaired venous outflow can cause congestion and result in hemorrhages along the distribution of the affected sinus.

4. B Sinus thrombosis does not have to present as an emergency. In this case, one of the transverse sinuses is affected, but the other remained patent. Venous drainage from the posterior fossa and the vestibular apparatus can be affected by thrombosis of the transverse and/or sigmoid sinuses. The transverse sinus is the second most commonly affect sinus in cases of thrombosis.

Case 37

1. A The inability to move the right eye suggests that multiple CNs are affected. This can be seen in the setting of local mass effect with compression of multiple nerves within the orbit. Possibilities include orbital tumor, orbital pseudotumor, and thyroid eye disease. Cavernous sinus syndrome is also possible, although the clinical presentation would likely be more severe. The vision is not disturbed, as would be expected with a lesion involving the globe. Sagittal sinus thrombosis and diseases of the optic nerve are not associated with proptosis.

2. B Disorders affecting a single CN are not likely to cause proptosis and orbital pain. Also, the inability to move the right eye suggests that multiple CNs are affected. The Tolosa-Hunt syndrome is an idiopathic granulomatous inflammatory condition, which begins in the superior orbital fissure and can present in this way. It is less common than orbital pseudotumor, a similar inflammatory process starting in the orbit itself. The associated mass effect compromises multiple CNs. Imaging studies and lumbar puncture are warranted to exclude other diagnostic possibilities. Anti-inflammatory therapy can be useful in this setting.

3. A Thyrotoxicosis is associated with inflammation of the soft tissue of the orbit, causing proptosis (exophthalmos). Thyroid eye disease is most likely to occur bilaterally. The other structures, when associated with proptosis, are more likely to be affected unilaterally.

4. D The maxillary division of the trigeminal nerve innervates the midface. It is the only CN branch in the cavernous sinus that does not enter the orbit or pass through the superior orbital fissure. Nerves passing through the superior orbital fissure mediate all the remaining functions listed.

Case 38

1. C Immediate initiation of appropriate antibiotic therapy is paramount when the diagnosis of bacterial meningitis is considered, because a few hours may make the difference between complete cure and death. Antibiotics should be given before head CT or lumbar puncture are obtained; head CT should precede lumbar puncture in the setting of an abnormality on neurologic examination to rule out obstructing masses. Ampicillin should be added to any young or elderly patient with suspected bacterial meningitis for coverage of *Listeria*. Bony cause of neck stiffness is much less likely than meningismus in this setting, making plain neck films of little use.

2. B A change in mental status after a fall in an elderly person should raise concerns for subdural hematoma. These will often attain a size that exhibits enough mass effect to cause confusion and possible focal neurologic signs without progressing further, whereas epidural hematoma is at greater risk of a mass effect because of the higher arterial pressure. Meningioma could create similar symptoms after a slow progression, not abruptly after a fall. Fungal meningitis is unlikely in a patient who is not immunocompromised, and it is less likely to be abrupt; Alzheimer's disease also does not have abrupt onset. Viral meningitis should not persist for 3 months, and it generally does not cause confusion (unless accompanied by encephalitis).

3. C This is a setup for an epidural hematoma, which is trauma to the temple with skull fracture, which may result in middle meningeal artery rupture. Her presentation is consistent with the "lucid interval" seen before mass effect from the expanding hematoma compromises consciousness. A cerebral contusion alone should not cause coma, and a subdural hematoma (answer B, crescentic mass) is less likely in a young person, particularly with such aggressive mass effect. No acute traumatic event results in a calcified mass (calcification is a chronic process), and cerebral edema, though a possibility, is also unlikely to cause such rapid deterioration of consciousness.

4. D This patient's clinical course is most consistent with viral meningitis because it has resolved spontaneously without treatment, now allowing an essentially normal examination without mental status changes. A bacterial, mycobacterial, or fungal meningitis, which are the most worrisome concerns, would not improve without treatment, and if he presented when his symptoms were acute, he would have deserved full empiric treatment for bacterial meningitis until the diagnosis could be made. Syphilitic meningitis is a theoretical possibility that may be addressed via a simple blood test. Therefore, antibiotics and head CT/MRI are not required, and a lumbar puncture is unlikely to give additional information (a resolving lymphocytic pleocytosis is anticipated) and runs the risk of complications. Should his symptoms worsen, he should return immediately for another evaluation.

Case 39

1. C The prompt states that tetrodotoxin acts by blocking Na^+ channels. In this way, it would be expected to have effects similar to myotonias in which Na^+ channels cannot open. Without Na^+ flow, signaling between neurons could not occur. The patient would have a resulting weakness or paralysis, an inability to move his limbs. Convulsions might be expected in a toxin that either affected the CNS or created a hyperexcitable state in which more ion flux increased signaling (answer A). Although the alteration in sodium flux would affect function, the quantities involved in neuronal signaling are quite small compared with overall in the body, and alterations in channel function would not create a noticeable change in urinary Na^+ (answer B).

2. B Ion channels are selective for specific ions. The question tells you the toxin acts on Na^+ channels; there is no information given to suggest it also affects K^+ channels (answers A and C). The toxin delays the inactivation of Na^+ channels, meaning the channel can remain open longer. Thus, the flow of sodium would be expected to increase rather than decrease or stop entirely (answers D and E).

3. E Strychnine is a competitive antagonist for glycine. Normally, glycine acts as a ligand trigger to open ion channels in the CNS. A competitive antagonist binds to glycine receptors, making their associated channels unable to bind glycine and therefore unable to open. Channel selectivity (answer A) is determined by an ion channel's structure; competitive antagonists do not change which ions can travel through the channel pore. Likewise, ligand-gated channels have a tertiary structure that requires ligand binding for opening; they are not reliant on membrane voltages (answer B). Because strychnine is stated to be a competitive antagonist for glycine, we know it binds to the same site glycine normally does. Thus, it cannot block the pore directly, because glycine does not block ion channels (answer C). Inactivation gates (answer D) are present in certain ion channels and generally are triggered as a function of voltage. They create a refractory period for ion channels and are not affected by ligand antagonists.

4. B By blocking voltage-gated sodium channels, the cell no longer has as many ion channels able to open and allow an influx of positive charge. Thus, depolarization is less likely; the threshold for excitation of the nerve has been raised. The result is a block in signaling along the treated fiber. As the question states, lidocaine is selective for voltage-gated sodium channels; it does not affect ligand-gated channels such as nicotinic receptors or $GABA_A$ channels (answers A and C). Normally, there is a higher gradient of sodium outside the cell; blocking sodium channels would maintain this gradient, not raise intracellular levels (answer D). Finally, the question specifies that lidocaine blocks sodium channels, which is the opposite of preventing their inactivation (answer E).

Case 40

1. E The signs of numbness and tingling indicate that normal action-potential generation and transmission has been disrupted. By blocking sodium channels, the toxin does not change the resting membrane potential, because this is a steady state established by transporters and not sodium channels. The toxin would, however, block the ability to form action potentials, because the first step is depolarization as a result of massive sodium influx through selective channels.

2. E In resting state, the membrane potential is about -70 MeV because of the relatively high concentration of potassium inside the cell, and the relatively high concentration of sodium outside the cell. Adding potassium to the external environment would lessen the gradient for potassium inside the cell, decreasing the overall charge across the membrane. Adding sodium to the external environment (answer A) would increase its gradient, or driving force into the cell, and thus increase the potential across the membrane, or hyperpolarize it. Chlorine is normally present in very small quantities and usually has minimal impact on membrane potential. However, adding large amounts of chlorine to the external milieu would make the environment outside the cell more negative, decreasing the relative potential charge separation across the membrane. This would decrease the membrane potential.

3. B ATP is used in the Na^+/K^+ transporter to maintain a higher gradient of sodium outside the cell, and more potassium inside the cell. Without the transporter, this gradient could not be maintained, and there would be nothing to drive the action depolarization of the action potential. Thus, firing would be inhibited. The effect would be to impair the generation of action potentials, not alter their dynamics once generated (answers C and E).

4. E After the initial depolarization and influx of sodium, potassium channels are opened. This allows positive charge to rush out of the cell, hyperpolarizing the recently active region. Normally the potassium channels quickly close and the ATP pump restores the resting potential. If the potassium channels were to remain open longer, the cell would remain hyperpolarized longer and refractory to another quick depolarization.

Case 41

1. E MS is a demyelinating disease of the CNS. Because oligodendrocytes are responsible for myelin in the CNS, their structure and function are expected to be impaired (answer A). The resulting deficit in conduction can result in faulty "UMN" input to the extremities, which is demonstrated as weakness or hyper-reflexia (answers B and C). The optic nerve is a part of the CNS and thus can also cause impaired vision in MS (answer D). Schwann cells provide myelin to the PNS, which is not a primary source of pathology in MS.

2. D Conduction velocity is the speed at which the action potential travels down the axon. It increases with ion channel density, degree of myelination, and axon diameter. Of these factors, myelination is the most critical. Although the length of an axon may affect the absolute time required for a signal to travel from one nerve to another, this does not affect the conduction velocity of the signal.

3. B As discussed in the Clinical Correlate section, gliosis, or glial scar formation, impairs neuronal signaling. Glial scars replace myelin and act as barriers to the transmission of action potentials. Myelin is the substance that would insulate the axonal membrane, not glial tissue (answer A). Although axons of larger diameter do have faster conduction velocities, glial deposition would not make the axon itself larger (answer C). Glial scars replace oligodendrocytes in the CNS; oligodendrocytes normally provide myelin to increase conduction velocity (answer D). Finally, glial scars do not increase the density of ion channels (answer E).

4. E This patient has a classic presentation of Guillain-Barré syndrome: after a viral illness, she subsequently developed weakness of the lower extremities, which is spreading upward. The finding of areflexia is particularly important, indicating that there is a problem at the level of the PNS (reflexes remain present and are often heightened in upper-motor lesions). Schwann cells provide myelin in the PNS, which is affected in Guillain-Barré syndrome. The axon hillock is the junction between the neuronal cell body and the axon in both the CNS and the PNS; it is not affected in Guillain-Barré (answer A). Likewise, nodes of Ranvier are present in myelinated axons in both the CNS and the PNS and are not the target of demyelinating disease (answer B). Axonal ion channels can be subject to autoimmune attack, but the presentation of such diseases is usually generalized and does not follow the "distal upward" pattern described here (answer C). Oligodendrocytes are solely in the CNS and are not affected in PNS disease (answer E).

Case 42

1. A Botulinum toxin is thought to inactivate proteins involved in exocytosis at the presynaptic terminal. Synaptic vesicles empty their contents into the cleft via exocytosis; when this process is impaired, there is no signal transmission across the synapse. Likewise, ACh cannot be released onto the muscular endplate, and so normal contractions cannot occur. Botulinum toxin has been used to treat severe muscle spasms and more recently to relax facial muscles in cosmetic applications. In our case, the infant will have diminished signaling at the neuromuscular junction and so will present with flaccid ("floppy") paralysis. Hyper-reflexia (answer B) would indicate increased transmitter at the NMJ, which could not occur here. Likewise, spastic paralysis (answer D) is rigidity that usually results from lesions of higher motor neurons, not from lack of transmission at the NMJ. Salivary gland activity is triggered by ACh signals from autonomic neurons; decreased ACh release would be expected to cause dry mouth, not excessive salivation (answer C). Finally, the danger of botulism is flaccid paralysis, which affects the muscles of respiration, quite the opposite of hyperventilation (answer E). Early treatment of botulism is administration of an antitoxin; in more advanced cases, artificial respiration is required until symptoms spontaneously reverse in days to weeks.

2. C The question states that aminoglycosides can induce paralysis by competing with calcium at the presynaptic terminal. Of the answer choices, only one directly involves calcium. The influx of Ca^{2+} through voltage-gated channels and increased intercellular calcium is directly responsible for vesicle fusion with the synaptic membrane, and neurotransmitter release (answer C). When aminoglycosides competitively inhibit calcium, transmitter release is blocked and paralysis results. Action-potential propagation along the axon (answer A) does require normal ion gradients but does not directly involve calcium. Neurotransmitter packaging in vesicles (answer B) can be interrupted by drugs such as vesamicol but does not involve calcium. Neurotransmitter in the synaptic cleft can be inactivated by a number of enzymes, but not by calcium directly (answer D). Finally, endocytosis of empty vesicles (answer E) is not a calcium-dependent process.

3. C By blocking NE transport, reserpine prevents the packaging of NE into vesicles. This has the effect of decreasing the number of functional vesicles and thus inhibits signaling at the presynaptic membrane. Likewise, blocking Ca^{2+} channels would block a necessary step that triggers release of neurotransmitter vesicles. Both would have a net inhibitory effect. To stimulate NE synthesis (answer A) would have the opposite effect by increasing available neurotransmitter. Likewise, presynaptic depolarization, vesicle fusion, and exocytosis are all normal steps in signaling at the presynaptic membrane (answers B, D, and E).

4. A The amount of neurotransmitter in each vesicle is relatively uniform. In fact, neurotransmitter release is directly related to the number of vesicles released; it is quantal. To increase the amount released into the synapse, a greater number of vesicles must undergo exocytosis. Vesicles at a presynaptic terminal do not vary greatly in volume, and neither does a longer duration of fusion cause more neurotransmitter to be released (answers B and C).

Case 43

1. D The dopamine in the striatum and the cortex is identical; the receptors determine the postsynaptic response. Which ion channels are opened or closed by a given receptor determines whether the postsynaptic effect is excitatory or inhibitory. Therefore, varying levels of dopamine release or degradation are not responsible for the different types of effects (answers A and E); they only determine the degree of effect. Ionotropic receptors are those that directly open ligand-gated ion channels; metabotropic receptors are those that act through a second messenger. Although these are different receptor types, both have excitatory and inhibitory subtypes. Whether a second messenger is involved does not determine what type of response a receptor evokes (answer B). (Furthermore, all dopaminergic receptors act through G-protein receptors; there are no known ionotropic dopamine receptors.) Likewise, the affinity of the receptors for their neurotransmitter ligand is unrelated to the type of effect it evokes (answer C).

2. D The spinal neuron in the question has both glutamate and glycine receptors on its membrane. While the glutamate receptors open Na^+ channels which cause EPSPs, the glycine receptor opens Cl^- channels which cause IPSPs. Glycine is an important inhibitory neurotransmitter in the spinal cord because activating its receptors causes a hyperpolarization, bringing the postsynaptic membrane far below threshold. Even simultaneous excitation is then insufficient to trigger an action potential. Glycine acts on its own receptors without directly interacting with glutamate at the synapse (answers A and B). Postsynaptic neurotransmitter receptors are specific for their ligand. Therefore, glycine does not act through direct competitive inhibition (answer C). Finally, glycine has no effect on glutamate reuptake mechanisms (answer E).

3. E ACh esterase is the enzyme that degrades ACh, clearing it from the synapse at the end of signal transmission. ACh esterase inhibitors block this enzyme and thus permit ACh to remain in the synaptic cleft longer. Without the clearing of the cleft between signals, new signals cannot be sent between neurons, and thus neuronal signaling overall is impaired. Although the other mechanisms described would inhibit signaling, none are the targets of ACh esterase inhibitors.

4. E SSRIs have the net effect of increasing serotonergic activity. They do this by inhibiting reuptake of serotonin from the synaptic cleft back into the presynaptic terminal (not the postsynaptic terminal, as in answer C). As a result, serotonin remains in the cleft longer and acts on postsynaptic receptors more. (This mechanism has been a USMLE favorite.) Although answers A, B, and D all describe ways to increase activity at the synapse, none are the targets of SSRIs.

Case 44

1. C Chlorpromazine and haloperidol are both antipsychotic drugs commonly prescribed for schizophrenia. Both selectively block D_2-receptors and are generally not used together because they have the same mechanism of action. In a subset of patients, particularly those using a high dose of these drugs, early in the course of treatment, a parkinsonism can arise. Most often this is reversible by either decreasing the antipsychotic or adding an antiparkinsonism agent. Symptoms can resolve over a few months. Even if you were unfamiliar with this syndrome, this question only requires you to know which of the listed enzymes directly acts on L-dopa. C is the only possible correct answer. Phenylalanine hydroxylase (choice A) acts to convert phenylalanine to tyrosine and is deficient in PKU. Tyrosine hydroxylase (choice B) is the rate-limiting step in natural dopamine synthesis, converting tyrosine to dopa. However, administering exogenous dopa bypasses this enzyme. MAO-A (choice D) metabolizes NE and serotonin; it is a target of antidepressants and not involved in dopamine synthesis. MAO-B (choice B) metabolizes dopamine in the brain, which would have the opposite of the desired effect. In fact, selegiline is an example of an MAO-B inhibitor which has been used with some success in treating parkinsonism.

2. D Parkinsonism results when dopaminergic cells of the substantia nigra compacta are lost. The cells of the substantia nigra reticulata are not dopaminergic; they primarily transmit GABA. As shown in Figure 44-2, The loss of dopamine from the substantia nigra compacta directly results in decreased activity in the putamen and caudate, collectively known as the *striatum.* Quieting the striatum has the effect of disinhibiting the internal segment of the globus pallidus, which subsequently "overinhibits" the ventrolateral thalamus. The result is decreased activity in motor cortex. Lesions to the cerebellum can result in movement disorders, such as in cerebellar stroke, but the cerebellum is not directly affected in PD.

3. D *Parkinsonism* refers to the syndrome of motor deficits such as rigidity, tremor, and bradykinesia associated with damage to the substantia nigra. Although most cases are idiopathic (of unclear etiology), anything that damages the substantia nigra or its connections can lead to parkinsonism. This includes viral encephalitis, trauma (as in dementia pugilistica, or boxer's dementia), or local ischemia.

4. A (See Figure 44-3.) The substantia nigra separates the cerebral peduncles from the tegmentum of the midbrain. It is not directly adjacent to the red nucleus, which lies dorsally, nor the cerebral aqueduct, also dorsal in the midbrain (answers B and C).

Case 45

1. A The serotonergic projections of the descending analgesia circuit inhibit pain signals in the spinal cord. The receptor must have an inhibitory effect on the postsynaptic membrane. Of the answers listed, only one would have an inhibitory effect: opening K^+ channels to increase K^+ efflux from the cell hyperpolarizes the cell, which inhibits action-potential generation at the postsynaptic membrane. Closing K^+ "leak" channels would depolarize the cell, creating an excitatory potential (answer B). Likewise, opening Na^+ channels would cause an influx of cations, and thus an excitatory depolarization (answer C). Chlorine channels must be opened to produce an inhibitory potential; closing them would not hyperpolarize the cell (answer D). Finally, increasing presynaptic Ca^{2+} conduction would increase neurotransmitter release from primary afferent neurons, which would not have the desired effect of inhibiting signaling (answer E).

2. D Although the enterochromaffin cells of the GI tract do contain large amounts of serotonin, the intestine has no direct innervation from the nucleus raphe. The other structures listed receive serotonergic inputs from the raphe.

3. D The area postrema is also known as the *medullary vomiting center;* serotonin acting at 5-HT$_3$ induces nausea and vomiting. Increased functional serotonin levels may have an antidepressant effect, but not through the area postrema (answer A). Serotonin normally causes vasoconstriction in cerebral and meningeal vessels, not vasodilation (answer B). Mimicking this effect is the mechanism of action of certain antimigraine drugs, such as sumatriptan. In this way, serotonin agonists relieve headache, rather than cause headache (answer C). Finally, although serotonin is involved in the descending analgesia circuit, this does not include the area postrema (answer E).

4. B The reticular formation is a dispersed network of neurons regulating sleep through inputs to the thalamus. The periaqueductal gray is a component of the descending analgesia circuit (answer A). The nucleus raphe in the pons and upper midbrain contains most serotonergic neurons in the brain and is a component of the reticular formation but does not receive the inputs controlling sleep (answer C). The hippocampus is generally associated with memory formation, not sleep patterns (answer D). The reticular formation indirectly affects cortical activity, but not through direct inputs to cortex (answer E).

Case 46

1. B Tyrosine is the amino acid precursor of NE. Reduced tyrosine intake has been shown to reverse the effects of antidepressants in depressed patients, presumably by lowering the amount of catecholamines in the brain. Cocaine and amphetamines (answers A and D) both increase the amount of NE in the synaptic cleft, causing increased arousal and even mania. Ingestion of a low-tryptophan diet has been shown to reverse the effects of serotonergic antidepressants but does not affect NE levels (answer C). MAOIs are themselves antidepressants and do not cause depression (answer E).

2. A There has been some evidence that heightened arousal at the time of trauma is linked to later development of post-traumatic stress disorder. Victims of post-traumatic stress disorder have been shown to have elevated NE levels and heightened activation of certain areas within the brain. Some studies have used NE blockers to dampen the immediate effects of the increase in NE and have found a subsequent decrease in development of post-traumatic stress disorder. Clonidine, an α_2-agonist, likewise decreases NE release by causing presynaptic inhibition at noradrenergic synapses. Paradoxically, antidepressant drugs such as TCAs and MAOIs, which increase NE in the synaptic cleft (answers B and D), have been used to treat existing post-traumatic stress disorder, alleviating symptoms through their antidepressant effects.

3. D VMA is the urinary metabolite of both epinephrine and NE. A patient with pheochromocytoma would have elevated blood levels

of catecholamines, which would be reflected by higher levels of VMA in the urine. 5-HIAA (answer A) is a metabolite of serotonin, which would not be elevated due to pheochromocytoma. Epinephrine (answer B) levels would be elevated systemically, but epinephrine is not a urinary metabolite of catecholamines and thus would not be useful measures. Tyrosine (answer C) is a precursor of NE and would not be expected to be elevated with pheochromocytoma. Dopamine is another precursor of NE and would not be elevated in this case.

4. E The marker would selectively bind to the locus ceruleus in the upper brainstem and lateral tegmentum, where the majority of the brain's noradrenergic neurons are located. The nucleus raphe (answer A) is predominantly serotonergic neurons. The substantia nigra (answer B) is composed of dopaminergic neurons. The periaqueductal gray (answer C) is a primarily serotonergic region involved in the descending analgesia circuit. The red nucleus (answer D) is a brainstem region involved in motor control, not particularly associated with NE.

Case 47

1. E The NMDA glutamate receptor is crucial for learning and strengthening new connections in the brain. Blocking NMDA receptors impairs memory formation; ketamine is an induction anesthetic that leaves patients with little or no memory of the events (or pain) that occurred while administered. In contrast, a drug that enhances glutamate activity would be expected to lower seizure threshold or even promote excitotoxicity (answers A and B). GABA formation is determined by the activity of the enzyme glutamic acid decarboxylase, not activity at NMDA receptors (answer C). Finally, ketamine decreases excitatory input and so does not increase the sensation or perception of pain (answer D).

2. A Benzodiazepines act on GABA receptors to increase the frequency with which the Cl$^-$ channels open. This causes more frequent hyperpolarization and more IPSPs. In a patient, overdose can manifest as severe and sometimes lethal CNS depression. These drugs do not affect glutamate or glutamate receptors, which can allow massive Ca^{2+} influx an excitotoxicity (answers B through D). Although some antiseizure drugs target GABA uptake to enhance normal activity, benzodiazepines act directly on the receptor to cause inhibition (answer E).

3. B Glutamate is the most prevalent excitatory neurotransmitter (answer A). Glutamine is the amino acid precursor. (Do not make the easy mistake of misreading these two on Step 1!) γ-Aminobutyric acid (answer C) is the full name of GABA, the major inhibitory neurotransmitter. Tyrosine (answer D) is the precursor of the catecholamines. Tryptophan (answer E) is the precursor of serotonin.

4. A Glutamate excitotoxicity occurs when too much glutamate accumulates in the synapse, leading to massive calcium influx and neuronal death. It is thought to underlie neuronal death in a number of diseases. Although glutamate deficiency might result in decreased excitation, it is not a characterized cause of cell death (answer B). GABA is an inhibitory neurotransmitter and is not the basis for excitotoxicity (answer C). Although GABA deficiency could result in high levels of excitation, this is not a known pattern leading to cell death in the aforementioned disorders (answer D). *Kindling* refers to lasting changes in neuronal activity resulting from chronic epileptic stimulation; it is not associated with stroke or HD (answer E).

Case 48

1. E Naloxone is an opioid antagonist primarily at the μ-receptor. By countering the effects of opiate agonists, it is particularly useful in the immediate reversal of opiate overdose, which may manifest as CNS or respiratory tract depression. Pain control often requires opiate agonists; and antagonist would only worsen pain in a patient requiring analgesia (answers A through D). Additionally, neurogenic inflammation is the result of substance P release, which would not respond to opioid antagonism (answer C).

2. D Of the substances listed, three act on opiate receptors. Dynorphins are endogenous opioids that are weak agonists at opiate receptors, supplying moderate analgesia. Morphine also binds to opiate receptors but is not an endogenous peptide (answer C). Likewise, naloxone is an antagonist at opiate receptors and is not endogenous (answer E). POMC is an endogenous molecule that is

a precursor to β-endorphin but does not itself bind to opiate receptors (answer A). Substance P is also an endogenous peptide but is active in pain signaling, not at opiate receptors (answer B).

3. E Capsaicin, a compound found in some plants and hot peppers, acts at sensory nerve endings to deplete substance P. Although the initial result is often a transient "hot" or "burning" sensation, the end goal is pain relief. With substance P depleted, sensory nerves cannot continue local pain signaling. Even without knowing how capsaicin acts, one can choose answer E by process of elimination. Substance P is best understood as a neurotransmitter in signaling pain but also causes vasodilation, mast cell degranulation, and attracts leukocytes (answers A through C). These are all components of neurogenic inflammation, which would not relieve pain. Likewise, cotransmitters with substance P enhance pain signals; they do not relieve pain (answer D). The only possible correct answer is E.

4. C POMC is a precursor of ACTH, β-endorphin, melanocyte MSH, and met-enkephalin. It is the most important precursor of peptide neurotransmitters. Proenkephalin is a precursor of several enkephalins, including leu-enkephalin. Prodynorphin is the precursor of the active dynorphin peptides.

Index

Index note: page references with an *f* or *t* indicate a figure or table.